EAT FAT, GET THIN

Why the Fat We Eat Is the Key to Sustained Weight Loss and Vibrant Health

Dr Mark Hyman

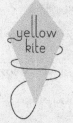

yellow
kite

First published the USA in 2016 by Little, Brown and Company
Hachette Book Group Inc

First published in Great Britain in 2016 by Hodder & Stoughton
An Hachette UK company

This edition published in 2016 by Yellow Kite Books
An imprint of Hodder & Stoughton
An Hachette UK company

1

A CIP catalogue record for this title is available from the British Library.

Paperback ISBN 978 1 473 63116 8
Ebook ISBN 978 1 473 63115 1

Printed and bound by Clays Ltd, St Ives plc

Hodder & Stoughton policy is to use papers that are natural,
renewable and recyclable   products and made from wood grown in
sustainable forests. The logging and manufacturing processes are expected
to conform to the environmental regulations of the country of origin.

This book is intended to supplement, not replace, the advice of a trained
health professional. If you know or suspect that you have a health problem,
you should consult a health professional. The author and publisher specifically
disclaim any liability, loss, or risk, personal or otherwise, that is incurred as a consequence,
directly or indirectly, of the use and application of any of the contents of this book.

Hodder & Stoughton Ltd
Carmelite House
50 Victoria Embankment
London EC4Y 0DZ

www.hodder.co.uk

*For the one in two Americans with chronic disease,
for those who struggle to answer the question, "What should I eat?"
this is for you.*

For the great enemy of truth is very often not the lie—deliberate, contrived, and dishonest—but the myth—persistent, persuasive, and unrealistic. Too often we hold fast to the clichés of our forebears. We subject all facts to a prefabricated set of interpretations. We enjoy the comfort of opinion without the discomfort of thought.

—John F. Kennedy

Contents

PART IV

EAT FAT, GET THIN COOKING AND RECIPES

EAT FAT,
GET THIN

Introduction

What is the single best thing you can do for your health, weight, and longevity?

Eat more fat!

That's right. Eat more fat to lose weight; feel good; prevent heart disease, diabetes, dementia, and cancer; and live longer.

How could that be true? Haven't we been told by every health and nutrition professional, leading medical associations, and our government to eat less fat because fat makes us fat and causes heart disease? We have faithfully followed this advice in America over the last 50 years and yet are fatter and sicker than ever.

It *is* true that the fat on our bodies is making us sick and causing us to die too soon. But the seemingly logical leap that the fat we eat creates the fat on our bodies and clogs our arteries is wrong.

It's an understandable mistake. The idea that if you eat fat, it turns to fat on your body makes sense. Fat equals fat, right? Same word. It looks and feels the same. Nutritionists have warned us that fat has twice as many calories (9 calories per gram) as carbs and protein (4 calories per gram), so if you eat less of it, you will lose weight and feel better. That seems like common sense. Except for one thing.

This whole idea, which we have bought wholesale, is scientifically untrue. In fact, the science shows the exact opposite. When you look closely at the data, it supports the idea that if you *eat fat, you get thin* (and reverse heart disease and type 2 diabetes, while preventing dementia, cancer, and other disease processes). The reality is that the more fat you eat, the more fat you lose and the better your body functions. Since

1980, the US Dietary Guidelines have warned us against the dangers of eating fat and implored us to eat less fat. But in a shocking reversal of this long-held dogma, the 2015 US Dietary Guidelines Advisory Committee exonerated cholesterol and removed any recommendation to limit dietary cholesterol or total dietary fat, except saturated fat (egg yolks are back on the menu!).[1]

If you are confused, it is not hard to understand why. I was confused myself, and I recommended low-fat diets to my patients for years. For decades, the advice from pretty much every doctor, nutritionist, professional society, and government agency had been to eat less fat to lose weight and prevent disease. Not only is this advice not working—it's actually doing us harm. It turns out that eating less fat results in *more* obesity and disease.

We have reduced fat in our diet from 43 percent to 33 percent of calories since 1970 and cut back even more on saturated fat. Yet we are sicker than ever, with the percentage of people getting heart disease increasing (although fewer people die from heart disease because we have better treatment). Type 2 diabetes and obesity rates around the globe are skyrocketing. In 1960, 1 out of 100 people in America had type 2 diabetes; today that ratio has changed to 1 out of 10 people, a tenfold increase. Since the 1980s, rates of type 2 diabetes have gone up *700 percent*. In 1960 only 1 in 7 Americans was obese; now it is 1 in 3, and it is projected that 1 out of every 2 Americans will be obese by the year 2050. In 1980, there were almost no cases of type 2 diabetes in children. By the year 2000, nearly 1 in 10 kids was pre-diabetic or had full-blown type 2 diabetes. By 2008, nearly 1 out of every 4 teenagers was pre-diabetic or had type 2 diabetes.[2] Where will it end?

Sadly, this isn't just a first world problem. Eighty percent of all type 2 diabetics are in the developing world. The single biggest health problem we face globally is the metabolic disaster that has led to a global epidemic of obesity, type 2 diabetes, and heart disease. More than twice as many people around the world go to bed overweight (about 2.5 billion) as go to bed hungry. And this affects more than just our health. It affects our global economic survival. Chronic preventable diseases will cost $47 trillion over the next 20 years.[3] That's more than the annual gross domestic products of the world's six largest economies combined. In America, the unfunded debt of Medicare and Medicaid dwarfs all other federal expenses; if health care costs continue to rise, they will consume 100 percent of our tax revenue by 2040, leaving no money for the military, education, justice, or anything else.

This is all deeply concerning, and we must collectively address the human, social, and economic issues caused by our diet and the diseases that result from what we eat. But first and foremost, let's start with you and your own health and weight. What most people want to know is very simple:

What do I need to do to stay healthy, lose weight, and reverse chronic disease?

That's exactly what this book will address—and it all starts with challenging what you believe to be true about fat. This book dispassionately reviews the evidence and uproots the conventional wisdom about fat — both the fat on our bodies and the fat we eat.

ABOUT THE PROGRAM

Eat Fat, Get Thin is divided into four parts. In Part I, I'll walk you through the fascinating (and at times unbelievable) story of how we got ourselves into this big, fat mess. You'll learn the truth about how dietary fat came to be unfairly and incorrectly demonized, and how and why it's finally being vindicated.

Part II is where I'll help you understand the often-confusing world of fats. What is a monounsaturated fat? Why are trans fats so bad? Doesn't saturated fat cause heart disease, as we've always been told? (And if not, what really does?) What's the story with cholesterol? Is it really the cause of heart disease? I'll help clear up some of our most common fallacies about vegetable oils, red meat, eggs, butter, nuts and seeds, and more. I'll also break down for you the specific reasons why eating fat is good for you. Most of all, I'll unpack the biggest myth of all when it comes to fat: that eating fat makes you fat.

Part III details the twenty-one-day *Eat Fat, Get Thin* Plan. This plan is a total reset for your body on every level. Food is the most powerful medicine there is, and by changing the way you fuel your body for twenty-one days, you're going to shut down your fat-storage hormone, reprogram your genes for weight loss and health, stop cravings in their tracks, and look and feel better than ever. You will shed unwanted pounds, alleviate or even eradicate health complaints, and reverse disease. Your skin will glow, your brain will feel sharp and clear, and you'll be filled with energy. You'll feel satisfied, happy, and—most of all— finally freed from your fear of fat!

WHAT YOU CAN EXPECT

Before I launch any program, I test it—not just on my patients, which I have done for decades (on more than 20,000 patients), but on people all over the country. I create a "beta program" for people to follow at home so that I can track the results and fine-tune the plan. We had more than 1,000 people do the *Eat Fat, Get Thin* beta program, and the results and stories were amazing. Throughout the book, you will get to read the testimonials of participants, not just about their weight loss but also about their radical health changes.

Here are the average results from the first group to go through the program:

- Weight loss: 7.1 pounds (some lost up to 46 pounds)
- Waist reduction: 1.9 inches (some lost up to 13 inches)
- Hip reduction: 1.7 inches (some lost up to 16 inches)
- Blood pressure reduction: systolic (top number) 9 points, diastolic (bottom number) 4.5 points
- Blood sugar reduction: 23 points

Before the program, 49 percent of participants reported they frequently had cravings; after the program that number dropped to only 1 percent! Before the program, a combined 89 percent reported they "frequently or sometimes" had cravings. After the program, 80 percent said they experienced cravings "rarely or never."

The program also simplified and clarified what people should eat so they didn't have to worry so much about their food choices. Before the program, 66 percent worried about meal planning because it was hard to make healthy choices. After the program, 75 percent rarely or never worried about their meal choices.

I also had people fill out the FLC Quiz (otherwise known as the Feel Like Crap Quiz, which measures the improvement of every aspect of their health and weight; you'll take this quiz yourself in Chapter 1). The results were astounding. The average score dropped from 68 to 21, or a 69 percent drop in all symptoms from all diseases. That is incredible. There is no drug on the planet that can create those results. Participants' digestion, energy, mood, joint pain, muscle aches, sinus problems and postnasal drip, allergies, skin, weight, mental health, sleep, sex drive, and more all dramatically improved. Why? *Eat Fat, Get Thin* is not really about weight loss. It's about providing the right information (food) for your body to create health. Then the symptoms and diseases— and weight—go away as a side effect. I never tell my patients to lose weight. I only tell them how to get healthy. When you get rid of the bad stuff and put in the good stuff, your body can heal and repair quickly. It doesn't take months or years. It takes days.

Let me share with you some of the results participants experienced on this program:

> *I have tried so many approaches to reclaim my health after decades of neglect resulting in heart disease, high blood pressure, sleep apnea, and being diagnosed with diabetes a year ago. This program has truly saved my life and has empowered me to take charge of my destiny at the age of sixty . . . to live a life of an adventure athlete and climb mountains and hike the Continental Divide Trail . . . all lifelong dreams that would never happen without Dr. Hyman's wisdom and insights and his creation of the EFGT program.* —Randy Davis

> *For over 20 years (I am thirty-five) I have been in daily pain. Over the years, I've been treated for depression, anxiety, back pain, joint pain, arthritis, post-traumatic stress disorder, spinal stenosis, irritable bowel syndrome, and PMS. I've been on a variety of medications. I've been in such*

physical/emotional pain that I have sat in the shower each morning, unable to stand, for over a decade. Since halfway into the EFGT program, I have stood in the shower every day. Although my sleep is still interrupted by a one-year-old, my sleep quantity and quality have improved. My joints feel remarkably better and I have more energy. Even at the end of the day, after the kids go to bed, I still have energy to do dishes or laundry. —Tara Foti

I have tried many diets and nothing worked. With this plan I lost thirteen pounds eating satisfying meals and lost my cravings for the bad stuff. The most important thing for me is the way I feel eating this way. I now sleep better, have more energy, and feel amazing! My aches and pains are gone. No more ibuprofen in the morning to get moving and three glasses of wine in the evening to relax. Thank you, Dr. Hyman . . . you have truly changed my life! —Jo Anne Matzuka

This opportunity came along at a time that I was nearly hopeless about ever being a normal weight again. I would go to bed at night exhausted from carrying an extra hundred pounds, and from being mentally worn out thinking about it. I lost thirteen pounds in three weeks, and now feel like I have the information and motivation I need to continue. I normally hesitate about going to the doctor, because my weight-related issues have been a problem for so long. However, I saw my doctor today, and I was actually excited to share with him the changes in my weight and my blood pressure. He was very supportive, and I actually feel like I'm partnering with him now. I'm hoping that the changes I make will be a testimony to my family and friends, and that I will have opportunities to share the principles I've learned with them. —Deborah Stine

I've been a critical care nurse for 30 years now and have been on every diet known to man. I've had great success, but the results never lasted. This is the first life plan where the cravings that caused the relapses are gone. I have no desire to "cheat" or "stray." I can honestly say that this is worth continuing because of the peace and harmony my physical body feels. I know that sounds corny but I don't know how else to explain how even my moods are, how regular my body feels. Wish I had this plan in my twenties; I think I'd be a different person now in my fifties! —Denise Pimintel

I was definitely in the nonbeliever camp upon starting. But then I started to see results almost immediately. The scale went down every day by some amount. The big question was how did this affect my lipid blood tests? I had a TIA [mini-stroke] a few years back and even with all the meds and my low-fat diet my numbers were not great. I tested after two weeks on the plan and found that all of my numbers were dramatically improved and my triglycerides were finally well into the normal range instead of high. I am a convert and intend to live my life with the principles of this plan incorporated into it! —Cheryl Schoenstein

This program contains the whole package for well-being. It helped me achieve the sleep I've been deprived of for so long. It improved my self-esteem and confidence (from not being embarrassed at the grocery store checkout to feeling deserving of a restful night of sleep). As a person who worries a lot and feels anxiety often, it significantly lowered that stress level. Never have I been addicted to a diet, but this is one that I don't want to give up. —Roxanne Ward

Besides losing eleven pounds, I am feeling less stress and calmer on the inside. I had heart palpitations, tingling in my hands and feet, and head-aches before this program, but now feel great! I know sugar has taken a toll on my body and am glad to have broken that addiction! —Cindy Victor

I feel great! My acid reflux is totally gone. My joints don't ache. I can move with fluidity and without any pain. My skin is smooth and well hydrated and I look younger because of that. I can bend down because my stomach is much smaller and softer. A world of difference from when I started. Before I started I felt like I was aging very fast and now I feel renewed, full of energy and young again. My brain fog has lifted and my mind is very sharp now. I feel like a new person, like someone who was given a new lease on life. Thank you, Dr. Mark Hyman, for showing me the way to better health and a better quality of life! —Katalin Vasko

EFGT is an awesome program! I never imagined how big a difference I would see in a mere three weeks and how much better I feel. Yesterday I even passed up dessert easily and without regret! Thank you for giving me the tools to make the changes I needed in life and for my health! —Pamela Barrett

While the *Eat Fat, Get Thin* Plan is based on very well-researched foundational principles, as we'll talk about in Part III, there is no one-size-fits-all approach to weight loss and health. This book will help you find the right long-term diet for *you*. The *Eat Fat, Get Thin* Plan is an initial reboot for your whole system. Then you will transition to a healthy eating plan for life that is best for you. In the quiz on pages 20 to 21, you can learn if you are carbohydrate intolerant and require very little carbs and more fat, or if you are more carbohydrate tolerant and can vary your diet a bit more after the twenty-one days. If your score is low, you may be able to include more carbohydrates, but if it is high, carbs will likely trigger more weight gain and other problems, so you can adjust accordingly.

Low-carb, higher-fat diets work for most people, but it is true that for some, that way of eating may not be optimal in the long term. Some may thrive on lots of saturated fats, but others may not have the same results. Big picture, this makes universal dietary recommendations a bit complicated. However, based on my research and hands-on experience with thousands of patients, I strongly believe *everyone* should try this way of eating for twenty-one days to see for themselves.

Finally, in Part IV, you'll find the specially designed, and delicious, *Eat Fat, Get Thin* recipes, which give you the optimal balance of fat, protein, and carbohydrates, along with simple cooking tips. You don't have to be a gourmet chef to be able to prepare fabulous, healthy meals for yourself and your family—it's easier than you think.

Welcome to your new world of eating and enjoying fats. In just twenty-one days, not only are we going to change how you think about fats—we're going to revolutionize how you eat and how you feel on every level.

PART I

HOW DID WE GET INTO THIS BIG, FAT MESS?

The truth is rarely pure and never simple.

—Oscar Wilde, *The Importance of Being Earnest*, 1895

1

The Demonization of Fat

Many of us have grown up in an era when we equated a low-fat diet with thinness and health. Doctors, nutritionists, scientists, the government, and the media have brainwashed us into believing that when you eat fat, it gets turned into fat in your body and, worse, it clogs your arteries. Except none of this is scientifically true. It is based on flawed science and ignores compelling evidence to the contrary. Our fear of fat has created a big, fat health mess.

It all started when—based on the seemingly sound advice of our government, our health care agencies, and the food industry—we cut out fat, which turns out to be the essential ingredient for health and weight loss. Then we replaced fat with sugar and carbs. In 1992, the US government published its Food Guide Pyramid. At the base of the pyramid were carbs, and we were told to eat six to eleven servings of bread, rice, cereal, and pasta a day. At the tippy top of the pyramid were fats and oils, which we were told to use only sparingly. The food industry jumped on board with the low-fat craze and created everything from low-fat salad dressing to fat-free yogurt to low-fat desserts (remember SnackWell's cookies?). And since they were low in fat (which we equated with "healthy"), you could eat the whole box—which many of us did!

Like good citizens, we listened to what our government advised, and now the average American consumes 152 pounds of sugar and 146 pounds of flour per year. Almost 20 percent of our daily calories come from sugar-sweetened beverages like soda, sports drinks, sweetened coffees and teas, and juice.[1] These liquid sugar calories are far worse than solid sugar or other carb calories because they go straight into fat production and storage. They are biologically addictive, increasing your craving for more sugar.[2] And since your body doesn't recognize these calories as food, you end up consuming more total calories than you would from solid food.[3] Sugar-sweetened drinks also wreak havoc on our health. In a dramatic study in the journal *Circulation*, researchers attributed 184,000 deaths each year to the effects of drinking these sugary concoctions. These drinks have been proven to cause obesity, heart disease, type 2 diabetes, and cancer.[4]

We now know from the research that sugars and refined carbs are the true causes of obesity and heart disease—not fats, as we've been told. Carbs turn on the metabolic switch, causing a spike in the hormone *insulin,* and this leads to fat storage (especially dangerous belly fat). Sugar and carbs, not fat, as you'll see in the pages to come, are also the main causes of abnormal cholesterol. Sugar and refined carbs are the culprits behind type 2 diabetes, many cancers, and even dementia.[5] As I have written about extensively in my books *The Blood Sugar Solution* and *The Blood Sugar Solution 10-Day Detox Diet*, the steep rise worldwide in type 2 diabetes and pre-diabetes directly resulted from the glut of refined carbs and sugar in our diet.

RETHINKING OUR FEAR OF FAT

When it comes to fat, we have a semantics problem. In other languages, the word for the fat we eat is different from the word for the unwanted stuff clinging to our midsections. And even within the world of fat we eat, there are many different kinds, some good and some bad. We don't have that confusion with sugar. Sugar is sugar is sugar. All forms of sugar (with small and relatively insignificant differences) have the same negative effects on your body. It doesn't matter if it is table sugar, high-fructose corn syrup, agave nectar, honey, or any of the other 257 names for sugar. It's all sugar.

But fat is not fat is not fat. There are saturated, monounsaturated, polyunsaturated, and trans fats, and even within each, there are different types. Saturated fats come in many flavors, as do polyunsaturated fats (I will explain in more detail soon). Bottom line: Not all fats are to be vilified, and eating liberal amounts of the right ones will *not* make you fat. In fact, the right ones are key to health and weight loss!

Our views on fat, thankfully, are shifting. Over the last five years, the scientific evidence has been mounting that high-fat diets outperform low-fat diets for weight loss and for reversing every single indicator of heart disease risk, including abnormal cholesterol, diabetes, hypertension, inflammation, and more.[6] In fact, the evidence has found no link between dietary fat, saturated fat, or cholesterol and heart disease.[7]

Joslin Diabetes Center at Harvard, one of the top diabetes centers in the world, was named after Dr. Elliott P. Joslin. In the 1920s he recommended a diet of 75 percent fat, 20 percent protein, and 5 percent carbohydrates to treat diabetes. After fat became demonized in the 1950s and 1960s, a low-fat, high-carb diet (55 percent to 60 percent carbs) was recommended by the scientists and doctors of the day. For decades, the American Diabetes Association (ADA) promoted this diet as the diabetes epidemic worsened year after year. Now researchers at Joslin Diabetes Center are once again recommending diets of up to 70 percent fat for the treatment of type 2 diabetes.[8]

As one example of how effective a high-fat diet can be, the head of the ADA in the Los Angeles region, Allison Hickey, had type 2 diabetes for 11 years. She followed the ADA advice, exercised, and was on injections and pills. Yet her diabetes was poorly controlled. After going on the diet I recommended of over 50 percent fat and slashing her carbohydrate intake, she got off her injections and most medications, and her blood sugar returned to normal. Her digestive problems and brain fog also disappeared.

Unfortunately, not everyone is getting the message about the importance of fat, and we still have a ways to go. The ADA is still pushing old and dangerous advice. It now recommends avoiding refined carbs but still pushes the low-fat message, even though studies have found that those who eat fatty nuts have a lower risk of developing type 2 diabetes,[9] and those who add a liter of olive oil a week and consume nuts on a daily basis have a significantly lower risk of heart attacks and death.[10]

For years, scientists pulled out their hair trying to understand the so-called French paradox. Why could the French eat so much butter and fat and be so thin and have lower rates of heart disease? They should have been paying attention to what I call the American paradox: how could Americans eat less and less fat and yet get fatter and fatter? How did they not wonder why Americans were eating less fat and yet getting more and more heart disease? Our paradigm was so entrenched we couldn't see it. The psychiatrist R. D. Laing said, "Scientists can see the way they see with their way of seeing."[11]

I am at the intersection of scientific research and clinical practice. My life's work has been dedicated to finding answers to my patients' problems and keeping them healthy for life. I wrote this book to clear up the confusion and give you the skinny on fat in our diet and fat in our bodies, and to outline a plan to help you figure out exactly what to eat to lose weight, reverse disease, and get vibrantly healthy.

In *Eat Fat, Get Thin,* I will take you on a guided tour of fat—both the fat we eat and the biology of it in our bodies—and show you how the fat you eat actually does not make you fat. Eating more of the right fats helps you lose weight and prevent dementia, heart disease, diabetes, and cancer, all while giving you the added side benefits of improved mood, skin, hair, and nails. Sounds crazy, for sure. For decades, I believed fat was to be avoided at all costs, too, until I dug into the evolving research. Based on what I discovered, I changed how I practiced medicine and saw with my own eyes the dramatic results in my patients' lab tests, bodies, and health. One patient, for example, increased the fat in his diet to about 50 percent of his overall food intake, and his cholesterol dropped 100 points. His triglycerides dropped 300 points in just 10 days, and his chronic asthma and reflux went away, while his energy soared.

I have uncovered some surprising facts in researching this book and testing and treating more than 20,000 patients over 30 years. I have documented my findings with many references throughout this book, so you can confirm them yourself if you find them hard to believe:

- Dietary fat speeds up your metabolism, reduces your hunger, and stimulates fat burning.[12]

- Dietary fat helps you reduce your overall calorie intake, not increase it.[13]
- Dietary fat, and saturated fat specifically, does not cause heart disease.[14]
- Dietary saturated fat raises the good kind of LDL (light, fluffy LDL) and raises HDL (the "good" cholesterol).[15]
- Diets higher in fat promote more weight loss than diets high in carbs, and they are easier to stick to.[16]
- Dietary fat reduces inflammation,[17] risk for clotting, and all heart disease risk factors.[18]
- Dietary fat improves blood vessel health.[19]
- Dietary fat improves brain function and mood and helps prevent dementia.[20]
- Diets very high in fat and low in carbs can reverse type 2 diabetes.[21]
- "Good" vegetable oils (such as soy, corn, sunflower, safflower) are harmful; they create inflammation and oxidize or make your cholesterol rancid, making it more likely to cause heart disease.[22]
- Dietary saturated fat (from butter or coconut oil) does not raise saturated fats in your blood.[23]
- Carbohydrates—not dietary fats—turn into saturated fats in your blood, the fats that cause heart disease.[24]
- Excess carbs stimulate your appetite and belly fat storage and slow your metabolism.[25]
- Carbohydrates turn on the fat production factory in your liver (called *lipogenesis*), causing high cholesterol and high triglycerides while lowering the good cholesterol (HDL) and creating small, dense, dangerous heart-disease-causing LDL particles.[26]
- Sugar and refined carbs—not fat—are responsible for the epidemic of obesity, type 2 diabetes, and heart disease[27] and the increased risk of dementia and premature deaths.[28]

MY OWN TRANSITION FROM FAT TO FIT

I went to medical school in the early eighties, in the heyday of the low-fat craze. I avoided fat and recommended my patients do the same in order to lose weight and prevent heart disease. I became a vegetarian, and for ten years I avoided any animal products except low-fat yogurt and egg whites. I kept oils to a minimum and ate lots of bread and pasta (then promoted as a health food). I knew too much sugar wasn't that good for you, but I ate plenty of whole-wheat low-fat cookies and low-fat frozen yogurt because I craved sugar and carbs. I was young and a runner, so I burned a lot of it off, but as I got older I noticed my body change. I developed love handles, my belly got a little bigger, my pant size increased two inches, and my body seemed flabby and less muscular. By the time I was thirty-five, I'd gained fifteen pounds. I studied nutrition and followed a healthy balanced diet—the same one I recommended to my patients—so I thought it was just normal aging. I didn't eat junk food; I never had soda or processed food. I ate a whole-foods diet rich in grains, beans, fruits, and veggies and didn't go overboard on sugar. I ate little fat. But my body just kept getting flabbier.

As the research started emerging on the dangers of sugar and refined carbs (even whole wheat bread), I cut down on sugar and carbs. But still, I feared fat, especially saturated fat, which I "knew," as a doctor, was the cause of heart disease. If I exercised a lot (like riding my bike thirty-five miles a day), I thought I could keep some of the excess weight off, but it wasn't sustainable.

Then, over the last ten years, as the tide turned, I began to change my own eating habits and my recommendations to my patients. I saw people lose one hundred or more pounds and reverse type 2 diabetes. I saw my patients get off insulin and optimize all their cholesterol levels not by eating *less* fat, but by eating *more* fat.

The changes in my own body were remarkable. Not only did I have more mental focus and clarity, but I lost the fifteen pounds, the love handles, and two inches off my waist, and at fifty-five years old I am more muscular and fit than I've ever been, while working out less; I feel younger and more energetic than ever.

Now I eat fat for breakfast without fear or guilt, with a big smile on my face and a deeply satisfied tummy. Sometimes I have whole eggs cooked in grass-fed butter or extra virgin coconut oil (high in saturated fat but super healthy), or a "fat" shake with a bunch of nuts, seeds, and coconut butter. For lunch I have a big salad with fatty sardines or wild salmon, doused in olive oil and sprinkled with fatty pumpkins seeds or pine nuts; and for dinner I might have grass-fed lamb without the fat cut off, and three or four veggie dishes cooked in olive oil, lemon, and spices and salt.

When I traveled to Tibet in my twenties, I was invited into the yurts of nomads and fed salty yak butter tea (actually it is *dri* butter—from the female yak), which was deeply satisfying and kept me going for a long time at high altitudes. And sometimes now I have the American version created by my friend David Asprey, Bulletproof Coffee—coffee blended with butter and MCT oil from coconut (a super fat that is a super fuel for your brain and your body). One close friend in medical school was an Arctic explorer who cross-country skied to the North Pole while living on sticks of butter for fuel. He was remarkably healthy and way ahead of his time.

Eating a high-fat diet—especially a diet high in "dangerous" saturated fat—sounds crazy, and up until ten years ago, I would have told you it was a health hazard. But my own body, my own blood work, and thousands of my patients and tens of thousands of others who have followed this approach in my online community all tell the true story. They all report the same benefits from welcoming fat back into our diets. And the emerging research on fat and health, which we will nerd out on in this book (sorry, I love the science...I can't help myself!), supports these benefits.

LET'S TALK ABOUT *YOU*

There are lots of fascinating findings and facts throughout this book that will surprise you, and I'm looking forward to sharing every one of them. But before we get to that, let's talk about the real reason you're here: You want to know how to lose weight and feel great. The program in this book will get you there, but before you embark on your journey—as with any journey—it's helpful to get a sense of where you are starting from when it comes to carbohydrates, fats, and your health.

As many of you know, I have written extensively about *diabesity,* which is the comprehensive term I use for the range of problems and diseases caused by blood sugar and insulin imbalances. Diabesity runs the gamut from having a pooch of extra belly fat to obesity, from moderately high blood sugar to pre-diabetes to full-blown type 2 diabetes. All the problems on this spectrum can have deadly consequences.

Diabesity is a disease of *carbohydrate intolerance.* Just as some people are gluten intolerant, many are carbohydrate intolerant. For those people, carbs drive a hormonal and brain chemical chain reaction that makes it almost impossible to lose weight or get healthy.

Diabesity affects 1 out of every 2 people in the US, 1 in 2 Medicare patients, and 1 in 4 teenagers. It affects skinny people, too! Twenty-three percent of adults look skinny but are what doctors call *metabolically obese normal weight,* or TOFI (thin on the outside, fat on the inside). Ninety percent of people with diabesity are not diagnosed . . . so there's a good chance that you have it and don't even know it. And it's the very thing standing in your way of losing weight and living a long, healthy life.

Are You Carbohydrate Intolerant?

If you answer yes to any of the following questions, you may be carbohydrate intolerant and already have diabesity or be heading in that direction. But the higher the score, the worse your carbohydrate intolerance, and the more you'll benefit from the *Eat Fat, Get Thin* program:

For questions 1 to 9, score 1 point for a "yes" response.
For questions 10 to 13, score 2 points for a "yes" response.

1. Do you have a family history of diabetes, heart disease, or obesity?
2. Are you of nonwhite ancestry (African, Asian, Native American, Pacific Islander, Hispanic, Indian, Middle Eastern)?
3. Do you have trouble losing weight on a low-fat diet?
4. Do you crave sugar and refined carbohydrates?

5. Are you inactive (less than thirty minutes of exercise four times a week)?

6. Are you overweight (body mass index, or BMI, over 25)? (Go to www .eatfatgetthin.com to calculate your BMI based on weight and height.)

7. Do you have heart disease?

8. Do you have high blood pressure?

9. Do you suffer from infertility, low sex drive, or sexual dysfunction?

10. Do you have extra belly fat? Is your waist circumference greater than 35 inches for women or greater than 40 inches for men?

11. Has your doctor told you that your blood sugar is a little high (greater than 100 mg/dl) or have you actually been diagnosed with insulin resistance, pre-diabetes, or type 2 diabetes?

12. Do you have high levels of triglycerides (over 100 mg/dl) or low HDL (good cholesterol) (less than 50 mg/dl)?

13. For women: Have you had gestational diabetes or polycystic ovarian syndrome?

If you score more than 5, you have advanced carbohydrate intolerance or diabesity and would do better on the *Eat Fat, Get Thin* Plan until your score improves to less than 5 (based on your labs, waist size, blood sugar, blood pressure, etc.). If you answer yes to any question but score less than 5, you may still have carbohydrate intolerance and benefit from the *Eat Fat, Get Thin* Plan. In fact, it is worth it for anyone to try because of all the plan's other benefits in addition to weight loss and reversing diabesity.

Even if you score 0, the plan is worth trying for all the plan's other benefits.

Do You Have FLC Syndrome?

In addition to carbohydrate intolerance, millions of Americans (and people around the world) have FLC syndrome—that's when you *feel like crap*! What most of us don't know is that this is directly related to the food we eat. Food can harm us or it can heal us. Whole, real, low-glycemic (low in sugar and refined carbs), high-fat (good fat), phytonutrient-rich food heals, while high-carb, low-fat, processed foods harm. And it is not just that you feel bad. The underlying inflammation and hormonal imbalance driven by eating the wrong foods drive not just symptoms but diseases and accelerated aging.

Take the following quiz to find out where you rate on the FLC scale. For the "before" part of the questionnaire, rate each of the symptoms based upon your health profile for the past thirty days. You'll take this quiz again after the twenty-one–day *Eat Fat, Get Thin* program. But without a baseline score, twenty-one days from now you may have a hard time believing just how different your "after" results are.

POINT SCALE

0 = Never or almost never have the symptom
1 = Occasionally have it; effect is not severe
2 = Occasionally have it; effect is severe
3 = Frequently have it; effect is not severe
4 = Frequently have it; effect is severe

DIGESTIVE TRACT

____ Nausea or vomiting
____ Diarrhea
____ Constipation
____ Bloated feeling
____ Belching or passing gas
____ Heartburn
____ Intestinal or stomach pain

Total before____
Total after____

EARS

____ Itchy ears
____ Earaches, ear infections
____ Drainage from ear
____ Ringing in ears, hearing loss

Total before____
Total after____

EMOTIONS

____ Mood swings
____ Anxiety, fear, or nervousness

____ Anger, irritability, or aggressiveness
____ Depression

Total before____
Total after____

ENERGY/ACTIVITY

____ Fatigue, sluggishness
____ Apathy, lethargy
____ Hyperactivity
____ Restlessness

Total before____
Total after____

EYES

____ Watery or itchy eyes
____ Swollen, reddened, or sticky eyelids
____ Bags or dark circles under eyes
____ Blurred or tunnel vision (does not include near- or farsightedness)

Total before____
Total after____

HEAD

____Headaches
____Faintness
____Dizziness
____Insomnia

Total before_____
Total after_____

HEART

____Irregular or skipped heartbeat
____Rapid or pounding heartbeat
____Chest pain

Total before_____
Total after_____

JOINTS/MUSCLES

____Pain or aches in joints
____Arthritis
____Stiffness or limitation of movement
____Pain or aches in muscles
____Feeling of weakness or tiredness

Total before_____
Total after_____

LUNGS

____Chest congestion
____Asthma, bronchitis
____Shortness of breath
____Difficulty breathing

Total before_____
Total after_____

MIND

____Poor memory
____Confusion, poor comprehension
____Poor concentration
____Poor physical coordination
____Difficulty in making decisions
____Stuttering or stammering
____Slurred speech
____Learning disabilities

Total before_____
Total after_____

MOUTH/THROAT

____Chronic coughing
____Gagging, frequent need to clear throat
____Sore throat, hoarseness, loss of voice
____Swollen or discolored tongue, gums, or lips
____Canker sores

Total before_____
Total after_____

NOSE

____Stuffy nose
____Sinus problems
____Hay fever
____Excessive mucus formation
____Sneezing attacks

Total before_____
Total after_____

SKIN

____Acne
____Hives, rashes, or dry skin
____Hair loss
____Flushing or hot flushes
____Excessive sweating

Total before_____
Total after_____

WEIGHT

____Binge eating or drinking
____Craving certain foods
____Excessive weight
____Compulsive eating
____Water retention
____Underweight

Total before_____
Total after_____

OTHER

____ Frequent illness

____ Frequent or urgent urination

____ Genital itch or discharge

Total before _____

Total after_____

GRAND TOTAL BEFORE _____

GRAND TOTAL AFTER _____

Key to Questionnaire

Optimal health: less than 10 points

Mild toxicity: 10 to 50 points

Moderate toxicity: 50 to 100 points

Severe toxicity: more than 100 points

If you scored not so great on either of these quizzes, don't panic. Here's the good news: You can reverse diabesity. You can get over FLC syndrome. And you can do all of that while delighting in the abundance of whole, rich foods. With the *Eat Fat, Get Thin* Plan, you will not be suffering or deprived. The promise of this book is that if you eat more of the right fats, you will feel good, get thin, look better, and get healthier than you've ever been, while enjoying delicious, savory, mouthwatering food.

2

Fleshing Out Our Fear of Fat

> A new scientific truth does not triumph by convincing its
> opponents and making them see the light, but rather
> because its opponents eventually die, and a new genera-
> tion grows up that is familiar with it.
>
> — Max Planck

Science is a veritable graveyard of closely held beliefs that once seemed obvious and completely in line with common sense. Certain ideas become so entrenched that they seem to be natural laws. That is, until they are proven false. Before Columbus, everyone believed the world was flat. It was true...until it wasn't. In the early seventeenth century, Galileo's idea that the sun did not revolve around the earth was so heretical that he was thrown in jail. But of course, he was right. Darwin postulated that species did not arise in their current form as sponta-neous creations of God, but evolved through natural selection. Even today, 150 years later, many still debate the theory of evolution.

And so it has been with fat. We've been told lots of falsehoods about fat over the past 50 years that have shaped what we eat, what we buy, how we diet—all of which has had huge and disastrous consequences for our health.

It all began with two big ideas about fat that have turned out to be wrong. Dead wrong, in fact. These two ideas seemed consistent with common sense, just like the earth looking flat. The first was that all calories operate the same way in your body. Since fat has more than twice as many calories as carbs or protein per gram, the natural conclusion was that if you ate less fat you would lose weight. That, in effect, the fat you ate turned to fat in your body.

The second idea was that since fatty cholesterol deposits caused heart disease, and dietary fat, especially saturated fat, raised cholesterol, then the fat we ate caused heart disease. Seems to make sense, except the body is more complex than this simplistic conclusion would suggest. Whole scientific careers and industries have been devoted to these false notions, based as they are on incorrect assumptions. Once people adopt a worldview, it is very hard to change.

In this chapter we'll examine how these two ideas became accepted facts in the scientific community—and why they are wrong. I'll explain how the government and the food industry jumped on the bandwagon to create a maelstrom of bad advice. It was the perfect storm of overzealous scientists leaping to premature conclusions, anxious government agencies eager to do something to stem the tide of obesity and heart disease, and a profit-hungry food industry that raced in to capitalize on the low-fat mania, leading, in fact, to a rise in obesity, heart disease, and diabetes.

This is the story of how fat became public enemy number one and triggered the biggest health crisis in human history: obesity and chronic disease caused by eating the wrong foods.

UNTANGLING THE RESEARCH ON FOOD

With literally millions of studies (more than 8 million in the National Library of Medicine database) performed over many decades on obesity, metabolism, type 2 diabetes, and heart disease, how could the scientific community have gotten this so very wrong, for so long?

Science is driven by hypotheses, ideas, and concepts that need to be proven or disproven. It should be simple. And in some cases, it is. But even in the face of clear evidence to the contrary, scientists get pretty stuck in their worldview. Edwin Friedman, a twentieth-century rabbi and family therapist, said, "The risk-averse are rarely emboldened by data."

For example, doctors long believed that stress caused stomach ulcers, even though they'd consistently find bacteria in patients with stomach ulcers; they'd dismiss the bacteria as insignificant. Even after Dr. Barry Marshall, a gastroenterologist from Australia, proved he could cure ulcers with antibiotics to kill the bacteria (called *Helicobacter pylori*), his theory was still dismissed for more than a decade. It was only after he drank a beaker full of bacteria, caused an ulcer in himself, and cured it with antibiotics that his theory was accepted. Dr. Marshall won the Nobel Prize for his discovery.

But biology (and human biology in particular) is infinitely complex. It's a web of genetic, hormonal, and biochemical reactions that vary dynamically under the influence of the environment. And food is the biggest "environmental" regulator of that complex system we call our bodies. Food, it turns out, is not just calories, but *information* that radically influences our genes, hormones, immune system, brain chemistry, and even gut flora with every single bite.

Yet there's an even bigger factor contributing to our confusion about food: the tricky business of nutritional research. How is it that we come to know what we know, and how can we determine what is accurate?

The first thing to understand is that all evidence, and all studies, are not created equal. As a young medical student and doctor, I believed in the infallibility of science. Science was objective and independent of bias and gave us clear answers to the questions we asked. But over time I learned to analyze data more carefully, to dissect the studies and look at methods and actual data to see what questions were actually asked, how the study was designed and if it was well done or not, and to dig into who funded the study to root out any conflicts of interest.

Dr. John Ioannidis, from the Stanford Research Prevention Center, has challenged the validity of most nutrition studies. Most studies that make conclusions from looking at diet in populations have been later proven in experimental trials to be wrong. Dr. Ioannidis writes, "Critics have focused on the poor track record of observational claims when tested in subsequent randomized trials (0/52 success rate in one review) and perpetuated fallacies."[1] Wait! Zero out of fifty-two population (observational) studies validated previous notions about what you should eat when those notions or hypotheses were subjected to actual human experiments!

There are different types of studies (for instance, observational studies vs. randomized controlled trials vs. animal studies), and the conclusions that can be drawn from each type are different: some prove cause and effect while others show only associations. Each type of study has its benefits and drawbacks, and it is impossible to draw definitive conclusions from any one study. It is important to look at the weight of all the evidence and how each type of study was done. For example, was it a study that asked people to eat a certain diet and hoped they would, or did the researchers supply food in their homes and expect they wouldn't cheat with ice cream? Clinical trials that simply provide participants with advice and guidelines about what to eat are also different from "metabolic ward studies," where people are locked in a hospital for a long period of time and have all their food provided and their metabolism directly measured.

It is also important to know what population was studied. Were they all white males who weighed 180 pounds, or was it a group of African American females or Asian children? There are tremendous differences in how populations with different genetics respond to different diets. If studies show an effect for one population, it might not be valid for another.

Another problem is that most nutritional research relies on large studies of populations and their dietary patterns, obtained mostly through dietary questionnaires or twenty-four-hour dietary recall. Do you really remember every single thing you ate over the last seven days or thirty days? And how closely does that represent what you have been eating over the last five years, or even 30 years? It is well described in the research that people often under- or overreport their habits depending on the recommendations of the day. For instance, if you think that eating meat is bad, you will likely underreport how much meat you actually eat.

Here's another piece we need to consider: Who is funding the study? Is there any conflict of interest? More than most doctors would like to admit, science is for sale. Researchers' work has to be funded, and it is often expensive (we're talking millions of dollars here). The funding generally comes from two sources: the government through the National Institutes of Health (NIH) and private industry (Big Pharma, or the food industry in this case).

We know that if a study is funded by a food company, it is eight times more likely to turn up positive findings for that food company's product.[2] If the National Dairy Council funds studies on milk, milk is more likely to be found beneficial. If Coca-Cola funds studies on soft drinks, they are likely to be found not linked to obesity and disease. It is very hard to find clean, clear, objective research in those cases, since the study was either designed to show a specific outcome or the data selection and emphasis were "spun" to get the desired impact. It gives a whole new meaning to the phrase "spin doctors."

You can see how this can get very confusing!

It's not easy to know for sure what is the "truth." Vegan diet studies show they help with weight loss, reverse diabetes, and lower cholesterol. Diets high in fat and animal protein seem to do the same thing. So should you be shunning animal foods and eating only beans, grains, and veggies, or should you eat meat and fat without guilt and give up all grains and beans? One respected scientist condemns saturated fat, while another equally esteemed scientist vindicates saturated fat. Whom should we believe?

Essentially, each scientist (or even each person reading the research) with a point of view adheres to his or her position with near religious fervor. And each can point to studies validating his or her perspective. We call this cherry picking. After reading thousands of studies on human nutrition over 30 years, even I get confused. But I can find my way through the headlines because I read between the lines. I read the methods and analyze the actual data to learn what the studies actually demonstrate — or, sometimes, what they *don't* demonstrate.

For instance, the first study linking saturated fats to heart disease, by Ancel Keys (on which 50 years of dietary policy to eat low-fat was based), looked at only about thirty men from Crete and their previous day's diet, and linked that to the fact that they had fewer heart attacks than people from countries where more saturated fat was consumed. Skimpy evidence at best!

It is very hard to tease out the factors that matter in population studies that are not real experiments. If I did a study on the link between your waking up and the sunrise, I would find 100 percent correlation. But that doesn't mean that your waking up caused the sun to rise. For example, when Asians move from Asia to the United States, they eat more meat and have more heart disease and cancer, but they also consume far more sugar. So it is the meat or is it the sugar? Hard to know. These types of population studies can show only correlation, not cause and effect. Yet, the media and consumers overinterpret the results and take them as gospel.

Many experimental nutrition studies often have only small numbers of people in them, making it hard to draw firm conclusions. Even worse: The diets they use for comparison (the control group) are not ideal alternative diets. Comparing a toxic vegan diet of chips, Coke, bagels, and pasta to a high-fat, whole-foods diet of healthy veggies, olive oil, nuts, and grass-fed meat won't be very helpful, nor would comparing a toxic, processed diet of feedlot meat, foods with trans fats, and no fresh veggies or fruit to a whole-foods, low-glycemic plant-based or vegan diet.

So how do you make sense of the contradictory, oftentimes confusing information, break past the unnecessary polarization in nutrition science, and find a path that forges an ideal weight and optimal health? You put all the pieces together like a puzzle, consider all the potential issues and conflicts, and see the story the data tells. I have spent hundreds if not thousands of hours combing through the research, reviewing thousands of scientific papers, and talking to dozens of experts. I have seen tens of thousands of patients, reviewed their blood work, and seen how they've responded to different dietary and nutritional interventions. I have spent the time wading through and deciphering all the geeky science so you don't have to do the hard work. I have done the homework for you to develop this program that gets you out of the dangerous fear of fat and into a sane, sustainable diet to rev up your metabolism and optimize your health.

> I love this program. The fats keep me full and remove cravings and eating real food is delicious. It doesn't feel like a diet; it feels like my new normal life.
>
> —Lisa Pelly

What gives me a unique perspective is one simple fact: I don't take money from any vested interests, nor have I spent my life proving one particular point of view, be it low-fat or low-carb, or pro– or anti–olive oil, or vegan or meat eater. In fact, I have been both a vegan and an omnivore over the course of my life. I have eaten low-fat, high-carb diets and low-carb, high-fat diets and have used all sorts of different diets with tens of thousands of patients over 30 years of medical practice. At points in my work I advocated for and prescribed low-fat vegetarian diets, but as the research emerged that convinced me that fat was good, I changed my recommendations. I am not married to a particular point of view. I am curious about what lies beneath the money and the egos behind the research. I am interested in one simple thing. What should we eat to stay fit, thin, and healthy? I want the same thing for myself as I do for you. I want to live long, be healthy, and avoid disease, and I would not eat things that I believe would threaten my health or longevity.

The Fallacy of Focusing on Nutrients Instead of Real Food

In this book, I will debunk some of the tightly held beliefs and myths that get in the way of our doing the right thing for our bodies and our health. Part of the confusion around nutrition is due to something called *nutritionism*. Nutritionism is the science of breaking down dietary components into their individual parts, such as one vitamin or one type of fat, and studying those components in isolation. This approach is helpful for studying medication, where there might be a single molecule designed to target one specific pathway and one specific disease. But it is not that helpful for studying individual nutritional components. Why? Because people eat food, not single components. They eat foods that contain often dozens of different ingredients, many different types of fat, proteins, carbohydrates, vitamins, minerals, phytonutrients, and more. For example, olive oil, which people think of as a "monounsaturated fat," also contains about 20 percent saturated fat and 20 percent polyunsaturated omega-6 fat and even a little bit of omega-3 fat. Beef also contains all different types of fat. The nutrition world is shifting away from focusing on individual nutrients and toward focusing on dietary patterns, whole foods, and complex assortments of foods, that is, the way we actually eat.

THE CREATION OF THE FAT FALLACY

In the beginning of our understanding of calories, weight, and metabolism, there were two competing ideas. The first was that all calories were equal. This was based in simple physics: Burn 100 calories from soda or from olive oil in a laboratory and they release exactly the same amount of energy. But think about this rationally when applied to human biology: If you eat the same amount of calories in kale or gummy bears, do they do the same thing to your body? Is your weight affected the same way, regardless of the source of the calories? We are continually told that the regulation of weight is as simple as calories in, calories out. Just eat less and exercise more, and we will lose weight. This is called the *energy balance hypothesis*. It seems like one of those fundamental self-evident truths, except we now know that it is false.

The calories in, calories out formula for weight maintenance became embedded in the halls of academia and in government policy, and the calorie counters won. Even the latest food-labeling regulations emphasize calories by making them big and bold on the label. New laws make it mandatory for fast-food restaurants to place calorie counts on menus. It stands to reason that if all calories are equal, and fat contains more than twice as many calories as carbs or protein (9 calories per gram vs. 4 calories per gram), then the best way to cut calories is to cut out fat. You could eat more food if you ate bread and pasta than if you ate butter, because butter is more energy-dense. This is what I was taught and what I believed until new research turned this idea upside down.

Dr. Frederick Stare, who founded the department of nutrition at the Harvard School of Public Health in 1942 and served as its chairman until he retired in 1976, helped to entrench the idea that obesity was nothing more than a matter of energy imbalance. He stated that all calories had an equal impact on weight gain, "regardless of whether they derive from eggs or eggplant, grapefruit or green beans, skim milk or scotch whisky or soda pop or sirloin steak." In his books, column, and writings, Stare encouraged the public to accept that "there are no 'fattening' foods or 'slimming' foods, just too much food." He wrote, "Calories are all alike, regardless of their source. Patients cannot be misled by a high carbohydrate or high protein or high fat fad if they are aware that surplus calories are surplus calories, whether the source is carbohydrate or protein or fat, or alcohol in various beverages."

The idea of energy balance naturally implies that willpower is the key to weight loss, that all one needs to do is limit calories and increase exercise. The logical conclusion of this distorted thinking is this: If you are overweight, it must be because you are a lazy glutton who shuns exercise and loves to eat. The subtle message here is that the overweight person *wants* to be fat. It is their fault they are fat. Yet, in treating more than 20,000 patients, I have never met a person who wakes up and says, "Hey, today I am going to see how much weight I can gain." On the contrary, most wake up with every intention of losing weight but can't, not because of a character defect but because of bad advice based on incorrect scientific assumptions.

When both the government (the Centers for Disease Control and Prevention) and the American Beverage Association's websites offer the same dietary advice for weight loss, we should be suspicious. In this model, there is no good or bad food. The answer to obesity and weight regulation is moderation. In fact, in testimony to Congress, under oath, the chair of the American Beverage Association said with a straight face, "In a well balanced diet we need two liters of liquids a day. Soft drinks can be a healthy part of that intake. I would reject any argument that they are in any way harmful." This is a staggering statement contradicted by mountains of research, including the 2015 study in the journal *Circulation* that found that sugar-sweetened drinks kill 184,000 people a year from obesity, heart disease, and cancer.

A CALORIE IS NOT A CALORIE

The conventional wisdom doesn't stack up against emerging research that shows us that a *calorie is not a calorie (when you eat it)*. In a vacuum or a lab, calories from all foods release the same amount of energy when burned—whether the food is coconut oil or honey. But when you eat, foods have to go through your body, and they can have profoundly different effects on your hormones, brain chemistry, and metabolism. Fat calories burn differently than sugar calories do. Fat calories speed up your metabolism. Fats have to be burned and are not easily stored because they don't spike insulin—the fat-storage hormone. Fat works on the brain to cut your appetite so you eat less overall during the day. On the other hand, sugar and carb calories do exactly the opposite: They spike insulin, promote fat storage, and are quickly laid down as dangerous belly and organ fat. They slow your metabolism and increase hunger and cravings. Mounds of scientific research support this perspective.

This *hormonal* or *metabolic hypothesis* of weight gain supports the idea that it is the composition and quality of the foods you eat (and the hormones and biochemistry they subsequently trigger) that determine whether you lose or gain weight. In other words, it is not *how much you eat* but *what you eat* that controls the metabolic switches. Food's inherent information—the messages and instructions it contains—is what drives your metabolism. Again, carbs shift

> I have lost both in belly fat and hip measurements. It has been many years since I have consumed this many calories while "dieting" and still lost weight!
> —Barbara Chitkara

your body toward fat storage (anabolism),[3] while fats shift your body toward fat burning (catabolism).

This idea was actually quite well described as early as the nineteenth century and was the basis for much of the dietary advice for the last part of the nineteenth and early part of the twentieth century. Leading medical experts in the late nineteenth century believed that the best strategy for treating obesity was carbohydrate restriction. It was in the medical textbooks of the day. The fathers of modern medicine, William Harvey, a nineteenth-century English physician, and William Osler, one of the founding physicians of Johns Hopkins, both advised low-carbohydrate diets for weight loss.

Despite historical evidence to the contrary, however, the idea of energy balance slowly took hold in the 1950s and 1960s. Dr. Frederick Stare at Harvard continued to heavily promote the idea, even while acknowledging obvious holes in the theory: He noted that chronically high blood sugar was looking more and more like a strong driver of weight gain. He called this "obesity of the metabolic type," caused by eating too much sugar. This is the crack in the theory that all calories are created equal.

Even if you consume less food and fewer calories, when you eat excess carbs or sugar, you trigger insulin, which turns on a fat-production factory in the liver and your fat-storage system, and you gain weight. Dietary fat, however, doesn't trigger insulin, and so you don't store fat. But despite understanding this perspective, which was advocated by other scientists at the time, Stare was unwilling to advocate for almost anything for weight loss but physical activity and calorie restriction.

At the beginning of the twentieth century, German diabetes specialist Carl von Noorden believed in the metabolic hypothesis, but he later changed his position. In his earlier work, he postulated that obesity was a pre-diabetic state and said, "Obese individuals of this type have already an altered metabolism for sugar, but instead of excreting the sugar in the urine, they transfer it to the fat-producing parts of the body."[4] This concept was pushed under the carpet and ignored despite evidence to the contrary, and the debate smoldered on for years.

In 1953, in a report in the *New England Journal of Medicine* titled "A Reorientation on Obesity," Dr. Alfred Pennington argued that obesity was caused by the hormonal effects of carbs and could be treated by restricting carbs, without worrying about fat and protein.[5] That was a radical departure from the idea that weight regulation was just a matter of calories in, calories out.

In 1977, a study published in the *American Journal of Clinical Nutrition* showed that the composition of your diet (high-carb, low-fat or high-fat, low-carb) could have profoundly different effects on human biology even though the calories consumed were identical. They kept ten obese men in a metabolic ward in a hospital and strictly controlled their diets. Even though there were only a few people in the study, these metabolic ward studies are relevant because of how carefully their food intake and energy expenditure was measured. For two weeks, these men consumed a high-carb diet of 70 percent carbs, 20 percent protein, and 10 percent fat. Then, after a 7-day rest period, the men were switched to a high-fat diet consisting of 70 percent fat, 20 percent protein, and 10 percent carbs. When the study subjects were on a high-fat diet they lost more weight than when they were on a high-carb diet, and had much greater drops in blood sugar, insulin levels, triglycerides, and cholesterol, even though they ate the same total number of calories.[6]

In 2002, Dr. Walter Willett, of the Harvard School of Public Health, summarized all the research on fat and obesity (as well as fat and heart disease) and found no connection. He stated that "diets high in fat do not appear to be the primary cause of the high prevalence of excess body fat in our society, and reductions in fat will not be a solution."[7]

DOES EATING FAT CAUSE HEART DISEASE?

Besides restricting fat for weight loss, the scientific community embraced and stridently promoted another hypothesis: that fat caused heart disease, our biggest killer. But the history of medicine is full of good ideas that turned out to be wrong and even dangerous. Thalidomide seemed to be a great idea and very effective at preventing morning sickness in pregnancy until it was discovered to cause severe birth defects. Hormone replacement therapy for women was thought to be so effective in preventing heart disease in women that it was considered malpractice not to prescribe it. More than 50 million menopausal women happily took hormones until a large study sponsored by the National Institutes of Health found that hormone replacement actually increased the risk of heart disease, stroke, and breast cancer.

Before you read any further, you need to know the truth: **Eating saturated fat does not cause heart disease.**[8] I know this might seem startling, given that we've spent the better part of a century avoiding everything from butter to egg yolks because we were told they weren't good for our hearts. But better to know the truth and make new and healthier habits going forward.

The theory that fat, and specifically saturated fat, is the cause of heart disease all started because of two main findings. First was that rabbits (which are obviously very different from humans) developed atherosclerosis (fatty deposits in the arteries) when they were fed cholesterol, which is completely absent from their vegetable diet. Second, countries that seemed to consume more saturated fat and the most fat generally (for example, Finland and the United States compared to Japan and Greece) had more heart disease. Since saturated fat raised blood levels of cholesterol, it was assumed that saturated fat caused heart disease. Suddenly, a weak hypothesis that was based on shaky observations, not on any real experiments, was taken as fact.

This idea, spawned in 1953, was the brainchild of a very outspoken, passionate scientist from the University of Minnesota named Ancel Keys. Many questioned Keys' scientific conclusions, but he was vigorous in criticizing anyone who challenged him. He was a dominant, persuasive, and charismatic man who convinced the world of his hypothesis.

The history and failure of Keys' diet–heart hypothesis, that fat is bad, is well documented in Nina Teicholz's book, *The Big Fat Surprise*.[9] Keys made his conclusions based on observations of heart disease, death rates, and fat consumption in six countries, even though data on twenty-two countries from the Food and Agriculture Organization of the United Nations and data from the World Health Organization (WHO) was available. The diet record keeping was questionable. He selected six countries that he felt had the best data (or perhaps that he knew would best support his ideas) and found a direct correlation between the amount of fat in the diet and heart disease. He ignored data from the other sixteen countries. A more recent 2010 review by the Food and Agriculture Organization found that "there is no probable or convincing evidence" that a high-fat diet causes heart disease.[10]

When all twenty-two countries were included in the analysis in 1957 by two who questioned Keys' conclusions, Drs. Herman Hilleboe, then New York State commissioner of health, and Jacob Yerushalmy, professor of statistics at the University of California, Berkeley, there was zero correlation between fat in the diet and heart disease.[11] Yet despite that fact, and the fact that observational or population studies cannot prove cause and effect, Keys' study took hold.

Dr. Keys followed up his six countries study with the famous Seven Countries Study, launched in 1956, in which he again carefully selected countries that supported his theory and conveniently omitted countries such as France and Switzerland that had high-fat diets and very little heart disease. He followed 12,770 people but evaluated diet intake for only 499, or 3.9 percent of them. This is poor science, insufficient to make broad conclusions. Yet draw "definitive" conclusions he did, and he further refined his theory to focus on saturated fat as the enemy.

The theory went something like this: Blood cholesterol was associated with (but not proven to be a factor in) increased risk of heart disease. Saturated fats increased cholesterol. So the enemy was saturated fat. While he did find a correlation between saturated fat and heart disease in the countries he picked, he did not find any reduction in death in countries with lower saturated fat intake. And though he found the correlation of saturated fat and heart disease between countries, when he looked at different regions of the same country—such as different regions of Finland or different islands in Greece, such as Corfu and Crete—he found that they had widely different rates of heart disease. Something didn't add up.

There were many problems with Keys' research, including the way in which he collected people's dietary history and how few people he had dietary information on for a population-type study, which usually requires thousands of participants to be able to draw any conclusions. He studied countries in postwar Europe, when diets were affected by wartime shortages, so they didn't represent the true diets of these populations. And there were many other severe limitations in his research. Basically, he set up his study to prove his hypothesis.

CHALLENGES TO THE DIET-HEART HYPOTHESIS

One of the voices Keys tried to silence was that of John Yudkin, the British physician and founding professor of the Department of Nutrition at Queen Elizabeth College in London. Dr. Yudkin was ahead of his time. As early as 1964, he challenged the unproved assumption that fat in the diet caused fat in the arteries. In the pre-Atkins era, he warned about the dangers of high sugar consumption and the risk of cardiovascular disease and promoted a low-carb, low-sugar diet in his popular 1972 book, *Pure, White and Deadly*. Dr. Yudkin carried out his own studies looking at the effects of sucrose on coronary risk factors and repeatedly published letters and reviews in leading medical journals arguing that the focus of public health efforts—at least as far as nutrition was concerned—should be on sugar.

In the *American Journal of Clinical Nutrition* in 1981, Dr. Yudkin wrote, "As long ago as 1957, it was suggested from epidemiological evidence that the current high sucrose [sugar] consumption in Western countries could be a cause of the high prevalence of coronary heart disease." He said that a high-sugar diet increases bad cholesterol and decreases good cholesterol, increases insulin and stress hormones (like cortisol), and even makes your blood more likely to clot—all tightly linked to heart attacks and strokes. High-sugar diets, he said, led to diabetes, blindness, and nerve and kidney damage and explained why diabetics have four times the risk of heart attacks as everyone else.

Dr. Yudkin went on to argue that the underlying cause of heart disease is sugar, not fat, caused by hormonal imbalances (from too much insulin). He said we should focus on getting rid of sugar, instead of the popular recommendation to substitute polyunsaturated omega-6 fats for saturated fats.[12]

The bottom line, according to Dr. Yudkin: Sugar is the bad guy here, not fat. He explained that the studies that linked fat and heart disease are the type of studies that cannot prove cause and effect and that actual scientific experiments proved that it was sugar that caused all the problems seen in heart disease (abnormal cholesterol, inflammation, thick blood, etc.).

This makes complete sense if you understand the biochemistry of cholesterol in the body. (See Chapter 5 to clear up the cholesterol confusion.) And even so, in 1961, based on Keys' work, the American Heart Association took up the mantra of fat as the cause of heart disease. *Time* magazine featured Keys on the cover and dubbed him "Mr. Cholesterol." They quoted him recommending we cut our dietary fat from 40 percent to 15 percent of calories and saturated fat from 17 percent to 4 percent, and his advice was cemented as fact. In the public consciousness, there was no turning back.

Despite the data that flooded in showing that cholesterol and dietary fat may not be the real drivers of heart disease—that sugar and refined carbs are the true drivers of heart disease,[13] weight gain,[14] and type 2 diabetes[15]—medical associations and the food industry pressed onward with the promotion of a low-fat diet for heart health.

Subsequently, in 1984, Keys published a follow-up study that reanalyzed the data and could not find any association between saturated fat and heart disease.[16] But by that time, the diet-heart hypothesis was so entrenched, policies set, and the food industry mobilized to produce fat-free (high-carb) foods that there was no going back.

The most important finding came in 1999, when all the data from Dr. Keys' Seven Countries study was analyzed again by the study's lead Italian researcher, Alessandro Menotti. He discovered a remarkable finding when he looked at all categories of food, not just fats.[17] He found that sugar had a higher correlation with heart disease than fat. Many others were on the trail of sugar and carbs as the driver of heart disease, including Dr. Pete Ahrens, one of the fathers of lipid research from Rockefeller University, and Dr. John Yudkin. In 1986, Dr. Yudkin said, "If only a small fraction of what we already know about the effects of sugar were revealed in relation to any other material used as a food additive, that material would be promptly banned." In others words, sugar would not be approved as a safe additive by the Food and Drug Administration (FDA).

THE LOW-FAT PLANT-BASED DIET AND HEART DISEASE

Some doctors and scientists have made observations and performed research that have shown that low-fat diets may be very effective in many diseases, including Drs. Dean Ornish, Neal Barnard, Caldwell Esselstyn, and Colin Campbell. Dr. Dean Ornish, a friend and colleague, has been a proponent of the diet-heart hypothesis. His Preventive Medicine Research Institute has done some impressive research on low-fat plant-based diets and heart-disease reversal, the reversal of prostate cancer, and the lengthening of telomeres (the ends of our chromosomes, which typically shorten as we age). Clearly, eating a whole-foods plant-based diet works. He has been a tireless and passionate advocate of lifestyle change for the prevention and reversal of chronic disease and has profoundly and beneficially impacted many lives.

The real question is how would this compare in effectiveness to all the same interventions but with a high-quality, high-fat diet that included organic or grass-fed animal products—or even with a high-fat, high-quality plant-based diet? That study has never been done so we can't know for sure. But Dr. Ornish took men who were eating the typical processed nutrient-poor standard American diet and put them on a whole-foods, low-fat, plant-based diet. Guaranteed that will improve anyone's health. It doesn't answer the question, though, of whether this is the best diet for weight loss and disease prevention. In fact in most studies of low-fat vs. low-carb diets for weight loss, the low-carb, high-fat diet prevails. In the A TO Z Weight Loss Study comparing the Ornish and Atkins diets (low-fat to high-fat) in 311 postmenopausal women for a year, the high-fat diet group achieved the quickest, most dramatic weight loss and had greater improvements in most cardiovascular risk factors.[18]

Some challenge the data in the A TO Z trial of only 311 women. However, in a recent review of fifty-three high-quality randomized, controlled trials that included 68,128 people and compared low-fat to high-fat diets lasting a year or more, the high-fat diets led to greater weight loss than the low-fat diets.[19] The researchers included only the best-quality studies (53 out of 3,517 studies). Some of the studies showed that when compared to the standard American diet (which is typically very bad), a low-fat diet did lead to weight loss. But in the studies that compared high-fat, low-carbohydrate diets to low-fat diets, the high-fat diets led to significantly greater weight loss. And in the studies where there was an even higher fat content, and where the triglycerides dropped the most, weight loss was even greater. Triglycerides go up in a high-carb diet and down in a high-fat diet, so by looking at the triglycerides the researchers were able to tell how well the study subjects adhered to the high-fat, low-carb diets. Bottom line: in the best review of the research to date, going head-to-head, high-fat, low-carb diets beat out low-fat diets for weight loss.

More studies are needed for sure. We need to compare high-fat to low-fat vegan diets. And we need to compare vegan diets to what I call a Pegan diet (more on that in Chapter 10), which is mostly plant-based with moderate amounts of clean animal protein. But the evidence is overwhelmingly pointing to the fact that it is our processed high-sugar diet, not the fat, that is driving disease and obesity, and that the key is to switch to a whole-foods diet rich in plant foods but also higher in good fats. Even Dr. Ornish recommends restricting refined carbs and sugar and adding omega-3 fats as part of his program.

Clearly Dr. Ornish's low-fat, whole-foods, low-sugar, plant-based diet worked when compared to a processed, high-sugar, and high-carb diet to reduce the burden of heart disease. What we don't know is how this diet compares to a higher-fat, whole-foods, mostly plant-based diet containing nuts, seeds, olive and coconut oil, and some healthy grass-fed, antibiotic-, hormone- and pesticide-free animal protein. We need to study this. There are significant genetic differences in how people handle fats and carbs and there may be some who do better on lower-fat diets, and others who do better on higher-fat diets; but all do better on a whole-foods diet that is the opposite of the standard American diet, the worst diet on the planet, which we are now exporting to every country in the world.

HOW COULD THE EXPERTS BE WRONG?

It seems implausible that the main associations and organizations entrusted with creating public health recommendations and policies and led by the world's experts could have gotten it so wrong. But they did, and that, too, plays a big part in how we got into this big, fat mess.

The American Diabetes Association (ADA), which for years recommended high-carb diets for type 2 diabetes, has moved toward advising people to limit their carb intake. But they still recommend that diabetics eat a low-fat diet,[20] despite overwhelming evidence that carb restriction combined with higher-fat diets (up to 70 percent fat) are profoundly effective in treating and reversing type 2 diabetes.[21] I have been at ADA meetings where the entire exhibit floor promotes diet, low-calorie, artificially sweetened low-fat goods in big booths sponsored by the food industry. Even though we know that artificial sweeteners actually cause type 2 diabetes[22] and weight gain, slow metabolism, increase hunger,[23] and alter gut flora or bacteria to promote obesity and type 2 diabetes,[24] they are still recommended by the ADA, diabetes doctors, and registered dietitians. That's right. Artificial sweeteners make you fat and diabetic!

The American Heart Association (AHA) partnered early with the National Institutes of Health (NIH) and funded most of the research on diet and heart disease. Their focus has been almost solely on the diet-heart hypothesis: the idea that fat, saturated fat, and dietary cholesterol were the cause of heart disease because they raised blood cholesterol. But even though in a long-term follow-up of the famous Framingham study, LDL (bad cholesterol) was the least associated cholesterol indicator of heart attack risk, on its website, at the time of writing the AHA continues to promote the same outdated recommendations to cut back on fat:

- Select fat-free, 1 percent fat, and low-fat dairy products.
- Choose lean meats and poultry without skin and prepare them without added saturated and trans fat.
- To lower cholesterol, reduce saturated fat to no more than 5 to 6 percent of total calories. For someone eating 2,000 calories a day, that's about 13 grams of saturated fat.
- Cut back on foods containing partially hydrogenated vegetable oils to reduce trans fat in your diet. (A good thing and something they got right!)

We should question whether the AHA's policies are shaped in part by the source of their funding. They get millions of dollars a year for giving their seal of approval to highly processed industrial foods like low-fat, high-fiber oat cereals, despite the fact that they often contain six different kinds of sugar.[25]

Despite recent multiple large and extensive reviews of the research that found no link between dietary fat, and especially saturated fat,[26] and heart disease,[27] these guidelines persist. Dr. Ronald Krauss, who chaired the guidelines committee of the AHA in the 1990s and is currently the director of atherosclerosis research at Children's Hospital Oakland Research Institute, challenged their fervent belief that saturated fat was the cause of heart disease. Despite his protestations, they continued to lower the acceptable limits of saturated fat in the diet, and he resigned from the committee. Dr. Krauss has proven that saturated fat actually improves the type of cholesterol (from small, dense, dangerous to light, fluffy, benign cholesterol).[28] He shows that it is, in fact, sugar and refined carbs that cause the most dangerous *atherogenic,* or heart disease–causing, type of cholesterol pattern.[29]

The Academy of Nutrition and Dietetics (AND), the organization for registered dietitians entrusted with providing nutrition advice to patients, is also on the low-fat bandwagon. I recently spoke at one of its annual meetings in Philadelphia and was shocked to see huge exhibits from the food industry promoting every type of high-sugar, low-fat processed food. A recent California chapter of AND had its lunch (which was mandatory for attendees) sponsored by McDonald's. AND had thirty-eight food industry funders in 2011, including Coca-Cola, PepsiCo, Nestlé, National Cattlemen's Beef Association, Mars, and many others. Corporate contributions are its largest source of income, generating nearly 40 percent of its total revenue.[30]

Makes you wonder: Why would they promote real food when they are funded by the food industry?

THE ROLE OF BIG GOVERNMENT

We can't lay all the blame on the scientific community for our fat phobia and the worldwide obesity epidemic it spurred. It is only one leg of the tripod that landed us where we are today.

In the 1970s, when it became evident that rates of obesity and heart disease were increasing, certain well-meaning politicians held hearings on diet and heath to determine how to advise Americans.

Mark Hegsted, a professor of nutrition at Harvard, led the group of scientists that in 1977—under the auspices of Senator George McGovern's Select Committee on Nutrition and Human Needs—issued the first Dietary Goals for the United States, the forerunner of the Dietary Guidelines for Americans. These guidelines, updated roughly every five years by the federal government, cemented the low-fat philosophy as the country's official diet, despite many scientists' testimony that the evidence for a low-fat diet was insufficient.[31] A recent review of all the randomized controlled studies (not population studies) that existed *before* the actual guidelines were developed in 1980 found no evidence linking fat to heart disease.[32]

Hegsted was fiercely against saturated fat. His research had shown that manipulating the levels of fat in a person's diet could drive the person's total cholesterol levels up or down. Hegsted found in his experiments that saturated fats raised the levels of total and LDL ("bad" cholesterol), that polyunsaturated fats lowered total cholesterol, and that monounsaturated fats did not seem to have much of an effect. But it wasn't proven that this was linked to heart disease, and at that time, we didn't know that HDL, triglycerides, and the size of your LDL (bad cholesterol) mattered more than total cholesterol.

The Dietary Goals report called for Americans to increase their carbohydrate intake to 55 to 60 percent of their daily calories, reduce their fat intake from 40 to 30 percent of their calories, and limit saturated fat consumption to no more than 10 percent of calories. It also advised them to limit their dietary cholesterol to about 300 milligrams a day. To its credit, the government did recommend a reduction in sugar (but not refined carbs) by about 40 percent from what Americans were eating at the time to account for 15 percent of calories.

Americans were told that they could protect themselves against cardiovascular disease, diabetes, and other chronic ills by eating more fruits, vegetables, poultry, fish, and whole grains, and by cutting back on the saturated fat in meat, eggs, butter, and whole-fat milk. They were told to eat low-fat foods like skim milk and to replace the saturated fat in animal products with polyunsaturated and monounsaturated fats from vegetable oils.

In 1992, the US Department of Agriculture issued the now-infamous Food Guide Pyramid. Carbs were firmly situated at the bottom of the pyramid and Americans were told to eat six to eleven servings of bread, rice, cereal, and pasta a day. Fats were at the tippy top, and we were warned to eat them sparingly. Suddenly pasta was a health food and fat was demonized.

In 2010, MyPlate, our government's new educational food icon, replaced the pyramid, and it was a slight improvement. But it still advises a low-fat diet and includes the recommendation that we eat more dairy, despite the fact that there is little scientific support for the health benefits that many people connect with dairy.[33] Walter Willett, the Harvard School of Public Health chair of the Department of Nutrition, criticized MyPlate, saying, "Unfortunately, like the earlier U.S. Department of Agriculture pyramids, MyPlate mixes science with the influence of powerful agricultural interests, which is not the recipe for healthy eating."[34]

The food industry has influenced governmental recommendations and dietary guidelines across the globe. In 2014 the *British Medical Journal* published a series of investigative reports that "uncovered evidence of the extraordinary extent to which key public health experts are involved with the sugar industry and related companies responsible for many of the products blamed for the obesity crisis through research grants, consultancy fees, and other forms of funding."[35]

In 2003 the World Health Organization (WHO) recommended the reduction of sugar to less than 10 percent of calories, and the sugar lobby descended on the White House. Tommy Thompson, the secretary of Health and Human Services under George Bush, flew to Geneva to intervene.[36] It wasn't until 12 years later, in 2015, that the WHO was brave enough to declare that "adults and children [should] reduce their daily intake of free sugars to less than 10 percent of their total energy intake. A further reduction to below 5 percent or roughly 25 grams (6 teaspoons) per day would provide additional health benefits."[37]

In a conversation with a former secretary of agriculture, Ann Veneman, I asked why we couldn't stop the use of $4 billion in food stamps to pay for sodas, or why we couldn't change the US Dietary Guidelines to more closely match current nutrition science. Her response was sobering. "The food industry has a lock on Congress and the White House." Unfortunately, the mission of the USDA is to set healthy nutrition policy and promote and market agricultural products to Americans, not necessarily provide the most accurate scientific recommendations.

This is an inherent conflict. It is a veritable revolving door of jobs between the USDA and Big Ag and Big Food. Americans should insist on the establishment of a new Department of Food run through the Department of Health and Human Services, which is paying for the consequences of harmful dietary recommendations through Medicare and Medicaid.

In 2015, the US Dietary Guidelines Advisory Committee quietly and with little fanfare ended the era of trumpeting low-fat diets for weight loss or health. After reviewing all the research, this group of scientists failed to find any reason to limit total fat or cholesterol in the diet. This was finally put into the official guidelines in late 2015.[38] A discussion of these recommendations in the *Journal of the American Medical Association* by Dr. David Ludwig of Harvard and Dr. Dariush Mozaffarian underscored these findings.[39] Dr. Mozaffarian said, "Low-fat diets have had unintended consequences, turning people away from healthy high-fat foods and toward foods rich in added sugars, starches, and refined grains. This has helped fuel the twin epidemics of obesity and diabetes in America. We really need to sing it from the rooftops that the low-fat diet concept is dead. There are no health benefits to it."

After six decades of fearing fat, ding-dong, the witch is dead!

BIG FOOD JUMPS ON THE LOW-FAT BANDWAGON

The food industry happily complies with any fad or recommendation of the day. With the low-fat wave of advice, the industry got busy creating a massive shift in their products. They replaced saturated fats with "healthy vegetable oils" like margarine and shortening. The grand irony, of course, is that hydrogenated fat (aka trans fat) has turned out to be one of the only fats scientifically linked to heart disease.

They took flawed research and the resulting flawed government recommendations and amassed a $1 trillion food industry that on the surface sounded healthy but was really anything but. They turned low-fat foods into an aspirational goal for most Americans: low-fat cookies, low-fat sweetened yogurt, low-fat salad dressing, and on and on. The biggest problem is that these foods are loaded with sugar. When you remove fat from foods, it tastes like cardboard, which is why they added sugar. This sugar, as you now know, is the main driver of obesity and heart disease, not fat.

Oops.

SUGAR BECOMES THE NEW FAT

In the late 1970s, in concert with Big Ag (the likes of Cargill and Monsanto) and fueled by new agricultural subsidies that promoted massive increases in the production of corn and soy, Big Food poured high-fructose corn syrup and hydrogenated fats into 600,000 industrial processed foods, 80 percent of which contained added sugar. These high-sugar, high-glycemic foods are highly addictive and spike insulin, which in turn leads to fat storage, hunger, a slow metabolism, and the cholesterol profile most linked to heart disease. Insulin is also the main cause of inflammation—now known to be the real driver of heart disease.

Eating low-fat foods became a virtue as we plowed through giant plates of pasta, oversized bagels, and muffins the size of softballs. But we paid a heavy price for demonizing fat and replacing it with sugar and foods that turn to sugar in our bodies. Ever since we went whole hog (or should I say whole bowl of pasta), dutifully following our government's misguided and harmful advice since the early 1980s and eating the foods the food industry inventively crafted for the low-fat craze, we went from not a single state having an obesity rate over 20 percent to not a single state having an obesity rate under 20 percent, and now with most states having rates over 25 and even 35 percent. And a full 70 percent of American adults and 40 percent of kids are overweight.

In the 1980s, our sugar consumption (including table sugar and high-fructose corn syrup) was 126 pounds per person per year (a lot). Now it is 152 pounds per person per year. Our consumption of flour, which raises blood sugar more than table sugar does, is about 146 pounds per person per year. That's a combined average of 1 pound of flour and sugar for every person in America every day! There are mountains of processed food products on the market, and nearly all of those products have added sugar. Your morning low-fat yogurt has more sugar than a can of soda, and your Prego tomato sauce has more sugar per serving than two Oreo cookies. This increase in sugar has tracked perfectly with our obesity epidemic.

Before the 1980s there was almost no high-fructose corn syrup in our diet. Now it is the biggest source of calories in our diet, with each American consuming more than 50 pounds a year. High-fructose corn syrup is especially dangerous because, unlike sugar, which is 50:50 glucose and fructose, high-fructose corn syrup may contain up to 75 percent fructose, which drives obesity, diabetes, cancer, fatty liver, and heart disease. While technically it is true that table sugar consumption has gone down because government subsidies make high-fructose corn syrup cheap and trade tariffs to protect American farmers make sugar more expensive, the total load of sweeteners in all forms has increased dramatically in the last 35 years, tracking exactly with our obesity and diabetes epidemic. It is high-fructose consumption that turns on fat production and storage in your liver through a process called *lipogenesis*.

According to new government surveys from the National Health and Nutrition Examination Survey, our sweetened beverage consumption (soda, sweetened coffees and teas, energy drinks, etc.) accounts for about 20 percent of our calories. That's bad news because sugar-sweetened beverages are the "foods" that are the number one cause of obesity and type 2 diabetes. One can of soda a day increases a child's risk of becoming obese by 60 percent. One can of soda a day increases a woman's risk of type 2 diabetes by 80 percent. Over the last few decades, sugar consumption surged in Mexico, mostly from soda. Today, 1 in 10 children in that country has type 2 diabetes (what used to be called adult-onset diabetes). What's remarkable is that soda companies still insist that sugar-sweetened beverages can be a part of a healthy diet as long as the total calories are balanced with the right amount of exercise. This flies in the face of mountains of scientific evidence to the contrary.

Sugar is a main cause of heart disease, too. Those with the highest intake of sugar have a 275 percent increased risk of heart attacks, and those with the lowest intake (which is still relatively a lot) have a 30 percent increased risk. If you think that soda is bad for you only if you gain weight from drinking it, think again. Even if you are skinny and drink sodas and never gain a pound, your risk of heart disease still goes up dramatically!

THE REDEMPTION OF FAT

So now you know the whole story of how we came to demonize fat and glorify sugar, and the price we paid. A few zealous scientists convinced the government to change policy, and the food industry followed right in step to fulfill the demand for low-fat foods. They took the fat out but replaced it with sugar and refined carbs. They were joined by policy makers who jumped on board, and a food industry that was all too happy to fill our plates with low-fat, sugar-laden foods.

But that's not the end of our story—far from it!

The evidence is now moving away from dietary fat as the root cause of both weight gain and heart disease, and shining a bright and damning light where it belongs: on carbs and sugar. The low-fat era is on its last breath. Even government guidelines are starting to change.

The 2015 US Dietary Guidelines have softened their view on reducing fat and have officially removed limits on dietary cholesterol from their advice. Eggs are back. And professional associations are backpedaling. Even the American Heart Association and the American Cardiology Association have abandoned the low-fat message and have told us to forget completely about worrying about dietary cholesterol.[40] Still they focus on saturated fat, but many scientists are questioning the purported dangers of saturated fat.[41]

Slowly, cautiously, the tide is turning to a more balanced view of what's good and what's not. In Part III we will dig into what we should eat, based on today's understanding. *Eat Fat, Get Thin* wades through all the confusing research and clears the muddied waters. You will learn which fats (and foods) promote health, help with effortless weight loss, prevent heart disease and cancer, improve your mood and brain function, and help prevent and even reverse dementia in its early stages.[42]

And all this while eating delicious, deeply satisfying food, because the thing that makes food the most satisfying is fat!

As I've said, I myself was confused for a long time about fat, but after reading more than 1,000 scientific papers and seeing more than 20,000 patients, I have a much better sense of the good, the bad, and the ugly fats. I will help guide you to understand the world of dietary fat so that you can make the right choices.

PART II

SEPARATING FAT FROM FICTION

There is nothing more difficult to carry out, nor more doubtful of success, nor more dangerous to handle, than to initiate a new order of things. For the reformer has enemies in all those who profit by the old order, and only lukewarm defenders in all those who would profit by the new order.

—Niccolò Machiavelli, *The Prince and The Discourses*

3

Eating Fat Does *Not* Make You Fat!

If you believe that all calories are created equal (and you now know they definitively are not), then it stands to reason that you'd also be quick to demonize fat and blame it for weight gain. It seems like simple math: If fat has more than twice as many calories per gram as carbs or protein, then if you eat less fat, you will eat fewer calories and lose weight. Sounds reasonable, doesn't it? Unfortunately it just doesn't work out that way for many reasons.

That all calories are the same in terms of effects on your weight and metabolism is one of the most persistent myths in medicine today. They are the same in a laboratory, when you burn them in a vacuum. But not when you eat them. New public policies require restaurants to list the calorie content of each dish, and food companies to label calories per serving in large, bold type. But this is the wrong strategy, because it implies that only calories matter. The truth is that different calories affect your gene expression, hormones, brain chemistry, immune system, metabolism, and even your gut flora differently. While it is helpful to track calories in processed and fast food (because they can be so loaded with bad calories)—it can deter you from eating that 1,200-calorie meal—if you eat real food, you don't need to track calories.

Metabolism is not a math problem. It's not about balancing "energy" or calories in and calories out. If it were, and you ate an additional 100 calories a day, which is about a big bite of food, after a year you would gain ten pounds. After a decade you would gain one hundred pounds. This just doesn't happen. Even if you were the world record holder in calorie counting, you couldn't get the math right to control your weight.

That's why weight and metabolism are not math problems. The quality of the food you eat matters much more than the quantity. If food were only about calories, it wouldn't matter what specific foods you ate, as long as you kept below a certain number of calories. But it does. Why?

Food is not just a source of energy or calories. *Food is information.* It contains instructions that affect every biological function of your body. It is the stuff that controls everything. Food affects the expression of your genes (determining which ones get triggered to cause or prevent disease) and influences your hormones, brain chemistry, immune system, gut flora, and metabolism at every level. It works fast, in real time with every bite. This is the groundbreaking science of *nutrigenomics*.

The whole idea that a calorie is a calorie is finally being intensely studied by the Nutrition Science Initiative,[1] headed by Dr. Peter Attia and Gary Taubes (author of *Good Calories, Bad Calories*). The institute is funding rigorous and larger studies by the world's best researchers to answer this question once and for all and quiet the naysayers — of which there are still many, despite adequate evidence. They are even enlisting scientists who disagree with their hypothesis that all calories are not equal so those scientists can prove themselves wrong.

This is not a new idea. Nutrition expert Ann Louise Gittleman, PhD, CNS, the former director of nutrition at the renowned low-fat, high-carb Pritikin Longevity Center, was the first in the country to write about the importance of fats in her bestselling *Beyond Pritikin*, released in 1988. For years, she has been a pioneer and the lone voice in promoting the importance of the right fats. She identified the flaws in the science back then and, in thirty of her books that followed, implored us to eat more fat. Sadly, we ignored her prescient advice.

More and more scientists are confirming that calories coming from fat are better for weight loss and improving metabolism. Kevin Hall, from the National Institutes of Health, has found that in a metabolic ward where every ounce of food and every movement and every calorie burned are carefully measured, those who ate more fat calories (compared to an identical number of calories from carbs) burned more than 100 additional calories a day. Over a year that amounts to a ten-pound weight loss. He also reported that in studies of brain imaging and function, eating more fat shuts off the hunger and craving centers of the brain.[2] It seems that the brain matters most in terms of controlling food intake, taste preferences, and metabolism. And that dietary fat can positively impact the whole calorie-burning process.

WHY WE OVEREAT

Most of us assume that overeating makes us gain weight. That sounds like a reasonable assumption, right? But in a brilliant paper in the *Journal of the American Medical Association,* Harvard professor Dr. David Ludwig lays out the case for a very different view of obesity and metabolism.

He says, simply, that we have it backwards. It is not eating more and exercising less that makes you fat, but being fat that makes you eat more and exercise less. Essentially your fat cells "get hungry" and drive you to overeat. He describes this process in detail in his book *Always Hungry?* When you are overweight, your hormones and brain chemistry make you hungry and tired.[3]

This turns all our thinking about weight gain upside down and contradicts every single established recommendation for weight loss. Rather than focus on calories and quantity, Dr. Ludwig suggests we focus on quality and the composition of our diet (amount and type of protein, fat, and carbs) to allow the body's natural intelligence to regulate hunger, activity, metabolism, and weight. Forget about willpower—use science to cut your hunger, give you energy, and speed up your metabolism!

Here's how this plays out in your biology.

First, when you try to restrict calories and exercise more, your body is hardwired to perceive a starvation situation. That makes you tired (so you move less and conserve energy) and hungry (so you eat more), and it slows down your metabolism (so you don't die!). This "eat less, exercise more" formula is not too successful for most people. It can work for a short time, certainly, but less than 10 percent of people lose weight and keep it off for a year;[4] you will almost always rebound and gain back the weight.

Second, when you eat carbs and sugar, insulin spikes and your blood sugar drops. The insulin drives most of the available fuel in your bloodstream into fat cells, especially the fat cells around your middle, otherwise known as belly fat. So your body is starved of fuel, and this stimulates your brain[5] to make you eat more.[6] You could have a year's worth of stored energy in your fat tissue and yet feel like you are starving.

The only thing that can stop this vicious cycle is eating a lot of fat and cutting out the refined carbs and sugar. A high-fat, low-carb diet leads to a faster metabolism and sustained weight loss.

WHY WE GAIN OR LOSE WEIGHT: THE BIOLOGY OF FAT CELLS

What makes our fat cells store fat? What makes them release and burn fat?

We are still learning how our bodies regulate our weight. At the heart of Functional Medicine is the concept of biochemical and genetic individuality. This concept is especially relevant in the world of body weight. There is not just one cause of weight gain. There is a wide range in how we respond to different foods—fats or carbs or protein. Even though we don't yet have all the answers, we do have enough "dots" to connect and can create the basic recommendations that will work for most of us.

Fat cells are known as *adipocytes*. Those plump little cells are not just there holding up your pants. They are busy producing all sorts of molecules that control nearly everything related to your weight, and they can drive pathways that promote heart disease, cancer, and dementia.

Hard as it is to imagine, your fats cells are actually endocrine cells that produce many hormones, just like your thyroid or ovaries or testes. Fat tissue is also part of your immune system because it contains white blood cells (macrophages), and the fat cells produce inflammatory messenger chemicals called *adipocytokines*. Your fat is also influenced by and regulates neurotransmitters—your brain messenger chemicals. It is a storage organ, providing a reservoir of energy when supplies get low (from starvation or low blood sugar). Your fat cells can even produce more fat from carbohydrates in your diet. The active little globules of fat are constantly communicating with your whole body—including your stomach, pancreas, brain, hormones, liver, and more. This complex web of interactions and feedback mechanisms can easily get disrupted.

But the most important thing I can tell you—the final dot in our connect-the-dots story that completes the picture—is that most of the biology of fat cells is controlled by the quality and type of food you eat. And this is why a high-fat, low-carb (low-glycemic), high-fiber, whole-foods diet—like the *Eat Fat, Get Thin* Plan—works for so many people. Almost everyone will benefit from trying this approach for twenty-one days, especially if you have diabesity. It is a perfect way to reset. Then, after you've completed the twenty-one-day program, you'll enter the transition stage, which you'll learn about in Chapter 14. During the transition stage, you can see how many metabolic degrees of freedom you have, and you may decide to include a few more healthy carbs, such as whole grains, starchy veggies, and beans, in your diet, all within the healthy eating parameters you'll learn throughout the program.

HIGH-FAT VS. LOW-FAT DIETS

There has been a lot of research done and much written about low-carb, high-fat diets for weight loss. And the conclusions seem clear: high-fat, low-carb diets work better than low-fat, high-carb diets. Let's review a few of the important studies that compare low-fat to high-fat diets so you can see exactly how and why I came to that conclusion.

I mentioned the A TO Z Weight Loss Study, published in the *Journal of the American Medical Association* in 2007,[7] in Chapter 2. It was a twelve-month study of 311 overweight, nondiabetic, postmenopausal women. Hands down, the high-fat group in this study did better in every way. They lost *twice as much* weight, and every cardiovascular risk factor improved. The cholesterol profile shifted from bad to good, with lower triglycerides, higher HDL, and lower total cholesterol to HDL ratio (the best predictor of heart attacks). LDL, or the bad cholesterol, went up a bit, but it shifted from small, dense, dangerous particles to light, fluffy particles — in other words, the total level was higher, but the type was not the kind that causes heart attacks. Blood pressure, insulin and insulin resistance, and blood sugar were all better on the high-fat diet.

Another important study, the DIRECT trial, published in the *New England Journal of Medicine* in 2008,[8] looked at 322 moderately obese people and gave each group a calorie-restricted low-fat diet, a Mediterranean diet, a calorie-restricted diet, or a low-carb, high-fat calorie-unrestricted diet. Guess what? The group that was told to not worry about calories and to eat the most fat lost more than 66 percent more weight. Even more surprising, the ratio of total cholesterol to HDL dropped 20 percent in the high-fat group but only 12 percent in the low-fat group. The high-fat group also had better results by a big margin for HDL, triglycerides, insulin and glucose, and inflammation, and even improvements in fatty liver.

The Diogenes Project found that a lower-carb, higher-protein diet worked better for weight loss maintenance.[9] Other studies[10] and large reviews of low-carb, high-fat diets all show that they are better at aiding weight loss[11] and cardiovascular health.[12] People also find it easier to stick with these diets because fat makes food more satisfying and taste better.

A very important study published in the *Lancet* by Dr. David Ludwig compared the effect of a high-glycemic diet vs. a low-glycemic diet on metabolism in rats.[13] He found that changes in dietary composition (high-glycemic or changing the ratios of protein, fat, and carbs) produced obesity in genetically normal animals, even when diets had exactly the same number of calories. He fed each group of rats the amount of food that would allow them to maintain identical body weights. The rats fed the high-glycemic diet (high in sugar and refined carbs) gained weight on an identical number of calories. In fact they gained 70 percent more body fat (mostly belly fat) than the rats fed the high-fat diet. They also had lower muscle mass, were hungrier, had higher levels of insulin, and had more cardiovascular risk factors.

Another study on rats fed a ketogenic diet (very, very low-carb and very high-fat) again found that weight loss was greater than in rats fed a high-carb diet, even though they ate exactly the same number of calories.[14] The genes that increase fat burning and reduced fat storage were all turned on. The rats on the high-fat diet also increased calorie burning and energy expenditure and reversed pre-diabetes.

That's great for the rats, sure, but what about people? In human experiments, those who ate the high-fat diets had a much faster metabolism. The low-fat, high-carb diets forced all the food energy into the cells (because of insulin spikes), and this slowed metabolism. The group that ate the higher-fat diet had a faster metabolism, even on the same number of calories.[15] That means they burned more calories even when watching TV or sleeping.

Another human study performed by Dr. Ludwig and his colleagues that compared high-fat, low-carb diets with high-carb, low-fat diets in a controlled feeding environment found the same thing.[16] This was a "crossover trial": For half the study participants ate a high-fat, low-carb, low-glycemic diet; then during the other half they ate a low-fat, high-carb, high-glycemic diet. There was also another group that ate a moderate-fat diet. This allowed the researchers to study the effects of different diets on metabolism for each person.

The low-fat, high-glycemic diet consisted of 60 percent carbs, 20 percent protein, and 20 percent fat; the low-glycemic, high-fat diet consisted of 60 percent fat, 10 percent carbs, and 30 percent protein. Calorie content was identical for each diet. The high-fat group ended up burning 300 calories more a day than the low-fat group. The high-fat group also had the most improvements in cholesterol, PAI-1 (which shows the likelihood of having blood clots and heart attacks), and insulin resistance.

We know that there is a lot of bias in the world of science. But the Cochrane Collaboration, a global independent network of researchers, professionals, patients, caregivers, and others interested in health who receive no money from industry and are not affiliated with governments, did a review of low-glycemic diets, which are typically high-fat.[17] They concluded that the low-glycemic, high-fat diets did much better than the low-fat, low-calorie diets for weight loss and health. And the final nail in the coffin proving that high-fat diets work better than low-fat diets for weight loss was a review by Harvard researchers of 53 different randomized controlled trials that lasted a year or more. They found that high-fat, low-carb diets, compared head to head with low-fat diets, worked much better for weight loss.[18]

EATING A LOW-FAT DIET MAKES YOU CRAVE BAD FOODS

When you eat a low-calorie, low-fat, high-carb diet, you want to eat more[19] and eat higher-calorie and higher-carb foods.[20] Higher-carb foods make you crave even more carbs.

What's fascinating is that even *before* people gain weight (and accumulate a lot of those greedy, lazy-making fat cells), they show significant metabolic changes as a result of consuming a higher-carb, lower-fat diet. These changes in belly fat cells start the whole process of weight gain. Body fat, especially belly fat, is not just a bunch of excess baggage storing calories for a later date. Body fat is a complex metabolic tissue that is critical in regulating your appetite, controlling the rate of calorie burning, and regulating weight.

In a clever experiment on a group of schoolchildren, scientists tested the effects of fat and carbs on eating behavior by giving sixth-grade kids either cheese wedges or potato chips. The kids were told they could eat as much as they wanted.[21] Both groups were equally hungry at the start of the study, according to standard hunger measures. Based on the idea that you will gain weight if you eat more fat-rich foods, like cheese, which contain more calories per gram of food (9 calories per gram of fat vs. 4 calories per gram of carb), the cheese-eating kids should have consumed more calories. Eat more calories (because fat is more calorie dense), gain more weight. Simple math, right? But it doesn't work that way in the complex world of biology. If carbs drive you to overeat, the potato chip group should have eaten more calories. What happened? The kids in the potato chip group ate three times as many calories as the kids in the cheese group! And kids who were already overweight consumed even more calories. More evidence that fat cells are "hungry."

When the cheese was combined with vegetables, the kids ate even fewer total calories. This was more notable in the kids who were overweight or obese. When we combine foods that are high in nutrients, we naturally eat less, even with hungry fat cells. The key here is that nutrient-dense foods (real whole foods) are satisfying, while processed empty foods (nutrient–poor foods) are less satisfying, even though they may contain more calories!

This is consistent with a review of research on carb consumption in kids showing that kids who ate more carbs ate more food and were overall hungrier.[22] If you eat a lot of carbs, you are hungrier and take in more overall food and calories in a day than if you eat fat.[23]

When taken as a whole, the science shows us a clear pattern of evidence that carbs make you fat, while fat makes you thin. Foods like white rice, potatoes, and sugary beverages promote obesity and related diseases. Fat- (and calorie-)rich foods, like nuts, oily fish, and olive oil, and even foods high in saturated fats, promote weight loss and reduce risk of these diseases when you cut out the sugar and refined carbs.

But Wait ...What About Studies That Show That Low-Fat Diets Speed Metabolism?

Recently, a study in *Cell Metabolism* by Kevin Hall from the National Institutes of Heath attracted a lot of buzz in the news and online, as it seemed to prove once and for all that low-fat diets work better for weight loss than low-carb diets. But it did no such thing. There were some real problems with the study, and things that were overlooked by the media reports.

Here are the important considerations:

- It was a very short-duration study (only six days) conducted on only nineteen people who were contained in a metabolic ward where all the food was provided; people did not self-regulate based on hunger or appetite, so it was not based on normal everyday experience. It showed what happened in a vacuum but not in real life.
- The low-carb diet wasn't low at all, actually, with 29 percent of calories coming from carbs, including refined carbs. A true low-carb diet would have less than 10 percent of calories from carbs.
- The low-fat study contained *very* low fat (about 7 percent of calories), which is incredibly hard to sustain in real life.

(Continued)

- The low-carb group actually did show an increase in fat burning, which is a good thing. But the low-fat group had a higher amount of body-fat loss, which also seems like a good thing. But it was such a short study; other studies show that it takes longer to adapt to a higher-fat diet. Also, other longer-term studies comparing fat and carbs show that a higher-fat diet leads to more weight loss.

- A new, big, long-term (one year vs. six days) trial of low-carb, higher-fat diets is currently under way (at the time of this writing) called the CENTRAL trial.[24] The preliminary data shows that the low-carb/higher-fat diet had major advantages over the low-fat diet. The high-fat diet improved body composition (more muscle, less fat). It also helped fix fatty liver and reduce dangerous belly or organ fat. The study actually provided part of the food so the study participants stuck with the diet.

Sorry it's so confusing, but looking at all the evidence and real-life experience, it is clear that in actual humans living in the real world (not as lab rats with their food intake completely controlled), lower-carb, higher-fat diets lead to greater satiety (feeling full), more weight loss, and faster metabolism.

CONCERNS ABOUT HIGH-FAT, LOW-CARB DIETS

My standing line about the Atkins Diet used to be that it works if you don't mind constipation, bad breath, and kidney failure (due to its high content of animal protein). Atkins focused on fat and protein and not enough on veggies and plant foods. It's true there are a few concerns worth mentioning if you don't follow the plan carefully by eating more fiber, vegetables, and salt, like constipation, electrolyte imbalances from low sodium (or salt), dizziness, and muscle cramps—but they are easy to prevent and manage.

When you cut out a lot of grains and beans and eat more fat, your fiber intake can drop. However, on the *Eat Fat, Get Thin* Plan you will be eating a ton of vegetables, nuts and seeds, and some fruit, all of which contain a lot of fiber. You will also be consuming extra fiber, called

PGX. You need to drink 8 glasses of water a day because you will lose a lot of fluid as you detox from all the sugar and processed foods. Those foods are inflammatory and make you retain water, so when you stop eating them you lose water. Also, when you eat less carbs, you burn up glycogen (the sugar stores in your muscle). Since glycogen makes you retain water, when glycogen gets burned up, you lose the water.

When you cut out the carbs you lower your insulin levels. That causes the kidneys to dump salt, or sodium, from your kidneys,[25] because insulin causes you to retain salt (and thus water). This can cause muscle cramps. The best solution is to add 1 to 2 teaspoons of salt to your diet every day. And you need more potassium, too (about 2 grams a day); you'll get this from the vegetable and bone broth I recommend in Chapter 13.

Some of you might worry that lowering your carb intake will affect your athletic performance. Many athletes "carb-load" before a race to replenish glycogen, glucose stored in muscles. However, many studies show that once you adapt to a lower-carb diet, endurance exercise is not affected at all. Anaerobic exercise like sprinting or weight lifting can be affected by lack of glycogen stores, but the carbs in the *Eat Fat, Get Thin* program will help you keep enough glycogen stores to prevent this problem. It takes a few weeks to adapt to lower-carb, higher-fat eating and to switch your body from carb burning to fat burning, which is what happens when you follow the *Eat Fat, Get Thin* program. And you need to make sure you eat enough protein—about 1.5 grams per kilogram (0.68 grams per pound) of body weight a day, or about 100 to 120 grams for the average person; eating protein at each meal helps to build muscle. However, too much protein can turn to sugar in your bloodstream if you are not active or exercising, so if you are not active you may need less protein. We'll talk about this more in Chapter 13.

In the next few chapters, I'll help dispel some of the other myths and clear up the confusion surrounding fat, both dietary and biological. We'll get to the bottom-line facts on everything from whether saturated fat causes heart disease (hint: it doesn't) to which oils are truly good for you and which unhealthy ones stole the spotlight thanks to clever marketing ploys. The way I see it, the way out of this big, fat mess we're in is through discovering the truth and embracing a way of eating that welcomes back fat as a critical component for weight loss and health.

Beyond Food: Other Causes of Obesity and Damaged Metabolism

John Muir said, "When we try to pick out anything by itself, we find it hitched to everything else in the Universe." And it is so with human biology. The framework of Functional Medicine is based on understanding the body as a dynamic system where everything is connected, where there is a web of interactions between the systems of the body. In each of these systems, imbalances can occur that contribute to disorders of weight regulation and metabolism.

A Functional Medicine doctor or heath care practitioner can help you figure out your own imbalances. In 2014 we started the Cleveland Clinic Center for Functional Medicine to help train doctors and health professionals and conduct the needed research in this field. I also have a practice with a wonderful group of Functional Medicine practitioners at The UltraWellness Center in Lenox, Massachusetts, who have helped thousands of people identify the root causes of their health issues. You can also find a certified practitioner through the Institute for Functional Medicine at www.functionalmedicine.org.

To help you sort through all the causes of weight gain and obesity I have created a special free e-book called *Beyond Food: Other Causes of Obesity and Damaged Metabolism*. You can download it at www.eat fatgetthin.com. There is also a free companion guide on testing and treatment, *How to Work with Your Doctor to Get What You Need*, where I explain how to assess and test for these causes and how to address them yourself or in partnership with your health care provider. In *Beyond Food*, I address the eight major causes of weight-loss resistance and what to do about them:

- Reason #1: Nutritional Imbalances: Over Fed and Under Nourished
- Reason #2: Gut Microbiome Imbalances: Bad Bugs and Weight Gain
- Reason #3: Inflammation and Immune Function: Fueling the Fires of Fat Storage
- Reason #4: Environmental Toxins: Poisoning Your Metabolism
- Reason #5: Trouble with Your Energy Producing System (Your Metabolism)
- Reason #6: Bad Communication: Fixing the Body's Hormone Messengers
- Reason #7: Is It My Genes that Prevent Me from Fitting in My Jeans?
- Reason #8: "Catching Obesity": The Role of Our Social Networks in Weight and Health

4

The Skinny on Fats

Fat is a complicated topic that inspires much debate among scientists and nutrition experts, but there's one thing everyone can agree on: There is no such thing as simply "fat." There are many different kinds of fats: some good, some good or bad, depending on certain factors, and some downright evil.

Foods often contain a wide variety of fats. For example, butter contains saturated fat, omega-3 fats, omega-6 fats, and monounsaturated fats. Some fatty foods such as nuts also contain protein and/or carbohydrates, which influence the effects of different fats on your body. Saturated fat, for instance, is bad when eaten with carbohydrates, but when eaten alone, not so much. See what I mean when I say it's easy to be confused about fat?

Because everyone looks at just part of the story, very smart scientists can have completely opposing views on fat. Some say omega-6 vegetable oils are healthy and others suggest they are lethal. Some promote the benefits of saturated fats, while still others declare their dangers. There is a way to think through these contradictory views.

There is a new framework for thinking about human biology. It tells a holistic story of how everything is interconnected. So much of our nutrition research is made up of population studies that suggest linkages but don't prove anything. For example, I could design a study to see if sex led to babies, but if I included only couples over fifty years old, I would conclude that sex does not result in babies. Silly, yes, but a lot of our research is done that way. Having an overarching theory allows us to make sense of the data. So what is that theory?

In *systems biology,* the dynamic real-time connections and interactions between environment, diet, and genetics can be mapped. The practical application of this approach is Functional Medicine. At its core it addresses the root causes of imbalances that drive disease — imbalances that result from the interaction of diet, environment, and genes. This is personalized medicine, medicine that understands we are all genetically and biochemically unique but are also hugely adaptable and as a species have thrived in diverse habitats and environments, on widely different diets. In Chapter 10 I will review what I have come to understand as the foundational principles of an optimal human diet, which can vary greatly from culture to culture and be adapted to different preferences but is guided by a basic theoretical framework of what makes sense from an evolutionary and historical perspective.

Science is discovering the multidimensional role of food in health. Food is not just calories; it is information that instructs your minute-to-minute functions, which control all aspects of your health and disease risks. We have co-evolved with the food in our environment and use it to regulate every single bodily process, including our gene expression, inflammation, oxidative stress (damage from oxygen, like when an apple turns brown or a car rusts—think of it like rusting on the inside), hormonal function, immune function, gut flora balance, detoxification, metabolism, and much, much more. Insights from our historical diet can help guide us in what range of foods we might do well on.

While *Eat Fat, Get Thin* is about fat, what it is, what types we should eat, and how much we should eat, there are wide differences in diets in different populations. For example, the Japanese consume 15 percent of calories as fat, the Mediterranean cultures consume 40 percent of calories as fat, and the Pacific Islanders and the Masai warriors consume mostly saturated fats. Yet none of these populations have the high rates of modern civilization diseases such as obesity, heart disease, diabetes, cancer, and dementia that we have in America.

The quality of our diet matters most. Real, whole, fresh, unadulterated, unmodified foods: Those must be the starting point. There are other things that contribute to weight gain and obesity besides what we eat—such as our genetics, activity levels, stress levels, gut flora, and environmental toxins and obesogens (toxins that cause obesity)—and that modify our risk of disease and even our response to different foods. But it is still true that the biggest determinant of our weight and our health is the food we eat.

And a review of the research shows that for many traditional cultures across the globe, fat is coveted, special, and necessary. Tibetans put butter in their tea. In China, pork fat is sold as a delicacy and preferred to the meat. Traditional cultures always preferred the organs of animals, high in fat. The Plains Indians ate the liver and organs of the buffalo first. And most of us thrive on higher-fat diets, especially those with pre-diabetes and type 2 diabetes, or what I like to call diabesity.

Our diets are so different today than they were 12,000 to 14,000 years ago when we were hunter-gatherers. The agricultural revolution and the advent of animal husbandry led to the replacement of traditional foods with cereal grains and dairy. However, all food was still organic, grass-fed, whole. Because of the Industrial Revolution, our diet has been transformed more in the last 100 years than it was in the previous 10,000. The Industrial Revolution has led to the manipulation of crop genetics through increased hybridization and genetic modification, intensive animal husbandry in confined animal feeding operations, the refining of vegetable and seed oils as well as cereal grains, the development of trans fats and high-fructose corn syrup, the dramatic decrease in omega-3 fats we obtained from wild foods, the increase in refined omega-6 oils, the use of chemicals (pesticides, herbicides, fertilizers, antibiotics, and hormones), and the depletion of nutrients in the soil. The quality of our diet has dramatically declined. From the perspective of food as simply a source of energy and calories, none of this would matter, but the science has peeled back this simplistic view to reveal a powerful understanding of the role of food in all of our biological processes, from the regulation of which genes get turned on or off, to the regulation of hormones, the production of immune messengers and neurotransmitters, the balance of gut flora, and even the structure and composition of our cells and tissues and organs.

Let's dig into the wide world of fats, so you can make sense of the different kinds and how they affect your biology.

A PRIMER ON FATS: THE GOOD, THE BAD, AND THE UGLY

So what is fat, anyway?

Fat can be thought of in two main ways. First, by its chemical structure, which is how we name and classify it (that's the easy part). Second, in terms of its biology and how it affects our health. Here comes the geeky science part, but it's super helpful to understand, so hang in there with me.

First, the chemistry. Fat, or as we call it in nutrition-speak, "fatty acids," is a chain of carbon, oxygen, and hydrogen atoms with a carboxyl group (more carbon, hydrogen, and oxygen atoms) on one end. Fatty acids are classified according to how many carbon atoms are in the chain, as well as how many double bonds exist within the molecule. There are short-chain and long-chain fats. And there are fats with lots of double bonds (polyunsaturated) or none (saturated). Fatty acid molecules are usually joined together in groups of three, forming a molecule called a *triglyceride*. Triglycerides are predominately made in our liver from the carbohydrates we eat.

These different chemical structures give fats different properties. For example, saturated fats are found in coconuts and in mammals and other warm-blooded animals. They are soft when they exist in the body of live animals but hard at room temperature outside the body, like butter or lard. Omega-3 fats are found in cold-water and Arctic fish. They are liquid at room temperature and can stay fluid when fish swim in very cold waters.

Fatty acids play a starring role in many important functions in the body, including regulating inflammation, hormones, mood, nerve function, and more. Most of us think of them as a form of energy storage. If glucose isn't available for energy, the body uses fatty acids to fuel your cells instead. Burning fat for energy is actually better and more sustainable for health; in fact, it's what your muscles and heart prefer. The ketones that are produced when you eat fat (especially the fat from coconut oil or MCTs) are better for your brain and can even be used in the prevention and treatment of Alzheimer's.[1] We have long believed that the brain could run only on sugar, but we now know that that is not true and that the brain can burn fat or ketones (produced from fat breakdown).

There are four types of fatty acids:

1. Saturated (SFA)
2. Monounsaturated (MUFA)
3. Polyunsaturated (PUFA)—omega-3 and omega-6
4. Trans fats (TFA)

What defines them is their structure: A saturated fat has zero double bonds (thus it is "saturated" with hydrogen), a monounsaturated fatty acid has one double bond, and a polyunsaturated fatty acid has more than one double bond. Trans fats are funny-shaped fats, not normally found as part of human biology; the double bonds are on the opposite side of the fat chain (or "trans") from where they are found in naturally occurring fats. Your body doesn't like them at all. The chemical structure of the double bonds found in polyunsaturated fats are unstable when they come in contact with a number of elements such as light, heat, and oxygen, and this makes them more likely to become damaged and toxic to our health.

It gets more complicated because there are many different subtypes of saturated fats, polyunsaturated fats, and even trans fats. Some polyunsaturated fats may be harmful, others healthful, and the same is true of saturated fats.

Adding to the complexity is the fact that most foods contain combinations of different types of fat. We say something is "saturated" or "monounsaturated," but the truth is that the fat content in foods is made up of many different types of fatty acids; we usually just focus on the most abundant type when referring to that food. For instance, coconut oil—which we call a saturated fat—is made of 90 percent saturated fat;

the rest is polyunsaturated and monounsaturated fats. We also call butter a saturated fat, but butter has only 60 percent saturated fatty acids, and the rest is monounsaturated and polyunsaturated fat.

Complexities aside, let's look more closely at each category of fat and how it affects our biology, our weight, and our health. (For an even more detailed review of fats, please see my free e-book called *The Fat Bible: The Whole Story on Fats,* which you can download at www.eatfatgetthin.com.)

A Brief Note on Cholesterol

Cholesterol is complex and confusing. We will go into it in detail in Chapter 5, but the important thing to know as you read this chapter is that what we thought of as "bad" cholesterol, or LDL, actually comes in two types, and only one of them is bad. There are big, light, fluffy, beach-ball LDL particles, and small, dense, hard, golf ball–like particles. The small, hard particles are the ones that cause heart disease. When you eat sugar and refined carbs, you get more of the small, bad LDL particles. When you eat saturated fat, you get more of the light, fluffy LDL particles, which are not associated with heart disease risk. The story is a little more complicated than that, but understanding it in this way is most useful and will help you make sense of the discussion about saturated fats that follows. New cholesterol tests can measure not just the total amount of cholesterol or LDL but the kind of particles you have — good or bad.

SATURATED FATS (SFA)

Since saturated fat has gotten such a bad rap, I want to get into the details so you understand it better. After all, it means the difference between a life with butter and a life without it!

Saturated fats are categorized based on their chemical structure. The key question is whether the carbons in the fatty acid chain add up to an even or odd number. This matters because odd-number-chain fats generally are good for you, while even-number-chain fats may carry some risk (although shorter even-number-chain fats like lauric acid from coconut are good). I know, it's complicated. Sorry. Please don't shoot the messenger!

The main types of saturated fats are *laurate, myristate, palmitate,* and *stearate,* which are even-chain fats (but there are more). Grain-fed meat and dairy are rich sources of palmitate. They also contain stearate, which is the saturated fat that has no negative effect on cholesterol levels. Palm oil is mostly palmitate. Cocoa butter is mostly stearate, and coconut and palm oil are mostly laurate and some myristate.

Each of these different saturated fats has different effects on the body. Lauric acid from coconut increases LDL the most (compared to other saturated fats), but it also increases HDL (good cholesterol) the most, which is a good thing. The net effect is to improve your cholesterol profile by lowering the total-to-HDL ratio (which is far more predictive of a heart attack than just your LDL level). It also increases the harmless light, fluffy LDL particles (whereas sugar and refined carbs increase the small, dangerous LDL particles, which are the real cause of heart disease). On the other hand, stearate has no effect on LDL (bad cholesterol) but raises HDL (good cholesterol), improving the overall cholesterol profile.

Where many people, including scientists, get confused is that we think that the saturated fats you eat become the saturated fats in your blood, but the shocking counterintuitive fact is that *dietary* saturated fats don't raise *blood* saturated fats. It is carbs and sugar (and excess protein) that cause your liver to produce the saturated fats found in your blood. Higher levels in the blood of stearate and palmitate are associated with increased cardiac risk. But these are produced mostly from eating carbs or sugar, not fat. In fact, eating foods with these types of fat—like meat or palm oil—has very little impact on your blood level of saturated fat; as it turns out, they are not associated with increased risk of heart disease.

Saturated fats are key fats that provide stiffness and structure to our cell membranes and tissues; they kind of keep the contents of our cells together. If we eat a lot of the very fluid and unstable refined polyunsaturated omega-6 oils (from seeds, grains, or beans—like corn, soy, or sunflower oils), our cells become too floppy and don't function as well. The worst fats for our cell membranes are trans fats, which are stiff and hard and literally embed themselves into our cell membranes, causing them to malfunction and creating disease. This affects the cell membrane's permeability (which allows cells to communicate with other cells). Basically, it makes your cells hard of hearing and a little blind!

Saturated fats play many critical roles in your body:[2]

- Saturated fats such as lauric acid (from coconut) and conjugated linoleic acid (from butter) strengthen the immune system and help your cells communicate better, thus protecting you against cancer.
- They help your lungs work better. Saturated fats in your body produce something called surfactant, which helps air cross over the lung membranes. Children given butter and full-fat milk have much less asthma than children given reduced-fat milk and margarine.[3]
- They are required for you to make hormones such as testosterone and estrogen.[4]
- They are critical for your nerves and nervous system to work properly.
- They help suppress inflammation, despite the common view about their causing inflammation. When eaten with a lot of sugar or refined carbs (think bread and butter, or cookies), saturated fats can cause inflammation. Or if you are deficient in omega-3 fats, they also can cause inflammation. The important thing to know here is that saturated fats *cause inflammation only when eaten with refined carbs or sugar or when you don't consume omega-3 fats.*[5]
- Saturated animal fats contain essential fat-soluble vitamins and nutrients that we need to be healthy,[6] including vitamin A, vitamin D, and vitamin K_2, the animal form of vitamin K. Compared to those eating the nutrient-poor standard American diet, hunter-gatherer societies, with very nutrient-dense diets, had levels of these nutrients that were ten times that of the average American.[7]

I could go on about the benefits of saturated fats...

Several important saturated fatty acids provide excellent energy sources for the body: lauric acid, found in coconut oil, myristic acid, found in coconut oil and dairy fats, and palmitic acid, found in palm oil, meat, and dairy fats.[8] Palmitic acid plays a part in the regulation of hormones, and both palmitic and myristic acid assist in cell messaging and immune function.[9]

Good brain function depends on saturated fats. In fact, most of your brain is made up of saturated fats and omega-3 fats. One study showed that consumption of saturated fats had the potential to reduce the risk of dementia by 36 percent.[10] Saturated fats also assist the brain in renewal and regeneration of nerve cells.

MONOUNSATURATED FATS (MUFA)

Here's the bottom line: MUFAs are good for you. Populations that consume a lot of olive oil and nuts, such as the people of Greece and Italy, have the lowest rates of heart disease in the world (except Japan, which has low MUFA intake).

The main dietary sources of MUFAs are whole olives, olive oil, avocados, lard, tallow (beef or sheep fat), certain types of fish, and many nuts, including macadamias, almonds, pecans, and cashews, to name a few. Monounsaturated fats are also found in dairy and animal foods.

For our pre-agricultural ancestors, MUFAs accounted for about half the total fat intake and 16 to 25 percent of total calorie intake from wild meat, bone marrow, and nuts. One of the only hunter-gatherer societies left on the planet, the Hadza, break open the bones of animals they hunt and suck out the fatty marrow, which is more than 50 percent monounsaturated fats. Modern grain-fed meat doesn't have much MUFA, but pasture-raised animals have as much as wild meats, which contain a lot of MUFA.[11]

Eating more monounsaturated fats greatly benefits your heart and cardiovascular system, which is why most cardiologists recommend the Mediterranean diet. Even the American Heart Association agrees. Higher intakes of MUFAs are associated with improved cholesterol numbers as well as lower levels of LDL oxidation (which is necessary for LDL to cause damage in the body) and less risk of blood clots and stroke.[12]

Monounsaturated fats are rich in vitamin E and other antioxidants. They improve insulin sensitivity and therefore reduce diabetes risk, reduce breast cancer risk, reduce pain in people with rheumatoid arthritis, promote weight loss, and reduce belly fat.[13]

However, some monounsaturated fats are produced in such a way that makes them unhealthy and even toxic to the body. For example, canola oil has been touted as a healthy oil for many years. The process of creating canola oil, and other vegetable oils, includes applying high heat and using harsh chemical solvents in the refining process. In an article titled "The Great Con-ola," the Weston A. Price Foundation states, "Like all modern vegetable oils, canola oil goes through the process of caustic refining, bleaching, and degumming, all of which involve high temperatures or chemicals of questionable safety. And because canola oil is high in omega-3 fatty acids, which easily become rancid and foul-smelling when subjected to oxygen and high temperatures, it must be deodorized."[14] Avoid canola oil and stick to extra virgin (and ideally organic) olive oil, avocados, and almonds.

POLYUNSATURATED FATS (PUFA): OMEGA-6 AND OMEGA-3 FATTY ACIDS

There are two main types of PUFAs: omega-6 and omega-3 fats. These fats are considered "essential." When scientists label a nutrient as "essential," they're not just saying that it's very important or nice to have. In nutrition-speak we call something essential if you get sick or can't live without it. It is essential because we can't make it in our bodies; thus, we have to eat it or take it as a supplement.

Polyunsaturated fats (PUFAs) play a key role in cellular, immune, and hormonal function. They are potent regulators of health and disease. Omega-3 fats, one type of PUFA, make up much of your cell membranes and regulate insulin function, inflammation, and even your neurotransmitters, which is why they are critical for preventing and treating diabetes, depression, and arthritis and autoimmune disease.

Soybean oil, canola oil, safflower oil, sunflower oil, flax oil, and fish oil are all examples of polyunsaturated oils, but not all of them are good. Other food sources high in PUFAs include walnuts; sunflower, sesame, pumpkin, and chia seeds; and fish.

But again, it's important to understand that, as with monounsaturated fats, the processing or cooking of polyunsaturated oils affects their ability to create health or disease. For example, PUFAs develop harmful free radicals when subjected to heat, and these can damage your tissues and promote disease of all sorts, especially age-related diseases such as heart disease, diabetes, cancer, and dementia. In fact, your LDL is harmful only if it is oxidized and damaged by free radicals.

So, the two essential fatty acids found in food are:

- LA—linoleic acid (omega-6): found in commercial seed and vegetable oils and certain nuts and seeds. We do need the LA omega-6 fats in moderation, but only from whole foods like nuts and seeds, or from cold- or expeller-pressed vegetable oils, but we should use these vegetable oils only in small amounts.
- ALA—alpha linolenic acid (omega-3): found in organ meats, pastured egg yolks, macadamia nuts, walnuts, and flax oil.

There are other longer-chain omega-3 and omega-6 derivatives that can be synthesized in the body, considered "conditionally essential fatty acids." But most people need to get them from dietary sources because their bodies are not effective at converting ALA into the active forms of the omega-3 fats called EPA and DHA. So I also consider these "essential":

- DHA—docosahexaenoic acid (omega-3 that can be made from ALA, but only about 5 to 10 percent of ALA can be converted to DHA): found in fish or algae or wild or pasture-raised animals.
- EPA—eicosapentaenoic acid (omega-3 that can also be derived from ALA, and a good anti-inflammatory fat): found in fish or wild or pasture-raised animals.
- AA—arachidonic acid (omega-6 fatty acid that can be derived from LA: found in animal foods like fish, poultry, eggs, and meat.

■ GLA—gamma linolenic acid (omega-6 fatty acid derived from LA): found in evening primrose, borage, or hemp oil.

Omega-6 Fats

Omega-6 fats typically get a bad rap, as they tend to cause inflammation in the body. But not all are harmful. Omega-3 fats are anti-inflammatory. The problem arises when the balance is tipped in favor of too many omega-6s compared to omega-3s.

We evolved to have a good ratio of omega-6 to omega-3 fatty acids of about 1:1 to 4:1. But our modern diet now provides far too many omega-6s (found in processed food, corn and safflower oils, and conventionally raised meat) and not enough omega-3s (found in wild-caught fatty fish, fish oil, and grass-fed meats).

When there are too many omega-6s and not enough omega-3s in the cell, things can start to go terribly wrong. An imbalance has been shown to depress immune system function, contribute to weight gain, and cause inflammation.[15] Dr. Artemis Simopoulos, one of the world's leading researchers on omega-3 fats, explains that "excessive amounts of omega-6 polyunsaturated fatty acids (PUFA) and a very high omega-6/omega-3 ratio, as is found in today's Western diets, promote the pathogenesis of many diseases, including cardiovascular disease, cancer, and inflammatory and autoimmune diseases, whereas increased levels of omega-3 PUFA (a low omega-6/omega-3 ratio) exert suppressive effects."[16]

In an article published in *Biomedicine and Pharmacotherapy,* Dr. Simopoulos reviews in detail the risks of going against our evolutionary balance of omega-3 and omega-6 fats.[17] The increased intake of omega-6 fats oxidizes your LDL (bad cholesterol), making it rancid and more likely to cause heart disease. It also makes your blood more sticky and likely to clot and blocks the uptake of the good omega-3 fats into your cell membranes. All bad news for your health.

Remember, food is information that influences the expression of your genes, and this is certainly true when it comes to foods containing omega-3 and omega-6 fatty acids. Omega-3 fats reduce the expression of inflammatory genes and molecules in the body, while omega-6 fats promote the expression of inflammatory genes. Omega-6 fats are heavily present in refined vegetable oils, like corn, safflower, and soybean oil. Although these oils have been considered the "healthy" alternative to saturated fats in the past, we now know the health dangers that come from refined oils (see Chapter 6 for more). They should not be part of your diet.

Unrefined oils are a better choice; however, the ratio of omega-6 to omega-3 fats is still important. The polyunsaturated unrefined oils that have the best ratio are flaxseed oil, walnut oil, and hemp seed oil, but make sure you don't heat them.[18] Unrefined oils are cold-pressed or expeller-pressed; neither of these processes uses the chemicals or solvents that are used in the oil-refining process.

Let's look at the omega-6 fats in more detail.

Medium-Chain Omega-6s: Linoleic Acid (LA)

Linoleic acid is now the most abundant fat in our diets and is highly concentrated in most vegetable and seed oils, especially soybean, safflower, sunflower, corn, and cottonseed oils. It has been consumed in unprecedented quantities over the last 100 years. Soybean oil consumption has increased 1,000-fold since 1900. Since soybean oil lowers the bad cholesterol, or LDL, most doctors love it and recommend that we swap it out for saturated fats. But the story is not so simple. Too many omega-6 fats from soybean and other vegetable or seed oils compete with omega-3s in your body and interfere with the heart-protective benefits of omega-3s. Even worse, these oils can be easily damaged by oxygen and become oxidized; in the body they can turn LDL rancid and dangerous.[19] These oxidized fats are called OXLAMs, or oxidized linoleic acid metabolites. Using these oils for frying, especially for frying carbs (like French fries), makes them even more harmful.

Linoleic acid, mostly from soybean oil, accounts for about 90 percent of all PUFA intake or about 7 percent of total energy intake. That's a lot of unstable oil in our diet. Pre-agricultural humans who lived in Africa consumed only about 3 percent of calories as LA from wild meat. Other ancestral humans living in coastal areas would have consumed less than 1 percent. There is no historical precedent for consuming our current amount of LA, and it has been called a "massive uncontrolled human experiment."[20]

Populations with traditionally low intakes of LA have a very low risk of heart disease. There are conflicting studies, but when separated out from diets that also include omega-3 fats, LA alone seems to increase the risk. The one large randomized controlled study that reduced LA to pre-industrial levels found a 70 percent reduction in heart disease and death.[21] LA should not be a significant portion of your diet, despite common recommendations to replace saturated fats with omega-6 linoleic acid from vegetable oils. See more on omega-6 fats in Chapter 6.

Long-Chain Omega-6s: Arachidonic Acid (AA)

Arachidonic acid is found in eggs, beef, poultry, pork, liver, and some fish. It is a component of all your cell membranes, including those in your blood vessels, platelets, and immune cells. It can be converted in the body into all sorts of metabolites, called *prostaglandins* and *leukotrienes,* some of which promote inflammation and clotting. These metabolites are needed to maintain a balance with the anti-inflammatory omega-3 fats. It is not as if omega-6 fats are only bad, or omega-3 fats are only good. It is all about balance. Wild and pasture-raised animals have a good balance of AA and omega-3s, whereas industrial animal production has led to more AA and almost no omega-3s. Some amount of AA is necessary, but too much is harmful.

GLA: A Long-Chain Omega-6

One beneficial source of omega-6 fats is gamma linolenic acid (GLA). GLA is a plant-derived omega-6 most abundant in the seeds of a Mediterranean flower known as borage, or from evening primrose. Although a member of the omega-6 family, it produces anti-inflammatory compounds. New research reveals this nutrient's power to combat chronic inflammation, eczema, dermatitis, asthma, rheumatoid arthritis, atherosclerosis, diabetes, obesity — even cancer.[22] GLA is rarely in our diet. Most people are deficient in it and would benefit from taking evening primrose oil supplements. You need just a little GLA to reap the benefit.

Omega-3 Fats

Considering that the body needs fewer omega-6 fats than are present in the standard American diet, and desperately needs more omega-3 fats, focusing on consistent intake of omega-3 fats is vital for good health. The best dietary sources of omega-3 fats are wild-caught cold-water fatty fish and seafood, high-quality fish oils, and grass-fed meat and dairy.

The benefits of omega-3 fats have been well studied and documented. Here is a list of conditions that these beneficial fats help:[23]

- High cholesterol
- High blood pressure
- Heart disease
- Diabetes
- Rheumatoid arthritis
- Osteoporosis
- Depression
- Bipolar disorder
- Schizophrenia
- ADHD
- Cognitive decline
- Skin disorders such as eczema and psoriasis
- Inflammatory bowel disease
- Asthma
- Macular degeneration
- Menstrual pain
- Colon cancer
- Breast cancer
- Prostate cancer

Diets high in good fat support your brain function. The brain is made primarily of phospholipids, the simplest form of fats. Omega-3 essential fatty acids provide proper fluidity for your brain cell membranes.

A study on the role of omega-3 fatty acids in depression showed that they were more effective than placebo for depression in both adults and children in small controlled studies and in an open study of bipolar depression.[24] A study done by Dr. S. Jazayeri published in the *Australian and New Zealand Journal of Psychiatry* comparing the therapeutic effects of EPA and fluoxetine (Prozac) in major depressive disorder showed that EPA is as effective as Prozac in treating major depressive disorder.[25] That's right: omega-3 fatty acid can alleviate the symptoms of depression as well as one of the most widely prescribed drugs in America today!

Here's a little more detail on each of the omega-3 fats:

Medium-Chain Omega-3s: Alpha Linolenic Acid (ALA)

Alpha linolenic acid is the main plant source of omega-3 fats. It is found in soybean oil, flaxseeds, hemp and chia seeds, walnuts, and canola oil, as well as a little in green leafy vegetables. Soybean-oil-based salad dressings and mayonnaise are the biggest source of ALA but are also accompanied by large amounts of omega-6 linoleic acid (LA), so I recommend avoiding soybean oil. Omega-3 fats from ALA are protective for health, and small amounts (5 to 10 percent) can be converted to the more beneficial long-chain omega-3s (EPA and DHA). However, in diets with lots of LA, the ALA cannot be converted to EPA and DHA. In one large study, ALA was associated with a 73 percent reduction in heart attacks and death, but only when the LA was reduced at the same time.[26]

Long-Chain Omega-3s: EPA and DHA

These essential fats were a critical part of our evolutionary diet and now more than 90 percent of Americans are deficient in them. They typically come from wild animal foods, although chickens fed foods containing omega-3 fat produce eggs with omega-3 fats. They are found in cold-water fatty fish, including sardines, mackerel, herring, trout, salmon, anchovies, oysters, and tuna (though tuna is best avoided because of high mercury content). There are also more in wild game such as deer, elk, and antelope. Lower amounts are found in grass- or pasture-fed cattle and shrimp, mussels, squid, and scallops. DHA is also found in algae, the only plant form of the long-chain omega-3 fats.

As discussed, these amazing fats have many beneficial effects. Most Americans are deficient in omega-3 fats, and up to 25 percent of Americans consume almost no long-chain (EPA/DHA) omega-3 fats. Most ancestors who lived inland consumed about 660 milligrams a day of EPA and DHA, about six times the amount the average American gets. Those who lived in coastal regions consumed much more. Populations with high intakes of EPA and DHA have low risks of heart disease, diabetes, and obesity. The benefits increase with intakes of up to twenty times that of the average American.

TRANS FATS (TFA)

In the wide world of fats, as you can see, very little is black and white. There's one exception, however, and that's trans fats. There is no room for debate on this one: Aside from one particular type, trans fats are evil, nasty stuff.

Also known as hydrogenated fats, trans fats are mostly man-made and found in processed foods, shortenings and margarines, fried foods, and commercially produced baked goods.

No one any longer doubts the dangers of trans fats, and in 2013 they were finally ruled as "not safe to eat" by the FDA. On January 1, 2006, the FDA required that any trans fat content had to be clearly declared on all foods. This declaration was an achievement, especially for the Harvard School of Public Health, which had been advocating since the early 1990s for transparency of trans fats in foods and supplements.[27] However, buyer beware! A product labeled "trans fat free" can still contain up to 0.5 gram of trans fat content. For example, Cool Whip, whose label says it contains zero trans fats, is made almost entirely from trans fats, but since it's mostly air, it has less than 0.5 gram per serving.[28] As of 2013 the FDA has begun the process to declare trans fats as no longer on the list of foods "generally recognized as safe,"[29] after a lawsuit was filed by Dr. Fred Kummerow, the ninety-nine-year-old researcher who first highlighted the dangers of trans fats in 1957. All these actions are good news and steps in the right direction, but unfortunately, trans fats won't be fully out of the food supply for a long time because there is a slow phase-in of the ban. Food companies have three years to remove them from their products, or they have to petition the FDA to permit them to use them. And there is no guarantee they will be replaced with better fats or compounds.

There is one type of trans fat that is fine to eat, though, and is even healthy. Dairy and beef contain CLA (conjugated linoleic acid), a different, naturally occurring trans fat that has beneficial effects on health and metabolism.

I Spy Trans Fats

It is important to be aware of the places trans fats may still be lurking: baked goods (crackers, cookies, cakes), snack foods (chips, microwave popcorn), frozen meals (pizza, TV dinners), Crisco, Pam spray, fake butter spreads, margarine, coffee creamer, pre-made frostings, and of course fast food.[30] Keep trans fats out of your body by avoiding processed and packaged foods, avoiding fast food, asking for your food to be cooked in butter or healthy oils like coconut or olive oil at restaurants, and checking ingredient labels for the words "partially hydrogenated oil." The good news is that many food producers are eliminating hydrogenated fats from their foods in an effort to keep business alive.

Historically we consumed about zero trans fat, and now in some populations in Western countries trans fat comprises up to more than 5 percent of calories. It was created around 1890 by scientists who developed the process of hydrogenation. It was cheap and thought to be healthier than butter, but it is far worse. It should never be consumed by humans or other living things. Even flies know better. They won't land on a tub of shortening!

According to the FDA, "Trans fat is created when hydrogen is added to vegetable oil (a process called hydrogenation) to make it more solid."[31] Making certain oils solid was helpful for both storage and transportation. In the early 1900s there was an abundance of soy and a shortage of butter. The creation of margarine from soybean oil solved this problem. "Hydrogenated fat such as Crisco and Spry, sold in England, began to replace lard in the baking of bread, pies, cookies, and cakes in 1920."[32] Food producers had found a fat that was inexpensive to produce and had a long shelf life.

By the 1960s, trans fat products were being used in industrialized food and were replacing animal fats (butter and lard) both in the United States and abroad. And since trans fats were considered *unsaturated fats*, "health" advocates promoted the idea that margarine was better for you than butter.

However, there were suggestions in the scientific literature as early as 1981 that trans fats could be linked to coronary artery disease. According to the Harvard School of Public Health, a study done in Scotland that year speculated on the fact that there was a correlation between trans fats and cardiovascular disease. Another study by Harvard in 1993 strongly linked partially hydrogenated oils and heart attack risk. This study calculated that if you simply replaced 2 percent of trans fats in the diet with healthy fats, you could cut the risk of heart disease by a third![33]

In 1994, it was estimated that trans fats caused 30,000 deaths annually in the United States from heart disease.[34] Even so, the consumption of hydrogenated fats has increased significantly over the past half century. It has only recently started to decline.

The danger of trans fats comes down to this: They cause increases in small, dense, dangerous LDL particles, and they reduce HDL (good cholesterol). This in turn causes inflammation, heart disease, diabetes, dementia, and sudden death. It also increases the risk of cancer.

Here's another unwanted gift from trans fats: obesity. There is a strong correlation between trans fats and weight issues. A study from Wake Forest Baptist Medical Center showed that diets high in trans fat increase belly fat and weight gain even without an increase in total calories. This study also further supported the link between trans fats and heart disease and diabetes.[35] Harvard studies over the last three decades, too, have proved that eating trans fats promotes obesity and insulin resistance, which leads to pre–diabetes and type 2 diabetes.[36]

The dark tale of trans fats doesn't end there. The link between cancer and trans fats is also of serious concern. A study on trans fatty acids and colon cancer showed that postmenopausal women who had high levels of trans fat in their diet doubled their risk of getting colon cancer.[37] A study published in the *American Journal of Epidemiology* found that eating trans fats leads to precancerous polyps.[38] Yet another study published in the same journal found that a woman's risk of breast cancer doubled if she had high levels of trans fats in her blood.[39]

So there you have it: the universe of fats in all its complexity. With your new knowledge in hand, you're now empowered to make healthier choices about which fats to eat and which to avoid. In the next few chapters, I'll give you even more insight and guidelines to help you answer, once and for all, the question, "What should I eat to stay healthy, prevent disease, and lose weight?"

5

The Surprising Truth About Fat and Heart Disease

For a long time, fat has been cast as the villain in the heart disease saga. The original assumption—that fat in general is bad for the heart—has since been replaced with the idea that saturated fat is bad and polyunsaturated and monounsaturated fats are good. The one thing we all agree on is that trans fats are evil, and monounsaturated fats (like olive oil) get to keep their top billing as good guys. But new evidence suggests that not *all* polyunsaturated fats (such as vegetable oils) are the heroes they originally appeared to be...and that saturated fat deserves some vindication.

WHAT DOES THE RESEARCH SAY?

Researchers from around the world, in both experimental and population studies, and in large reviews of all the research on this topic, consistently come up with the same conclusion. In 2015 leading fat researchers Patty Siri-Tarino, Ronald Krauss, and others reviewed all the latest data in an article titled "Saturated Fats versus Polyunsaturated Fats versus Carbohydrates for Cardiovascular Disease Prevention and Treatment."[1] They addressed all the controversies about saturated fat and polyunsaturated fats and carbs and found *no link between total dietary fat or saturated fat and heart disease.* This was in the context of the typical unhealthy diet consumed by most Americans. There is some data that swapping out polyunsaturated fats for saturated fats may be beneficial, but the studies are contradictory.

A large randomized controlled study named PREDIMED (Prevención con Dieta Mediterránea), reported in the *New England Journal of Medicine* in 2013, showed that added fat actually reduced the risk of heart attacks and deaths by 30 percent.[2] That's as much as statin medication. This was one of the largest and best-performed nutritional experiments ever done. Some say that the low-fat group wasn't low-fat enough, but the fact remains that added fat was beneficial.[3] The researchers studied more than 7,000 people who were at risk for but had never had heart attacks. The control group was told to eat a reduced-fat diet. One group got an extra liter of olive oil a week, and another was told to eat a combination of walnuts, almonds, and hazelnuts (30 grams a day). They didn't restrict calories to compensate for the extra fat. They had to stop the study after almost five years because it became clear that depriving the control group of fat was increasing their risk of heart attacks and death; the groups eating fat were protected against heart attacks.

Many other studies came before this that showed no link between fat and heart disease, including the Lyon Diet Heart Study, published in 1999.[4] It showed that a higher-fat Mediterranean diet rich in omega-3 fats reduced death from both heart disease and all causes, including stroke, cancer, and so on. In this study, the group that lowered the omega-6 fats the most and increased the omega-3 fats the most did the best. In another small controlled trial performed on 264 men who had had heart attacks, the low-fat group ate a third less fat and 500 fewer calories per day and achieved a lower cholesterol and weight than the control group, and still there was no benefit in reducing repeat heart attacks or death.[5]

The Women's Health Initiative was another study that showed no benefit in preventing heart disease from reducing fat in the diet. One of the largest diet studies ever conducted, it tracked 49,000 women over eight years and cost hundreds of millions of dollars. It showed no benefit in preventing heart disease from reducing fat in the diet. The study began in 1991, when everyone was still riding high on the low-fat bandwagon, and was designed to lower fat from 38 percent to 20 percent of daily calories. The women in the low-fat group reduced their fat only to 29 percent of their diet (because it is so hard for people to cut fat from their diets and still be satisfied), but still, there was no improvement in the low-fat group in rates of heart disease (despite significant reductions in LDL, or bad cholesterol),[6] breast cancer,[7] colon cancer,[8] and obesity.[9] Some say these women didn't lower fat enough to have the desired effect, but if there was going to be an effect, this study should have shown something. It showed nothing. Zip. Nada.

This was similar to an earlier, very large study called the MRFIT (Multiple Risk Factor Intervention Trial), which was also designed to study the effects of saturated fat on heart disease. Again, there was no difference in outcomes for heart disease in the group that cut saturated fat.[10]

The proof that saturated fat isn't the heart disease threat we thought it was just keeps rolling in. The famous Nurses' Health Study also found no connection between fat and heart disease or fat and weight gain in more than 80,000 women studied over 20 years.[11] There was an increased risk of heart disease with trans fats, and a decrease in risk from polyunsaturated fats, but it was unclear if it was the omega-3 or the omega-6 that was beneficial.

A group of independent scientists, the Cochrane Collaboration, reviewed the effect of dietary fat on heart disease and found no correlation.[12] Another long-term large prospective study, of 43,000 men, the Physicians' Health Study, found no link between total fat or saturated fat and heart disease.[13] This study concluded that the connection between high-fat and saturated-fat diets and heart disease was not because of the fat, but because people who followed high-fat diets ate fewer vegetables, less fiber, more sugar, and more refined and processed foods. The study also found that higher amounts of omega-3 fats were associated with reduced risk of heart disease.

These large studies, done over decades and costing hundreds of millions of dollars, certainly would have found a connection between fat and heart disease if there were one. The only culprit they found was trans fats.

The current scientific consensus is that total fat in your diet does not affect your risk of heart disease or being overweight, and yet many doctors and dietitians still hold on to this outdated idea. It is still embedded in our popular culture, too, with thousands of low-fat foods still on grocery store shelves and menus. I recently had a patient who struggled with weight for 30 years. She was a low-fat fanatic. Her diet consisted of low-fat, high-sugar salad dressings, low-fat yogurt, and bread (naturally low-fat). She steamed her veggies and didn't add olive oil, and ate lots of fruit. She avoided nuts, seeds, avocados, and all other fatty foods, all with no results. I recommended healthy fats like avocados and coconut oil, and despite her fat phobia, she followed my plan. In just four days, she lost six pounds and her energy skyrocketed, her brain fog disappeared, her joints didn't hurt, and her postnasal drip stopped. She continued to lose weight on the program without starvation, deprivation, or fat or calorie restriction.

The American Heart Association, the American College of Cardiology, and the US Dietary Guidelines Advisory Committee have all given up on the low-fat message. The 2015 Dietary Guidelines Committee said that "reducing total fat (replacing total fat with overall carbohydrates) does not lower CVD risk." But then things get a bit fuzzier. These organizations still cling to two big ideas about fat that aren't supported by science: first, that saturated fat causes heart disease, and second, that polyunsaturated fats (vegetable oils) are protective and we should increase their intake.

Should we be eating animal fat, like butter, or not? For more than 60 years, saturated fat has been the bad guy because it does indeed raise your LDL and your total blood cholesterol level. The whole idea that LDL or total cholesterol led to heart disease came from a very few early, poorly done studies. But even as early as 1996, at the height of the high-carb, low-fat craze, in a 10-year study of 43,757 people, Harvard researchers found no link between diets high in saturated fat and cholesterol, if they accounted for the amount of fiber in the diet. In other words, when saturated fat was consumed with lots of fiber and low levels of sugar and refined carbs, there was no correlation with heart disease; it was only a problem when consumed with lots of sugar and carbs.

Unfortunately, we can't rewrite history, and the poorly done studies condemning saturated fat led Americans to buy into the "butter is bad" dogma. So we switched to margarine, made from vegetable oil—until we realized that the trans fat it contains is, in fact, the only fat conclusively proven to cause heart attacks. We were also told to swap out saturated fats with polyunsaturated fats (like vegetable oils) because they lower cholesterol. But lowering cholesterol is not the most important consideration in reducing heart attack risk (more on that soon). And the research didn't distinguish between omega-3 and omega-6 polyunsaturated fats, which have different effects on the body. New analysis proves the benefits of PUFAs come from the omega-3 fats in fish, nuts, and seeds, not refined omega-6 vegetable oils.

THE BREAKTHROUGH ON SATURATED FATS

Then came one big study that changed everything. A comprehensive review in 2014 led by Dr. Rajiv Chowdhury looked at seventy-two of the best studies on fat and heart disease (more than 600,000 people from eighteen countries) and came to the conclusion that there was no link between total fat or saturated fat and heart disease. The study also did not support the heavily promoted policy and guidelines to increase polyunsaturated fats (vegetable oils).[14] It did find, however, that trans fats increased and omega-3 fats decreased heart disease.

The researchers looked at three different types of studies. They reviewed thirty-two population studies with 512,420 people for dietary habits; seventeen studies with 25,721 people that measured blood levels of different fats, a very good indicator of what people are actually eating rather than their recall of dietary intake; and twenty-seven randomized controlled trials including 105,085 people assessing dietary supplements of omega-3 fatty acids. For a geeky guy like me, finding this study was like hitting the jackpot.

Let me weed through for you what was buried in this groundbreaking study, because it tells so much about what is truly going on in the fat and heart disease story. The most beautiful part of this study was how it broke down all the different types of saturated fat and polyunsaturated fats and how they impact heart disease. This was radical. Often all saturated fats are lumped together as one big evil type of fat.

The truth is that saturated fat comes in lots of varieties, each with different effects. There are odd- and even-chain saturated fats and different types of polyunsaturated fats, not just omega-3s and omega-6s but different types of omega-6s. And the fact that these were actually measured in the blood of real people and not just based on shakier dietary recall records (do you really remember what you ate for lunch a week ago?) makes these really important to pay attention to.

What story do these blood levels of fatty acids tell us? Hang in there with me; this is where all the nuggets of insight are that explain what's really at the root of this whole cholesterol, fat, saturated fat, and polyunsaturated fat story.

First let's look at what they found out about saturated fats. As you know by now, there are different types of saturated fats: myristic acid, pentadecanoic acid, palmitic acid, margaric acid, stearic acid, lauric acid, and so on. They are classified as odd- or even-chain. Some come from diet; some are produced mostly in the liver. Here's where it gets interesting. The kinds of saturated fats circulating in the blood that were associated with heart disease were even-chain palmitic and stearic acid. And guess what: Most palmitic and stearic acids in the body are produced in your liver when you eat carbohydrates. They don't come from eating fat. That's right. Carbs and alcohol (a form of sugar), not saturated fat, trigger high blood levels of stearic and palmitic acid. This is kind of shocking news. (Just a note about alcohol: It doesn't trigger much insulin secretion, and small amounts may be protective against heart disease.)

Another interesting finding was that the odd-chain fats, such as margaric acid, that come from dairy fat like butter actually showed a reduction in risk of heart disease. Yes, you read that right: Butter showed a reduction in heart disease risk! Grass-fed animals have more of these odd-chain protective fats.

This study also showed no benefit from the omega-6 fats in vegetable oils; in fact, it showed that these tend to cause heart disease. It also showed that omega-3 fats from fish or supplements were the most protective against heart disease.

On the other hand, the omega-6 fat called arachidonic acid was the only omega-6 found to reduce risk of heart disease. It is not in vegetable oil, but instead is made by the body and is also found in the highest amounts in poultry, eggs, and beef. One of the main authors of the study, Dariush Mozaffarian, from Tufts University, had previously published a study that recommended swapping out saturated fats for polyunsaturated vegetable oils.[15] Now he moved toward this conclusion: "Current evidence does not clearly support cardiovascular guidelines that encourage high consumption of polyunsaturated fatty acids and low consumption of total saturated fats."

This turns things upside down, doesn't it? Let's review.

- Saturated fats (palmitic acid and stearic acid) in your blood that cause heart attacks come from eating sugar and carbs, not fat.
- Saturated fats (margaric acid) that come from dairy and butter show a reduced risk of heart disease.
- Omega-6 fats from vegetable oils show no benefit and may increase risk of heart attacks.
- Omega-6 fats from poultry, eggs, and beef (arachidonic acid) seem to be protective.
- Omega-3 fats from fish are the most protective.

The conclusion? Avoid most vegetable oils. Eat more butter, fish, chicken, eggs, and meat. And stay away from sugar and carbs. Boy, did we get this wrong!

This was far from the only study that redeemed the sullied reputation of saturated fat. There have been a slew of studies that have been mostly ignored by policy makers and medical associations. In a review of twenty-one studies done with almost 350,000 people over the span of 23 years, saturated fat was not shown to be associated with increased risk of heart attacks, stroke, or death.[16] One of the lead authors of this review, Dr. Ronald Krauss, was formerly the head of the Dietary Guidelines Committee at the American Heart Association. He fought their fervent belief in the dangers of saturated fat and ultimately left the association because of this difference of opinion. Other scientists have spoken out, noting that the current recommendations do not reflect the scientific evidence. Dr. Robert Hoenselaar from the Netherlands found that the "results and conclusions about saturated fat intake in relation to cardiovascular disease, from leading advisory committees, do not reflect the available scientific literature."[17]

A diverse group of scientists published a review in the journal *Open Heart*. They went way back and looked at all the randomized controlled trials comparing high- and low-fat diets done up to 1983—around the time the government recommended that Americans cut the fat, saturated fat, and cholesterol from their diets. None of these randomized trials showed that if you lowered total fat, saturated fat, or cholesterol, there was a reduction in heart disease. They stated that the governments of the United States and UK were guilty of telling their citizens (276 million altogether) to cut total and saturated fat in their diets without having any evidence from the gold standard of studies, randomized controlled trials.[18]

Our dietary recommendations are based on the idea that saturated fats in our diet cause elevated cholesterol levels. But even this is being called into question. In one review published in 2014, the authors noted that there was very little data to show that saturated fats in the diet caused elevated cholesterol.[19] What they found was striking. Only in the case of omega-3 deficiency (which affects more than 90 percent of the population) do saturated fats cause a problem. To put this another way: When you have enough omega-3 fats in your diet, the effect of saturated fat on your cholesterol is either neutral or beneficial.[20]

This conclusion was confirmed by a dramatic study published in *Lipids* in 2010 that compared the effects of a very low-carb, high-fat diet with either high amounts of omega-6 or high amounts of saturated fats. The researchers examined blood levels of fats, cholesterol, and inflammation before and after different dietary changes.[21] They controlled diets by providing all the food (remember, in studies where participants provide their own food, there are unknown variables). When they then measured blood levels of important markers of cardiovascular health (including blood levels of saturated fat, cholesterol, and inflammation markers), they found that more than doubling the dietary intake of saturated fat had no impact. That's right: ingesting twice as much or more saturated fat had no impact on blood levels of saturated fat. Even more striking, the group that ate more dietary saturated fat, in the absence of sugar or refined carbs, had lower levels of inflammation across the board. Remember, this wasn't a study of populations, but a true experiment where researchers provided all the food and measured true and immediate responses of the body to different diets, so these are highly reliable results.

SATURATED FATS AND INFLAMMATION

There is evidence that saturated fats cause inflammation in humans and animals, and that is not a good thing because inflammation is an underlying cause of heart disease, obesity, type 2 diabetes, cancer, and dementia. But there are some important caveats. It seems that saturated fats cause inflammation only in the context of two things: *low levels of omega-3 fats* and *high levels of carbohydrates*. Take out the high-carb foods and add omega-3-rich foods or supplements, and saturated fat is not a problem.

The data on omega-3 fats and how they interact with saturated fat is interesting. It is estimated that up to 90 percent of Americans have insufficient levels of omega-3 fats. I do omega-3 testing in my office and see this almost every day. When you don't have enough omega-3 fats in your diet and you eat saturated fat, the saturated fat stimulates the production of arachidonic acid, which turns into inflammatory molecules called eicosanoids. (There are both inflammatory and anti-inflammatory eicosanoids.) *No omega-3s and too much saturated fat is bad news.*

But add a little omega-3 into your diet and the saturated fats actually *reduce* inflammation by inhibiting or turning off genes that produce *cytokines* (inflammatory molecules), and they promote the production of anti-inflammatory eicosanoids. When consumed with a diet rich in omega-3 fats, saturated fat leads to lower triglycerides[22] and an increase in HDL, or good cholesterol, and it promotes the formation of large, light, fluffy, less harmful LDL particles.[23]

In one study of overweight men and women, researchers found that even in the face of a high-fat diet (55 percent) and high saturated fat (25 percent of calories), there was no impact on inflammatory markers or oxidative stress, two things we know drive heart disease and aging in general.[24]

In other studies, saturated fat seems to promote inflammation only in the presence of too many carbs or too little fiber, or there is no connection at all.[25] (The key to eating more fat, as you'll learn in Part III, is also eating more fiber.) In one study where the same people were given either butter or soybean oil at different times, there was no increase in inflammatory markers.

Even more striking, only saturated fat was able to reverse liver damage caused by inflammation in rats when they consumed sugar in the form of alcohol.[26] Polyunsaturated fat had no effect. In this study, saturated fat—mostly MCT, or medium-chain triglycerides, from coconut oil—was found to be therapeutic in reversing liver damage even in the face of continued alcohol intake. (But that doesn't mean you can drink as much as you want—it's still sugar!) Considering that nonalcoholic steatohepatitis (NASH—commonly known as fatty liver), caused by too much sugar and carbs, is now the most common liver disease and the leading cause of liver transplants, cutting the carbs and boosting the saturated fats may be part of the solution.

The take-home message here: Saturated fats lower inflammation when consumed with a low-carb, high-fiber, omega-3-rich diet. And lowering inflammation is key to healing and weight loss.

Does Saturated Fat Cause Strokes?

One study of 60,000 people in Japan showed that higher intakes of saturated fat led to a reduced risk of stroke.[27] So based on this study we should be recommending saturated fat to reduce heart disease risk and stroke, not warning against it.

SATURATED FATS AND CARBOHYDRATES

As we've reviewed, the saturated fats you eat don't increase blood levels of saturated fats. Doubling or even tripling saturated fat in your diet has no impact on saturated fat in your blood. It's the carbs that spike your blood levels of saturated fats. Many studies confirm that blood levels of saturated fat (palmitic, stearic, and palmitoleic acid) are significantly correlated with the development of type 2 diabetes[28] and heart disease.[29] But these fats in the blood are not coming from the fat you eat. They are produced by the liver in response to the carbs in your diet.

A group of researchers from Ohio State University did a very elegant study that tested this idea in a group of overweight pre-diabetic people.[30] They gave the study participants six different diets, each three weeks long. In the first part of the study, they increased the amount of carbs, starting at 50 grams a day and going up to 350 grams a day, and decreased the saturated fat. In the other part of the study they increased the saturated fat and reduced the carbs. There was *no difference in blood levels of saturated fats* despite a doubling of saturated fat from 46 to 84 grams a day. Only when the participants got to the high-carb part of the study did the researchers find higher levels of saturated fats in the blood, specifically palmitic acid.

The liver formed these bad fats even when the participants lost weight. So it was carbs, not fat, that raised the levels of saturated fat in the blood. These well-done studies show over and over again that in the face of low-carbohydrate diets, saturated fats are harmless and may be beneficial.

Another interesting study found that saturated fats consumed in a low-carbohydrate diet had no impact on blood cholesterol levels or profile, but in a high-carb diet, they made things worse.[31] So we should skip the bread and eat the butter. At least our cholesterol would improve.

I've put thousands of patients on a high-fat, low-carb diet and have seen for myself beneficial changes in all the important known risk factors for heart disease, including overall cholesterol profile, blood sugar, insulin, inflammation, liver function, hormones, and belly fat.

SATURATED FATS AND CHOLESTEROL

The obsession with cholesterol and LDL in particular as the only thing that drives heart disease is completely misguided. Why are we all so focused as doctors and patients on LDL? Simple. There is a multibillion-dollar drug industry behind the number one selling class of drugs on the market: statins. And the main effect of statins is to reduce LDL (bad cholesterol), which turns out not to be the most important thing in preventing heart disease. More on statins in a minute. First, let's dispel one of the biggest myths we have in medicine today: the connection between cholesterol and heart disease.

Saturated Fat Facts

- They have not been linked to heart disease, despite more than half a century of this belief and billions of dollars of research.
- They actually improve your overall cholesterol profile in the face of a low-carb diet by lowering triglycerides, raising HDL, and decreasing the small, dangerous LDL particles.
- They are a problem only in the face of a high-carb, low-fiber, omega-3-fat-deficient diet.
- They seem to be neutral or improve inflammation in many studies.
- When compared with higher-carb low-fat diets, higher-fat and saturated-fat diets do better in improving every single risk factor for heart disease (and promoting weight loss).
- Some dietary saturated fats (from dairy) may reduce the risk of heart disease.
- Blood levels of certain saturated fats are associated with heart disease, but it is carbs that increase those blood levels of saturated fat, not the saturated fats we eat.

The fact that saturated fat raises cholesterol is the biggest reason we have vilified meat and butter. The logic went that if high blood cholesterol causes heart attacks, and saturated fat raises cholesterol, then reducing saturated fat in the diet should reduce heart attacks and death. Sounds sensible. Except for one thing. The overwhelming body of research doesn't support this.[32]

We need a little biochemistry lesson here to understand cholesterol metabolism in the body. Hang in there with me; this is super important.

Most of the cholesterol floating around your blood is made in the liver. The liver gets triggered to produce fat and cholesterol in response to sugar and carbs. This is called *lipogenesis*. Everyone who has taken a biochemistry course knows this (or should know it); it is basic science. But somehow this fact has been completely ignored by most doctors and scientists studying cholesterol.

High-carb diets increase the production of triglycerides, lower the good cholesterol (HDL), and increase the number of LDL particles.[33] They also reduce the size of your cholesterol particles, or the small LDL particles.[34] It's not the LDL that's bad, but the small LDL. This kind of lipid profile is called atherogenic — in other words, it causes atherosclerosis, or hardening of the arteries, the very thing at the root of heart disease, stroke, and many cases of dementia. If you reduce fat, you may lower LDL (bad cholesterol), and that may seem like a good thing, but in fact it is a bad thing. Lower cholesterol is not always better cholesterol.

Shifting your diet from fat to carbs shifts you from light, fluffy, harmless LDL particles to small, dense, dangerous ones. In one study, a low-fat diet was compared to a higher-fat diet of exactly the same number of calories. The low-fat (high-sugar and refined-carb) diet led to dramatically higher triglycerides in both thin and overweight people.[35] In another analysis of more than sixty studies, researchers found that increasing saturated fats in the diet raised both LDL (which is not bad if it is large particles) and HDL while lowering triglycerides and increasing LDL particle size.[36] All these changes are beneficial, not harmful. In fact, it isn't the typical LDL value (which is the weight of your cholesterol measured in milligrams per deciliter) that correlates with heart disease at all. It is the LDL particle size and number.[37]

The LDL number your doctor measures is simply the weight of LDL

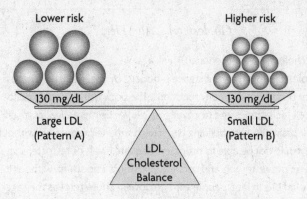

You can have the exact same LDL value (130 mg/dl), which is the weight, but it can be made up of many dangerous small particles (pattern B) or a few large, light, fluffy particles (pattern A).[38]

in your blood (in milligrams per deciliter). Think of it as a box that weighs a certain amount. Inside that box there can be many small golf balls (small, dangerous LDL particles), or a few large, light beach balls (large, benign LDL particles). Most doctors never measure that, but that is what is most correlated with heart disease. Doctors should order the NMR (nuclear magnetic resonance) lipid test, offered by LabCorp or the Cardio IQ test offered by Quest Diagnostics. It puts your cholesterol in a mini MRI machine to examine the number and size of the particles. The other cholesterol tests should be left in the twentieth century. Demand the NMR lipid or Cardio IQ test instead!

The main factor that stimulates your liver to produce these small, dense cholesterol particles and to produce many of them is sugar and refined carbs. It seems hard to believe that we got the whole story wrong for more than half a century, but it is true. It is sugar, not fat, that is the big driver of heart disease (as well as stroke, obesity, type 2 diabetes, and dementia). In fact, our whole effort to reduce heart disease by lowering LDL (bad cholesterol) by reducing saturated fat and prescribing statin drugs has had unintended consequences.

Cholesterol . . . the Hero?

Think cholesterol is the enemy? Think again!

Cholesterol is a fatty substance produced by the liver that is necessary for thousands of bodily functions. The body uses it to help build your cell membranes and to cover your nerve sheaths as well as much of your brain. It's a key building block for hormone production; without it you would not be able to maintain adequate levels of testosterone, estrogen, progesterone, and cortisol. Even more important, without it, you would die. In fact, people with the lowest cholesterol as they age are at highest risk of death. Under certain circumstances, higher cholesterol can actually help to increase life span.

In terms of cholesterol, the *type* of fat that you eat is more important than the *amount* of fat. Trans fats or hydrogenated fats and refined vegetable oils (omega-6 PUFAs) promote abnormal cholesterol, whereas omega-3 fats from fish and monounsaturated fats found in nuts and olive oil actually improve the type and amount of cholesterol your body produces.

In reality, the biggest source of abnormal cholesterol is not fat at all—it's sugar. The sugar you consume converts to fat in your body. And the worst culprit of all is high-fructose corn syrup. Consumption of high-fructose corn syrup, which is present in sodas, juices, and processed foods, is the primary nutritional cause of most of the cholesterol issues we doctors see in our patients. Fructose is a problem because when ingested in high amounts (without the associated fiber found in whole fruit) it turns on the cholesterol production factory in your liver, called lipogenesis.[39]

A study published in the *American Journal of Clinical Nutrition* looked at the impact that sugar intake has on cholesterol. The researchers carried out a meta-analysis of thirty-nine randomized controlled trials on sugar intake. Overall, it showed that people who ate higher amounts of sugar had significantly higher levels of triglycerides and LDL and total cholesterol. This effect occurred even if there was no change in weight with higher-sugar and carb diets. In other words, it was not weight gain that made the cholesterol worse; it was sugar.

So the real concern isn't the amount of cholesterol in your blood, but the type of fats and sugar and refined carbohydrates in your diet. Of course, many health-conscious people today know that total cholesterol or LDL is not as critical as the following factors or numbers:

- Your levels of HDL (good cholesterol) vs. LDL (bad cholesterol) (HDL ideally greater than 60 mg/dl)
- Your triglyceride levels (ideally less than 100 mg/dl)
- Your ratio of triglycerides to HDL (ideally less than 1:1 or 2:1)
- Your ratio of total cholesterol to HDL (ideally less than 3:1)

Another concern is whether or not the cholesterol in your blood is rancid or oxidized. If it is, the risk of arterial plaque is real. Rancid or oxidized cholesterol results from oxidative stress and free radicals, which trigger a vicious cycle of inflammation and fat or plaque deposits under the artery walls. This can occur more often when consuming omega-6 fats because they are unstable and more easily oxidized. Cholesterol is like the body's Band-Aid, and when there is inflammation it tries to patch things up. That is the real danger: When small, dense LDL particles are oxidized, they become hazardous by starting the buildup of plaque or cholesterol in your arteries.

It is fine to enjoy dietary cholesterol from the right type of fat in any amount because it has no impact on your blood cholesterol or heart disease risk. In Europe, Australia, Canada, New Zealand, Korea, and India, there is no upper limit on the amount of cholesterol considered safe in the diet, and America is finally catching up. The 2013 American College of Cardiology/American Heart Association Task Force on Practice Guidelines did not recommend lowering total fat, only saturated fat.[40] And they completely gave up on decades of advice to reduce dietary cholesterol, which had us all eating tasteless egg white omelets and avoiding shrimp and lobster. In fact they noted that dietary cholesterol had no impact on blood cholesterol. In about 25 percent of people it raises the LDL (bad cholesterol), but it also raises the HDL, or good cholesterol, resulting in a neutral effect on your cholesterol profile.[41]

The government's own 2015 Dietary Guidelines Advisory Committee (DGAC) Report also did not make any recommendations to lower total fat content, only saturated fat. And for the first time since the guidelines were established in 1980, dietary cholesterol was exonerated: "Previously, the Dietary Guidelines for Americans recommended that cholesterol intake be limited to no more than 300 mg/day. The 2015 DGAC will not bring forward this recommendation because available evidence shows no appreciable relationship between consumption of dietary cholesterol and serum cholesterol, consistent with the conclusions of the AHA/ACC (American College of Cardiology/American Heart Association Task Force) report. Cholesterol is not a nutrient of concern for overconsumption."[42]

I love that: "not a nutrient of concern." What an unceremonious death for the tarnished reputation of dietary cholesterol!

THE BIG BUSINESS OF STATINS

Drug company marketing has convinced us all that statin drugs are God's gift to humankind and that they are essential to lower your risk of heart attacks and death. Think about how many feel-good commercials and magazine ads you've seen for cholesterol-lowering drugs. But do statins live up to all the hype? What does the science really prove?

Most doctors now know that inflammation and oxidative stress are the biggest causes of heart disease, not cholesterol. A landmark paper in the *New England Journal of Medicine*[43] lays out the science of why inflammation, not cholesterol, is the root cause of atherosclerosis. It explains how macrophages (white blood cells) are driven into the walls of your arteries to protect you against rancid or oxidized cholesterol. They soak up the toxic oxidized or rancid cholesterol (not all the cholesterol), and that is what causes the plaque that clogs your arteries and leads to heart attacks. It turns out that the reason statins have any effect at all is not because they lower cholesterol, but because they lower inflammation and also act as antioxidants. So they do have some benefit, but there are a lot better ways to reduce inflammation and get antioxidants with many fewer side effects!

However, a recent study found that using statins did not lead to lower heart attacks or death. In 2011, a group of Swedish researchers looked at the relationship between statin prescriptions and heart attacks in their country. They found that between 1998 and 2002, the rate of statin use among Swedish men and women between the ages of forty and seventy-nine roughly tripled. Yet this had no impact on the corresponding rate of heart attack incidence or mortality. Stunning, isn't it? A tripling of statin use and no impact on heart disease! This is not a randomized trial, and just shows a correlation, but it still worries me.

Roger Williams, a twentieth-century American biochemist who discovered vitamin B_5, once said something about research that rings true: "There are liars, damn liars, and statisticians." We see prominent ads on television and in medical journals for statins that report a 36 percent reduction in the risk of having a heart attack. But we don't look at the fine print. What does that really mean, and how does it affect decisions about who should be using these drugs?

Before I explain that, here are some interesting findings to ponder about cholesterol and statins:

- If you lower bad cholesterol (LDL) but have a low HDL (good cholesterol) there is no benefit to statins.[44]
- If you lower bad cholesterol (LDL) but don't reduce inflammation (marked by a test called C-reactive protein), there is no benefit to statins.[45]
- If you are a healthy woman with high cholesterol, there is no proof that taking statins reduces your risk of heart attack or death.[46]
- If you are a man or a woman over sixty-nine years old with high cholesterol, there is no proof that taking statins reduces your risk of heart attack or death.[47]
- Aggressive cholesterol treatment with two medications (Zocor and Zetia) lowered cholesterol much more than one drug alone but led to more plaque buildup in the arteries and no fewer heart attacks.[48]

- Older patients with lower cholesterol have a higher risk of death than those with higher cholesterol.[49]
- Countries with higher average cholesterol than America, such as Switzerland and Spain, have less heart disease.
- Recent evidence shows that it is probably the ability of statins to lower inflammation that accounts for the benefits of statins, not their ability to lower cholesterol.[50]
- About 20 percent of people who take statins have side effects, including muscle damage and pain,[51] neurologic problems, memory issues,[52] sexual dysfunction,[53] and more.[54]
- Statins have been linked to a dramatically higher risk of diabetes. In one study of almost 26,000 healthy people, those taking statins to prevent heart attacks were 87 percent more likely to get type 2 diabetes.[55] In another randomized controlled trial of 153,840 women, those who took statins were 48 percent more likely to get type 2 diabetes.[56] Large reviews of all the studies show about a 10 percent increased risk. But if all the people who are currently advised to take statins did so, that would mean we would have another 4 to 5 million diabetics in the country!

Winston Churchill said—and I am paraphrasing—that men occasionally stumble over the truth, but most of them pick themselves up and hurry off as if nothing happened. This is precisely what happened with a dramatic study published in 2009 in the *American Heart Journal,* which found that 75 percent of patients admitted to hospitals with heart disease had normal cholesterol levels.[57] The authors looked at 231,836 hospital admissions from 541 hospitals, accounting for 59 percent of all heart attack admissions in the country from 2000 to 2006. A very big sample! They assessed cholesterol levels within the first 24 hours of admission. Their findings were shocking. About 75 percent had normal LDL (bad cholesterol) levels (under 130 mg/dl) and more than 50 percent had "optimal" LDL levels (under 100 mg/dl). For those who argue that this means we need to lower LDL benchmarks even further, the study also found that more than 17 percent had LDL levels below 70 mg/dl.

There is still some data showing that high LDL is a problem, but it is only one of many other factors, not necessarily the most important one.[58] I have seen many eighty-five-year-olds with cholesterol of over 300 mg/dl and normal HDL and triglycerides, with no heart disease at all and clean arteries. What they did find in the study of heart attacks and hospital admissions was not surprising if you understand the link between sugar, carbs, and heart disease. The pattern most associated with heart attacks was low HDL and high triglycerides (not the LDL level), which is caused by sugar and refined carbs.

Years ago I had a chance to snowshoe through the Berkshires with Dr. Peter Libby from Harvard, one of the world's most renowned cardiologists. I asked about all these patients I had, especially women, who had cholesterol levels over 300 mg/dl but also had very high HDL levels and low triglycerides, were slim, and had no other heart disease risk factors. I wondered if I should treat them with statins. He said that there was no evidence I should treat them, even with their high cholesterol levels.

People with the lowest cholesterol as they age are in fact at highest risk of death. In a study of more than 3,500 elderly men, those with the lowest cholesterol had a 64 percent higher risk of death. Under certain circumstances, higher cholesterol can actually help increase life span. It's all in the spin of the statistics and numbers. And it's easy to get confused.

I have tested thousands of patients on statins. I measure particle size, and despite statins' ability to lower total LDL, I often see very high LDL particle numbers and very small LDL particle sizes in these patients, the pattern most associated with heart attacks.

This is not to say that statins don't work. In fact, they help prevent heart attacks in people, especially men under seventy, who have already had heart attacks. And they work slightly for middle-aged men who have many risk factors for heart disease, like high blood pressure, obesity, and diabetes. But for most people to whom they are prescribed— people who have never had a heart attack—they don't provide real benefit and come with a whole host of side effects and risks.[59]

You might ask why then did the 2004 National Cholesterol Education Program guidelines expand the previous guidelines to recommend that more people take statins (from 13 million to 40 million), and why did they recommend that people who don't have heart disease take them to prevent heart disease (known as primary prevention)? Could it have been that 8 of the 9 experts on the panel who developed these guidelines had financial ties to the drug industry? Thirty-four other non–industry-affiliated experts sent a petition to the National Institutes of Health to protest the recommendations, saying the evidence was weak. Having industry-funded scientists make the guidelines is like having a fox guard the chicken coop.

Worse, more recent guidelines from the American College of Cardiology and the American Heart Association have recommended that even *more* people take statins, based on a 10-year risk calculation. That means 56 million Americans could be taking statins, up from 43.2 million.[60] Many experts challenge the assumptions made in these guidelines.[61] Do we really think that heart disease is a statin deficiency? Shouldn't we be addressing the root causes? Is there other research that contradicts these guidelines? When you look under the hood of the research data you find that the touted "36 percent reduction" in heart attacks attributable to statins means a reduction of the number of people having heart attacks from 3 percent to 2 percent. Yes, it's a reduction, but not as big a reduction as it sounds. But drug companies would rather ignore the distinction between absolute risk reduction (1 percent) and relative risk reduction (36 percent) when they market their products.

That data also shows that treatment works only if you already have heart disease. In those who *don't* have documented heart disease, there seems to be no benefit. A group of independent scientists (with no links to or funding from pharmaceutical companies) reviewed the data on the benefits of using statins for preventing a first heart attack (their review is known as the Cochrane Database Systematic Reviews). They found that researchers looking at heart attacks and deaths in the statin treatment studies were selective in what they reported; they didn't report bad outcomes, and they included people who had already had heart attacks (even though they weren't supposed to). The independent experts concluded that only limited evidence existed that statins could prevent first heart attacks, reduce health care costs, or improve quality of life. As they stated, "Caution should be taken in prescribing statins for primary prevention among people at low cardiovascular risk."[62] And yet 75 percent of statin prescriptions are for people at low risk.

In 1954, Darrell Huff published an influential book called *How to Lie with Statistics*. It seems to have been well read by many drug researchers.

UNTANGLING THE STATS ON STATINS

There is a little-known concept in medicine called NNT or "number needed to treat." This is a way of looking at the real benefits and risks in research. An independent group of doctors and scientists who receive no industry funding have created a platform for reviewing the literature on various medical topics. Their work can be found at www.thennt .com. And they have taken a deep look at statins and their pros and cons.

What they report is a bit shocking considering the hype and passionate promotion of statins by most doctors. In patients with no preexisting heart disease who took statins for five years, no lives were saved. In that group, statins helped prevent a heart attack in only 1 in 104 people (1.6 percent). And they helped prevent stroke in only 1 in 154 (0.37 percent).[63] Not a very effective drug. Worse, 1 in 10 people had muscle damage and pain, and 1 in 50 developed diabetes. More people were harmed than helped by the medication. So it seems the risks outweigh the benefits.

But what if you already have heart disease, or have had a heart attack? The results for those who take statins are better, but not much. Statins helped prevent death in 1 in 83 people who already had heart disease (1.2 percent); they helped prevent a nonfatal heart attack in 1 in 39 (2.6 percent); and they helped prevent a stroke in 1 in 125 (0.8 percent).[64] One in 50 got diabetes and 1 in 10 had muscle damage.

Just to put that in perspective: If a drug works, it has a very low NNT (number needed to treat). For example, if you have a urinary tract infection and take an antibiotic, you will get nearly a 100 percent benefit. The number needed to treat is 1, because every person treated will benefit. But if you have an NNT of 104, like statins do for preventing heart attacks in 75 percent of the people who take them (those without heart disease), it is basically a crapshoot and the side effects are serious (muscle damage, diabetes, memory loss, and even sexual dysfunction).

Here's what the NNT group had to say about the state of statin research: "Virtually all of the major statin studies were paid for and conducted by their respective pharmaceutical company. A long history of misrepresentation of data and occasionally fraudulent reporting of data suggests that these results are often much more optimistic than subsequent data produced by researchers and parties that do not have a financial stake in the results. Also, harm from these drugs is difficult to predict, partly because harms are often difficult to anticipate and are often poorly tracked. Such findings often come up years after new drugs have been on the market."

Yet at a cost of more than $28 billion a year, 75 percent of all statin prescriptions are for unproven primary prevention. Simply applying the science over 10 years would save more than $200 billion in health care costs.

PREVENTING AND TREATING HEART DISEASE

So if lowering cholesterol is not the great panacea that we thought, and statins aren't effective, how do we treat heart disease? And how do we make sure we have the right kind of blood cholesterol—high HDL, low LDL, and low triglycerides, and cholesterol particles that are large, light, and fluffy rather than small, dense, and hard?

Our current thinking about how to treat and prevent heart disease is at best misguided, and at worst harmful. Most doctors believe they are treating the causes of heart disease by lowering cholesterol, lowering blood pressure, and lowering blood sugar with medication. But the real question is, "What causes high cholesterol, high blood pressure, and high blood sugar in the first place?"[65] It is certainly not a medication deficiency.

Don't go blaming your genes entirely, either. It is the environment working on your genes that determines your risk. What you eat, how much you exercise, how you deal with stress, and how your body handles environmental toxins[66] are the underlying causes of high cholesterol, high blood pressure, high blood sugar, and therefore heart disease.

The EPIC (European Prospective Investigation into Cancer and Nutrition) study of more than 500,000 people in ten countries, published in the *Archives of Internal Medicine*, reviewed a subset of 23,000 people's adherence to four simple behaviors—not smoking, exercising three and a half hours a week, eating a healthy diet (fruits, vegetables, beans, whole grains, nuts, seeds, and limited amounts of meat), and maintaining a healthy weight (body mass index of less than 30). In those adhering to these behaviors, 93 percent of diabetes, 81 percent of heart attacks, 50 percent of strokes, and 36 percent of all cancers were prevented.[67] And the INTERHEART study, published in the *Lancet* in 2004, followed 30,000 people and found that changing lifestyle could prevent at least 90 percent of all heart disease.[68]

These studies are among a large evidence base documenting how lifestyle intervention is often more effective in reducing cardiovascular disease, hypertension, heart failure, stroke, cancer, diabetes, and deaths from all causes than almost any other medical intervention.[69] A healthy lifestyle doesn't only reduce risk factors such as high blood pressure, high blood sugar, or high cholesterol; it influences a fundamental biological mechanism—gene expression, which modulates inflammation, oxidative stress, nutrient levels, and metabolic function. These are the real reasons we get sick.

Disregarding the underlying causes and treating only risk factors is somewhat like mopping up the floor around an overflowing sink instead of turning off the faucet. When the lifestyle causes are addressed, patients are often able to get better without medication or surgery.

In order to control these key biological functions and keep them in balance, you need to look at your overall health as well as your genetic predispositions. Your genes, lifestyle, and environment ultimately determine your risks—and the outcome of your life.

The good news is that your genes are under your control if you feed them right and treat them right. The science of how food acts as information to turn on or off genes that control health and disease is called *nutrigenomics*. And many other things affect your gene expression and function besides diet, including stress and activity levels.

The biggest risk factor for heart disease is pre-diabetes or type 2 diabetes—diabesity. Diabesity, an insulin and blood sugar problem caused by high doses of sugar and refined carbs, now affects 1 in 2 Americans and 1 in 4 teenagers. I have written extensively about this problem in my books *The Blood Sugar Solution* and *The Blood Sugar Solution 10-Day Detox Diet*.

Right up there with diabesity as a top risk factor is inflammation. What causes inflammation?

- A poor diet (high-sugar, refined carbs, processed food, low-fiber, etc.)
- A sedentary lifestyle
- Stress
- Food allergies (like gluten and dairy)
- Hidden infections (such as gum disease)
- Toxins (such as mercury or pesticides)

Finding and addressing all the causes of inflammation is critical to preventing heart disease (and almost all the diseases of aging, including obesity, cancer, diabetes, and dementia).

Many of these factors are synergistic and at play at the same time if there is inflammation. I recommend that people undergo a comprehensive medical evaluation to see what their risk really is and evaluate the presence and causes of inflammation. For example, gluten sensitivity (not even full-blown celiac disease) can trigger heart attacks and death and is often undiagnosed.[70]

A major study done at Harvard found that people with high levels of a blood test that measures inflammation called C-reactive protein (CRP) had higher risks of heart disease than people with high cholesterol. Normal cholesterol levels were *not* protective to those with high

CRP. The risks were greatest for those with high levels of both CRP and cholesterol.

There is another easily treatable risk factor for heart disease. There is a blood test that measures homocysteine (which is related to your body's levels of the key heart-protective nutrients folic acid and vitamins B_6 and B_{12}). High levels of homocysteine trigger oxidative stress and inflammation, which may cause heart disease. It's easily fixed by taking the right forms of folic acid, and vitamins B_6 and B_{12}.

GETTING THE RIGHT TESTS

There are special tests that can identify imbalances in blood sugar and insulin, inflammation, nutrient levels such as homocysteine (folic acid), clotting factors, hormones, and other factors that affect your risk of cardiovascular disease. If you want to test your overall risk, you can consider asking your doctor to perform the following tests. (To learn more about testing and how to interpret these tests, you can also download my free e-book, *How to Work with Your Doctor to Get What You Need*. See www.eatfatgetthin.com.)

Total Cholesterol, HDL (Good Cholesterol), LDL (Bad Cholesterol), and Triglycerides

- Your total cholesterol should be under 200 mg/dl (this depends on your overall profile and risk factors)
- Your triglycerides should be under 100.
- Your HDL should be over 60 mg/dl.
- Your LDL should ideally be under 80 mg/dl (although this matters less than the LDL particle number and size; see the following section on NMR and Cardio IQ test). This also depends on your overall profile and risk factors.
- Your ratio of total cholesterol to HDL should be less than 3:1.
- Your ratio of triglycerides to HDL should be no greater than 1:1 or 2:1; this ratio can indicate insulin resistance if elevated.

NMR Lipid Profile or Cardio IQ Lipoprotein Fractionation (Ion Mobility)

▪ The NMR test (available from Labcorp) looks at your cholesterol under an MRI scan to assess the size of the particles; particle size is the real determinant of your cardiovascular risk. The Cardio IQ uses a different technology and is available from Quest Diagnostics. It is important to track this as you change your diet. These are really the *only* cholesterol tests you should have. You should have less than 1,000 total LDL particles and no more than 400 small particles (although ideally you shouldn't have any!).

Glucose and Insulin Tolerance Test

▪ Measurements of fasting and one- and two-hour levels of glucose *and* insulin after taking a 75-gram load of glucose help identify pre-diabetes and excessively high levels of insulin, and even diabetes. You can also just do a fasting and thirty-minute test after drinking glucose; this can be almost as good an indicator of diabesity. Your fasting sugar should be between 70 and 80 mg/dl and your one- and two-hour sugars should be less than 120 mg/dl. Your fasting insulin should be less than 5 and one- and two-hour insulin levels should be less than 30. Most doctors just check blood sugar and not insulin, which is the first thing to go up. By the time your blood sugar goes up, the train has left the station. Be sure to ask that your insulin, not just your blood sugar, gets measured.

Hemoglobin A1c

▪ This test measures your average blood sugar level over the previous six weeks. Anything over 5.5 percent is high. Just measuring your fasting blood sugar is not enough to detect early problems.

Cardio or High-Sensitivity C-Reactive Protein

▪ This marker of inflammation in the body is essential to understand in the context of overall risk. Your high-sensitivity C-reactive protein level should be less than 1.0 mg/L, and ideally less than 0.7 mg/L.

Homocysteine

- Your homocysteine measures your folate status and should be between 6 and 8 micromoles per liter.

Oxidized LDL

- This test looks at the amount of oxidized or rancid cholesterol in the blood. This should be within normal limits of the test. It is available through LabCorp.

Fibrinogen

- This test looks at clotting in the blood. It should be less than 300 mg/dl.

Lipoprotein(a)

- This is another factor that can promote the risk of heart disease, especially in men. It is mostly genetically determined. It should be less than 30 mg/dl.

Gluten Antibodies

- Testing IgG and IgA anti-gliadin and IgA and IgG tissue trans-glutaminase antibodies measures immune response to gluten found in wheat, barley, rye, spelt, and oats and can help you identify this hidden cause of inflammation and heart disease (and many, many other health problems). Any level of antibodies indicates you may have a reaction to gluten. Your body should not make autoimmune antibodies to gluten. There really is no "normal" level.

Genes or SNPs

- Genetic tests may also be useful in assessing your heart disease risk factors. A number of key genes regulate cholesterol and metabolism:
  - Apo E genes
  - Cholesterol ester transfer protein gene
  - MTHFR gene, which regulates homocysteine

High-Speed CT or EBT Scan

- This high-speed X-ray of the heart can help determine if you have cardiovascular disease. It may be helpful in assessing overall plaque burden and calcium score and can inform how aggressive you need to be in terms of prevention. A score higher than 100 is a concern, and a score higher than 400 indicates severe risk of cardiovascular disease.

Carotid Intimal Thickness

- This test is done through ultrasound and looks for plaque in the arteries in your neck, which correlates with heart disease and stroke risk.

SHOW YOUR HEART SOME LOVE

Okay, so here's what we know: Heart disease risk is linked to a variety of factors, including inflammation, insulin resistance, metabolic syndrome, low levels of HDL, high triglycerides, increased LDL particle number and decreased particle size, belly fat, thickness of your blood, blood pressure, smoking, stress, environmental toxins, and age.

Phew…that's a long list! But here's the bright spot: Other than age, environmental toxins, stress, and smoking, all of these can be corrected by eating a lower-carb, higher-fat diet. If eating a certain way moves things in the right direction, then that gets my attention.

While it is true that we have cut the death rates from heart disease in middle-aged people because of better drugs and treatments, we have not been winning the war on the increase in the number of new people getting heart disease. In fact, heart disease is spreading like wildfire across the globe and is now the world's number one killer.

That is why, more than ever, we need to give up on the dietary myths about saturated fat and cholesterol and focus our attention and efforts on addressing the *real* causes of heart disease, as outlined in this chapter.

6

Vegetable Oils — A Slippery Subject

As you know by now, right on the heels of the "eat less saturated fat" message has been the message to eat more PUFAs, or polyunsaturated fats, especially omega-6 fats. We know these oils well. They are the common "vegetable" oils we all grew up on, including corn oil, soybean oil, canola oil, safflower oil, and sunflower oil—clear, tasteless oils that are highly refined and processed. Advisory groups such as the American Heart Association, the National Cholesterol Education Program, the National Institutes of Health, the government's dietary guidelines, and many well-respected scientists have been recommending that we substitute polyunsaturated fats for saturated fats.[1]

Thanks to farm subsidies and the power of Monsanto's global soybean monopoly, Americans now consume about 18 billion pounds of soybean oil a year. About 10 percent of our calories come from soybean oil, which is 50 percent linoleic acid, an inflammatory omega-6 fat.[2] Check your grocery store labels; soybean oil is in almost everything.

At the turn of the century, vegetable oils were almost unknown in the food supply. After the Industrial Revolution, we learned how to process seeds, grains, and beans into refined oils. What's surprising to most people is that meat and chicken are big sources of omega-6 fats. How can that be? Because industrial farming practices have led farmers to switch their feed from grass to corn and cereal grains, and now those omega-6 vegetable fats comprise a significant portion of "animal" fat. You are what you eat. Or more accurately: You are what your food eats.

With the introduction of refined oils and our shift away from grass-fed and wild animals to industrial animal production, our dietary omega-6 fats have skyrocketed, while omega-3 fats have declined. Now we eat about ten times as much omega-6 as omega-3 oils, and some people eat up to twenty-five times as much. While it is not clear what the exact ratio should be, we do know it's now way out of whack.

Balance is critical. The omega-6 fats fuel inflammatory pathways in the body, while omega-3 fats are anti-inflammatory. Most important, omega-6 fats reduce the availability of anti-inflammatory omega-3 fats in our tissues (leading to more inflammation) and prevent the conversion of plant-based omega-3s (ALA) into the active forms of omega-3s (EPA/DHA) in the body by 40 percent. That means that even if you eat omega-3 fats, in the presence of excess omega-6 fats, the omega-3 fats don't work as well.

IS IT OMEGA-3S (FISH OIL) OR OMEGA-6S (VEGETABLE OILS) THAT PREVENT HEART DISEASE?

The first, largest, and most important study I want to review, the Lyon Heart Study, found that increasing omega-3 fats in the diet resulted in a 70 percent reduction in heart attacks and death. This study is often quoted to support the idea that polyunsaturated fats are good. The thing is, PUFAs, or polyunsaturated fats, are not created equally. Omega-3 is protective and omega-6s are harmful in excess.[3] And the Lyon Heart Study actually reduced the amount of omega-6 fats, while increasing the omega-3s. It is hard to explain why this fact is ignored when this study is used to promote the benefits of omega-6 oils.

We know it is hard to attack entrenched ideas. But we have to have a deeper look to understand the advice to stop saturated fats and eat more polyunsaturated fats. The standard policy line is that saturated fats are bad and polyunsaturated fats are good. The only way to figure this out is to dig into all the research on this topic. A number of brave scientists have ventured into this hallowed territory and changed the status quo. They are from the National Institutes of Health (NIH) and have no conflicts of interest. Many other scientists in this fight get funding from the food industry.

Two of the leading voices are Dr. Chris Ramsden and Dr. Joseph

Hibbeln from the NIH, who have taken a deep view into this controversy. In a series of papers[4] they reviewed all the research on this topic, digging deep into history, going all the way back to data hidden away from the 1960s. There are two major kinds of studies, as we have discussed. The first is population or observational studies, which can show correlation but do not prove cause and effect. These can be helpful to highlight correlations among things (like fat and heart disease) but can also lead people down the wrong path because, even though they might show a correlation, they don't prove cause and effect. That is why we need the second type of study, or experimental studies, often called randomized controlled trials. When these are well done, they can prove cause and effect. Most of our advice about fat in the diet comes from the population-type studies because dietary interventions on a large scale are often very hard to do. But there are some important experimental studies, and Drs. Ramsden and Hibbeln have reviewed them all and taken a look at the long history of fat and saturated fat. They paint a picture of omega-6 fats that contradicts the conventional wisdom.

Here's what they found:

1. In a review of studies where people consumed a mixture of omega-3 and omega-6 fats, there was in fact a 27 percent reduction in heart attacks and death.
2. If studies increased only omega-6 fats, there was a 13 percent *increase* in heart attacks.
3. Randomized trials that used omega-6 fats alone (without any omega-3 fats) while reducing saturated and trans fats also showed an increased risk of death.
4. Many of the current recommendations and the analysis on which they were based omitted a number of important studies and didn't distinguish between studies in which people only consumed omega-6 fats from those in which people consumed a combination of omega-3 and omega-6 fats.

For example, one highly cited study that many scientists consider critical in supporting the recommendations for more PUFAs (which is translated into more omega-6 vegetable oils in food policy) is the Oslo Diet-Heart Study. The participants were told to substitute meat and eggs for fish, shellfish, and "whale beef," all rich sources of omega-3 fats. They were even given considerable quantities of Norwegian sardines canned in cod liver oil as a "bread spread." This is about the equivalent of sixteen fish oil pills, about five times the amount given in an Italian study that showed a reduction in sudden cardiac deaths by 40 percent and total deaths by 20 percent.[5] The study participants were also told to cut out trans fats and limit refined grains and sugar. All these things reduce the risk of heart disease. This study never proved that high levels of omega-6s were beneficial. They showed only that eating more omega-3 fats and eating less trans fats and sugar and refined grains are protective.

The only trial mentioned in the big recent analysis that is used as the basis to recommend a higher amount of PUFAs from omega-6 in the diet that looked only at an increase in omega-6 fats was the Minnesota Coronary Survey of 4,393 men and 4,664 women. The women in this study more than doubled their risk of heart attack in the first year. This showed an increased risk of heart attacks! In other studies that used corn and safflower oil (mostly omega-6 linoleic acid), participants had a 4.64-fold increased risk for heart attacks and death from all causes. That is a 464 percent increase in bad outcomes from eating too much omega-6 oil.

The Lyon Heart Study, the randomized controlled trial mentioned previously that showed a 70 percent reduction in heart attacks, was the only study that reduced the amount of omega-6 fats below 5 percent of calories while increasing the omega-3 fats.

The final death knell for omega-6 PUFA being touted as a health food was the Sydney Diet Heart Study.[6] Drs. Ramsden and Hibbeln went back and dug into all the original data on this big randomized controlled trial done from 1966 to 1973. This study was designed to find out if using more omega-6 oils from safflower oil and cutting out saturated fat would impact heart disease risk. Participants were told to increase safflower oil to 15 percent of calories, while decreasing saturated fat to less than 10 percent of calories and cholesterol to less than 300 milligrams a day. Safflower oil is a concentrated source of linoleic acid, the fat that leads to inflammation in the body. The study did instruct participants to include some margarines, which may have increased trans fats, but both groups had trans fats in equal amounts, so this probably didn't affect the results. Also the safflower oil margarine was soft and didn't contain as many trans fats as hard margarine or shortening.

So what did the study show? Compared to the group that ate more saturated fats and cholesterol, the linoleic omega-6 fat group had an increased risk across the board of death from all causes, heart attacks and cardiac deaths. In fact, the omega-6 group had a 37 percent increased risk from heart attacks, despite significant lowering of their cholesterol.

How could this be? Well it turns out the omega-6 fat, linoleic acid, can create a lot of havoc in the body, the kind of havoc that leads to heart disease.

First, omega-6s easily oxidize or go rancid, which makes any cholesterol you do have much more likely to cause heart disease. Even if your cholesterol is low, if it is oxidized or rancid, it is much more likely to cause heart attacks. These fats are called OXLAMs, or oxidized linoleic acid metabolites; think of them as rancid fats. They are what make up the cholesterol plaques in your arteries. Things that increase oxidative stress—such as smoking, excessive drinking, and low intake of dietary antioxidants such as fruits and vegetables—all increase heart disease (and all chronic illnesses).

And these NIH scientists are not alone. A recent review of all the literature published in the *Mayo Clinic Proceedings* in 2014 pointed out the flawed basis of our current recommendations to lower saturated fat and increase omega-6 fats.[7] Unfortunately this advice still has not penetrated the recommendations coming from any advisory group or the government.

What's clear is that we have been given completely wrong advice over the last 50 years. We were told to cut saturated fat and cholesterol, increase omega-6 PUFAs, and increase our carb intake. This has been a massive failure of public policy and has provided us a window into the challenges of nutrition research. The time has come for a change.

THE FLAWED AMERICAN HEART ASSOCIATION ADVISORY ON OMEGA-6 FATTY ACIDS

The American Heart Association (AHA) recommends that adults get no more than 5 percent of their calories from saturated fat, and urges people to use linoleic-rich (omega-6 polyunsaturated fats, or PUFAs) vegetable oils instead. The AHA advises people to eat at least 5 to 10 percent of their calories in the form of omega-6 PUFAs. The rationale for this is that linoleic acid, unlike saturated fat, lowers LDL (bad cholesterol) levels.

As a result, the average intake of linoleic acid (an omega-6 fatty acid) has risen sharply since the 1960s, and even more dramatically since the early 1900s. Americans consume at least twice the amount of linoleic acid today that they did in the 1960s (at least 7 percent of daily calories, up from 3 percent in 1960).

In 2010, Philip C. Calder, a scientist at the University of Southampton's Institute of Human Nutrition, published an analysis of the recommendations on linoleic acid.[8] Based on the evidence, he warned that while linoleic acid lowers LDL, it also makes cholesterol more vulnerable to oxidation (going rancid) and inflammation, which can increase atherosclerosis, or cholesterol deposits in the arteries. There is also some evidence that it promotes cancer. As one expert UK committee warned, "There is reason to be cautious about high intakes of omega-6 PUFAs, and we recommend that the proportion of the population consuming in excess of about 10 percent of energy [as n-6 PUFAs] should not increase."

There are many reasons why linoleic acid should be consumed only in moderation, Dr. Calder argues. But the most important are that it increases arachidonic acid, which is pro-inflammatory, and perhaps more importantly acts as an antagonist of omega-3 fatty acids.

Recently, the American Heart Association published an advisory that declared the benefits of increasing omega-6 fatty acids but didn't address the potential harm. The advisory argued that concerns about inflammation, thrombosis, and LDL oxidation were unsubstantiated.

But Dr. Calder argues that the AHA advisory was flawed. Most of the evidence for the advisory came from observational studies. It also included randomized controlled trials, but the majority of those trials had design flaws. "Although these limitations appear not to have been considered in developing the advisory, they may have influenced its major scientific conclusion (replacing saturated fatty acids with PUFAs lowered cardiovascular events), which is clearly not an omega 6 fatty acid (or linoleic acid) specific summary statement, and so somewhat blurs the boundaries between PUFA [which includes protective omega-3 fats], omega-6 PUFA and linoleic acid," Dr. Calder wrote.

The AHA advisory and recommendations are based on randomized controlled trials that often did not address the question of omega-6 PUFA or linoleic acid in isolation, "but rather included mixtures of omega-6 and omega-3 PUFA." And for that reason—and others— Calder wrote, Americans should be cautious about following any recommendations to increase omega-6 PUFA intake. In fact most other studies that separated out the omega-3 and omega-6 fats found that without the omega-3 fats there was no benefit and that the omega-6 fats caused increased risk of heart attacks and death. Let's look at some of the other risks of the increase in omega-6 fats in our diet.

HOW EXCESS OMEGA-6 FATS AFFECT OUR HEALTH

Dr. Joseph Hibbeln from the National Institutes of Health has researched the impact of omega-6 oils on our health.[9] He explains that the overconsumption of omega-6 fats and the underconsumption of omega-3 fats have led to increases in the following:[10]

- Cardiovascular disease
- Type 2 diabetes[11]
- Obesity
- Metabolic syndrome (pre-diabetes)
- Irritable bowel syndrome and inflammatory bowel disease
- Macular degeneration (age-related blindness)
- Rheumatoid arthritis
- Asthma

- Cancer
- Psychiatric disorders
- Autoimmune diseases

Dr. Hibbeln found that the increase of linoleic acid, mostly from soybean oil, in the diet from 1960 to 1999 in five countries studied predicted a 100-fold increase in the risk of homicide deaths.[12] Not only do these vegetable oils result in more heart attacks, obesity, and cancer, but they may make people murderers! Considering omega-3 fats make up much of your brain tissue, this makes sense because high intake of omega-6 fats interferes with the benefits of omega-3 fats. Another study on ulcerative colitis showed a 250 percent increased risk of inflammatory bowel disease in the group that consumed the highest amount of linoleic acid.[13]

Dr. Hibbeln says in his review that the "increases in world LA (linoleic acid) consumption over the past century may be considered a very large uncontrolled experiment that may have contributed to increased societal burdens of aggression, depression, and cardiovascular mortality. It's quite likely that most of the diseases of modern civilization, major depression, heart disease, and obesity are linked to the radical and dramatic shift in the composition of the fats in the food supply."

He goes on to say that "increasing tissue concentrations of omega-3 fats on a population level may result in a substantial decrease in health care costs by reducing the illnesses that account for the largest burden of disease worldwide."

In Part III, you'll learn what I recommend when it comes to which fats to eat and which to stay away from. Here's a quick sneak peak:

- Cut out refined oils except extra virgin olive oil.
- Use extra virgin coconut oil and a little grass-fed butter or ghee.
- Stop fearing animal fat, but stick with grass-fed, pasture-raised, and organic.
- Get fats from whole foods like avocados, nuts, and seeds.

Are Genetically Modified Crops a Health Danger?

Most vegetable oils are made from genetically modified crops (genetically modified organisms, or GMOs).[14]

While GMOs are highly controversial and may not be all bad, there are some concerns in the science. The American Academy of Environmental Medicine (AAEM) reported that "several animal studies indicate serious health risks associated with GM food," including infertility, immune problems, accelerated aging, faulty insulin regulation, and changes in major organs and the gastrointestinal system. The AAEM asked physicians to advise patients to avoid GM foods.[15]

Soybean oil, our most abundantly consumed oil, is high in omega-6 fatty acids. Ninety-four percent of US soybean crops are genetically modified. A recent survey showed that most Americans use Wesson vegetable oil, which is now made from GMO soybeans.

Genetically engineered soybeans are called Roundup Ready soybeans because they are "ready" to not be harmed by the herbicide called *glyphosate* (Roundup) used to selectively kill the weeds. There are many adverse health effects, including increased infertility rates with each passing generation.[16] New research shows that the GMO Roundup Ready soybeans, made by Monsanto, produce formaldehyde (which is toxic) and deplete glutathione (a powerful natural antioxidant).[17] The genes in these soybeans that produce these effects can be transferred into the bacteria in your gut. This means that long after we stop eating genetically modified foods, we may still have their genetically modified proteins produced continuously inside us. Do you really want to experiment with your health and your children's health?

An Austrian government study published in November 2008 showed that the more genetically modified corn fed to mice, the fewer babies they had, and the smaller the babies were.[18] Researchers at Baylor College of Medicine accidentally discovered that rats raised on GMO corncob bedding "neither breed nor exhibit reproductive behavior."[19]

(Continued)

While the data is still coming in about the health effects of GMO foods, and there may be some benefits to these modified plants from an agricultural perspective (including a means to feed our ever-increasing human population), there are still some real concerns. At the very least, we need to be informed so we can make personal choices about what we eat and what we don't.

Research published in 2015 in *Lancet Oncology* and based on a review of the literature by seventeen independent experts from eleven countries found that Monsanto's herbicide Roundup has been linked to cancer.[20] The World Health Organization released a statement that glyphosate (Roundup) is a "probable carcinogen" in humans.[21]

We need labeling and transparency in the US — something that is required in sixty-four countries, including the European Union (where GMOs are banned), Japan, Australia, Brazil, Russia, and even China.[22] In Argentina, 30,000 doctors and health professionals represented by the Federation of Health Professionals of Argentina have called for an outright ban on glyphosate (Roundup) because "glyphosate not only causes cancer. It is also associated with increased spontaneous abortions, birth defects, skin diseases, and respiratory and neurological disease."[23]

Monsanto, the company that brought us some of the most of the most toxic products over the last fifty years, including Agent Orange, PCBs and dioxin, DDT, saccharin, and aspartame, came out swinging against the World Health Organization and demanded they retract their position statement that Monsanto's glyphosate "probably" causes cancer.[24] It's time to let Americans decide what they want to eat and provide clear labeling of GMO foods. The GMO soybeans are a problem for two reasons. They are the number one source of omega-6 oils in our diet and they contain harmful residues of glyphosate.

7

Meat — Doesn't It Cause Heart Disease and Type 2 Diabetes?

Fat is a controversial subject, but meat is an emotional one. It is hard to separate the scientific facts about the health effects of meat from the ethical concerns and environmental impact. What's the truth: Is meat good or bad? Will it cause heart disease, obesity, and cancer and lead to a shorter life, or is it the key to health and longevity? The Plains Indians lived on buffalo and had the highest number of centenarians per capita, while the Seventh-day Adventists are vegetarians and are among the longest-lived people on the planet. What gives? Meat or veggies? Maybe we're asking the wrong question.

The answer seems to be that it is not the meat or veggies, but the sugar and refined carbs that are part of the typical meat eater's diet and our highly processed inflammatory diet that we should be concerned with.

There are so many questions about meat. Some are concerned about the saturated fat and cholesterol in meat, others about its potential to cause inflammation. Yet others worry about a possible link to changes in gut bacteria that produce a compound linked to heart disease called TMAO. Some stay away because of carcinogens such as polycyclic aromatic hydrocarbons or heterocyclic amines, formed when you grill or cook meat at high temperatures, or advanced glycation end products, which are formed when proteins and sugars combine in cooking to form that crispy outside. It's enough to make you swear off steak forever.

The topic of meat is complex for sure (and could take up a whole book). I will put on hold for a moment the very real ethical considerations that motivate some to become vegans, and the serious environmental impact of factory farming of animals. We will get to these issues shortly. First, I want to tackle the question of animal protein in general — and red meat in particular — as it relates to health.

THE PROBLEM WITH RESEARCH ON MEAT

Even after reviewing most of the research on meat and health, it's going to be hard to give a definitive answer on whether meat is good or bad. Why? Simply because, as we've discussed, good research on diet is very hard to do. And no one has done any really good studies on meat. The right type of studies (direct experiments comparing different diets, where all food is provided and all variables controlled, not association studies) would cost billions of dollars, take decades, and be almost impossible to conduct. We have to make do with the limited data we have — associations, not causes.

Let's look at the seemingly impressive National Institutes of Health–AARP Diet and Health Study of more than 500,000 men and women from fifty to seventy-one years old followed for 10 years. Researchers assessed their diet through a food frequency questionnaire. Do you really remember what you ate over the last year? How about even last week? That's the first problem with the study. Food recall is not the best way to assess intake (though it is pretty much all researchers have to work with, which is why they use it).

Then there is the problem of the population they were studying. They didn't study the Plains Indians living on buffalo, berries, roots, and nuts. They studied an average American population that ate a highly processed, high-sugar diet with very little fruits and vegetables, a population that smoked too much and exercised too little and drank too much alcohol. Those who ate less meat were healthier, yes — but why? It may be because of something called the *healthy user effect.*[1] That's when people who want to be healthy avoid the things that our culture says will make them sick (meat, processed food, sugar, smoking, etc.) and do the things that make them healthier (exercise, eat more fruits and veggies, sleep, etc.). It's their overall lifestyle that makes them healthier, which makes it hard to attribute their good health specifically to less meat.

Take the case of hormone replacement therapy for women. The women who cared about their health went to the doctor more often, ate better, exercised more, and didn't smoke. They were the healthy users of the hormone replacement. When their doctor told them to take hormones to prevent heart disease, they took the hormones. They wanted to do everything they could to get and stay healthy. This was why population studies showed a connection between hormones and health — it was the healthy user effect at work.

Then along came the Women's Health Initiative, which found, in fact, that the women who took the hormones had more heart attacks, strokes, and cancer. Overnight we did a scientific about-face. Experiments that prove cause and effect trump studies that find only associations (which could be explained by other factors). Studies that can't prove cause and effect are plagued by what are called "confounders," variables that confound or confuse the question.

The National Institutes of Health–AARP Diet and Health Study did find a correlation of meat, heart disease, cancer, and death. But they also found that the meat eaters, on the whole, were a very unhealthy bunch. These people smoked more, weighed more, consumed on average 800 more calories a day, exercised less, ate more sugar, drank more alcohol, ate fewer fruits and vegetables (and thus less fiber), and took fewer vitamin supplements. Are you really surprised they had higher rates of heart disease, cancer, and death? Sadly the only headline the media grabs is "Meat Kills."

The question is not, Do people who eat industrially produced meat, lots of refined sugar and carbs, and very little fruits or veggies, and who smoke, are overweight, don't exercise, drink too much alcohol, and don't take vitamins have more heart disease? The real question is whether grass-fed meat eaters who eat lots of healthy food, don't smoke, exercise, and take vitamins have more heart disease.

Thankfully, some researchers have asked this question. Scientists studied 11,000 omnivores (57 percent) and vegetarians (43 percent) who were health conscious; in other words, meat eaters and vegetarians who shopped at health food stores.[2] This is a more conclusive study because other than their meat intake, the two groups were similar in their overall lifestyle and health habits. The researchers found that the overall rates of death were cut in half for both health-conscious meat eaters and vegetarians when compared to the average person eating a Western processed-food diet. No benefit was found for vegetarians or harm for meat eaters in terms of risk of heart disease, cancer, or death. Most studies on meat eaters vs. vegetarians do not compare "healthy" meat eaters who eat only grass-fed meat without hormones, antibiotics, or pesticides; who eat no processed food; who enjoy lots of fruits, veggies, nuts, and seeds; who eat a diet that is very low in sugar and refined carbs and high in fiber; and who exercise, don't smoke, and take vitamin supplements to vegetarians who shared the same health habits (with the exception of eating meat). As was found in the study just cited, I suspect there would be very few differences between these groups.

In most studies, the meat consumed is industrially raised from confined animal feeding operations. Industrial grain-fed meat is full of hormones, antibiotics, and pesticides and has more inflammatory omega-6 fats (from corn feed) and fewer anti-inflammatory omega-3 fats than grass-fed meat. So it's very hard to get an accurate reading on meat's effects on the body.

There is stronger data on processed meats such as bacon, hot dogs, bologna, and luncheon meats, showing them to be harmful. The EPIC study of nearly 500,000 people found no association between unprocessed fresh meat and heart disease or cancer, but it did show a link between processed meat and cancer and heart disease.[3]

As I said, I could fill an entire book with the subject of meat. But for now, let's just zero in on the most common—and toughest—questions people have about meat.

DO SATURATED FAT AND CHOLESTEROL IN MEAT CAUSE HEART DISEASE?

We have covered the debate about saturated fat and cholesterol already. The bottom line is that everyone, including the American Heart

Association and our government's Dietary Guidelines Committee, have debunked any connection between dietary cholesterol and heart disease. Saturated fat is still under debate. Part of the confusion is that elevated saturated fat levels in our blood do in fact cause heart disease. But—and pay close attention, because here's the key point—the types of saturated fats in the blood that cause heart disease, stearic and palmitic, *don't come from eating meat*. They are produced in your liver when you eat sugar and carbs. I know I'm probably beginning to sound like a broken record, but for the vast majority of questions out there about whether fat is harmful, the "uh-oh" needle repeatedly points instead to sugar and carbs.

There is no consistent evidence that saturated fat in our diet from meat raises our blood cholesterol.[4] In fact, there is plenty of evidence that eating meat actually improves our cholesterol profile when consumed in the absence of sugar and refined carbs. How? By raising the good cholesterol and boosting protective, or large, LDL particles.

In randomized controlled studies on what some call the Paleolithic diet—a diet more like that of our caveman ancestors, of good-quality fresh meat, eggs, lots of fruits and vegetables, nuts and seeds, but no grains, dairy, beans, or processed food—heart disease and diabetes risk factors and blood tests got better, not worse.[5]

In one amazing experiment, a researcher sent ten Australian aborigines with obesity, diabetes, high blood pressure, and high blood sugar back into the bush to hunt kangaroo and alligator and gather roots, nuts, and berries. In seven weeks, all their numbers normalized, enabling them to come off their medications, and they lost significant amounts of weight.[6]

In study after study,[7] feeding obese, diabetic, or heart disease patients a diet higher in fat and high-quality animal protein resulted in better outcomes for everything, including weight, body fat, waist circumference, muscle mass, metabolism, blood pressure, triglycerides, HDL, and LDL. People on diets such as these found them much more satisfying and were less hungry than when on high-carb, low-fat, low-meat diets, even when the number of calories was exactly the same.[8] These effects are profound.

DOES RED MEAT CAUSE HEART ATTACKS BY PROMOTING BAD GUT BACTERIA?

In science we often try to pick apart one thing and blame it for the problem. However, in medicine and health there are many variables that may explain the observations we make.

In a recent elegant study published in the journal *Nature Medicine*,[9] researchers from the Cleveland Clinic linked red meat to a chemical called TMAO (trimethylamine N-oxide), which has been associated with heart disease. These researchers wondered whether it was something in meat besides saturated fat and cholesterol that seemed to link it to heart disease. They measured levels of TMAO in meat eaters and vegans, and it was higher in meat eaters. They fed meat eaters a steak and found that their TMAO levels went up. The researchers then managed to convince an individual vegan to eat a steak and found the TMAO did *not* go up. Then they gave the meat eaters antibiotics and found their TMAO levels did not go up after eating meat.

To follow this up, they gave a group of long-term vegans and vegetarians carnitine (a compound derived from dietary amino acids in protein that is important in fat and energy metabolism) and found that this group "had markedly reduced capacity to synthesize TMAO from oral carnitine." Vegans seem to have healthy gut bacteria, and meat eaters do not. And the antibiotics can kill the bad bugs that make the TMAO in meat eaters. So is the solution to cut out meat or live on antibiotics? Probably neither.

Interestingly, in a subsequent study with mice, some of the same researchers found that mice with gut bacteria that protected against atherosclerosis (the plaques that cause heart disease) didn't show any plaque in the arteries on the high-choline diet even though the choline caused super elevated levels of TMAO.[10] Together these findings indicate that we should be cautious about jumping to conclusions about TMAO. We have already learned this lesson from our belief that saturated fat causes heart disease. In fact, since we have replaced saturated fat in our diets with refined carbohydrates, the rates of heart disease have gone up.[11] What these studies do seem to provide strong evidence for is the importance of gut bacteria in heart health.

Let's look at how this theory about meat and gut bacteria and TMAO holds up and what we should do about the findings: First, if red meat increased the risk of heart disease, then we should have better epidemiological evidence—but we don't, as we have just reviewed. Yes, if you are a smoking, drinking, non-exercising, potato-eating, soda-consuming meat eater, the evidence is there, but otherwise not so much. If red meat were really the problem, we should have seen it in the research. Yet in a study of over 1.2 million people, no link was found between red meat and heart disease, stroke, or diabetes.[12] Some studies show a link,[13] but as we learned earlier, there are a lot of confounders. Also, if eating meat caused more heart disease, we should see lower risks in vegetarians and vegans. We do see this a little, but it is likely because they are more health conscious in general. Remember the healthy user effect. In meat eaters who shop at health food stores, there is no difference in heart disease or death rates between them and vegans and vegetarians. Eating meat in the context of an overall healthy diet does not increase the risk of heart attacks or death as shown in a study of more than 65,000 health-conscious meat eaters and vegetarians.[14]

When the effects of increasing meat intake was studied in Asian countries—using a sample of almost 300,000 people who generally have healthier diets heavy in fish and vegetables and light in processed sugary foods—they found red meat was actually associated with a lower risk of heart disease in men and cancer in women.[15]

A key insight from this study is that your gut bacteria matter and can produce compounds that cause heart disease and, more importantly, that what you eat influences your gut bacteria. If a vegan who eats a steak is safe, then how do we all get this protective gut bacteria? The answer is simple: Eat mostly plant foods, then the meat won't be a problem. Don't be a meat eater who drinks too much alcohol, smokes, doesn't eat veggies, and has very little fiber and more refined oils, sugar, and refined carbs. Those behaviors are a perfect prescription for growing a very toxic inner garden.[16] The problem isn't the red meat. It *is* the

ia. Eating the right fibers (like resistant starch), taking probi-
avoiding antibiotics are part of a good plan to cultivate your
inner garden.

And there's another sticky issue. The level of TMAO in meat is far
less than that in fish.[17] So we should see big increases in heart disease in
fish eaters. In fact it is just the opposite. Fish eaters have the lowest risk
of heart disease.[18] The data around TMAO is interesting yes, but doesn't
prove that meat causes heart attacks, only that the average American
meat eater has a crappy diet and lifestyle that leads to a very bad gut
environment. And we know that a bad gut is connected to bad health.

The right way to design a research study would be to test two
groups, the first being health-conscious meat eaters who have an overall
healthy diet and lifestyle and perhaps even take probiotics, the second
being healthy whole food vegans. My guess is there wouldn't be much
difference in each group's risk of heart disease.

To learn more about how gut flora is connected to your weight and
the risk of heart disease, diabetes, and cancer (and how to get good bacteria and cultivate a healthy inner garden), see my free e-book *Beyond
Food: Other Causes of Obesity and Damaged Metabolism* and follow the
section on "How to Tend Your Inner Garden." You can download it at
www.eatfatgetthin.com.

DOES RED MEAT CAUSE TYPE 2 DIABETES AND WEIGHT GAIN?

There have been some studies linking meat intake to type 2 diabetes.[19]
The Health Professionals' and Nurses' Health Study of more than
400,000 people followed for decades was based on food questionnaires.
Researchers found that a 50-gram serving of processed red meat, like
hot dogs and deli meats, increased the risk of type 2 diabetes by 51 percent, and the same serving of fresh red meat increased the risk by about
20 percent. But these numbers show relative risk, not absolute risk. In
other words, if you reduce the risk from 3 percent to 2 percent, that's a
30 percent "relative" risk reduction, but it is only a 1 percent reduction

in actual risk. So in the Nurses' Health Study the actual risk (or absolute risk) increase for fresh red meat was from 7 percent to 8.4 percent. But again, the meat eaters in the study were also not so healthy overall. They exercised less than the non–meat eaters; smoked more; drank soda, sugar-sweetened beverages, and more alcohol; ate more sugar, processed food, fried foods, and trans fats; and ate fewer vegetables but more potatoes. So was it the meat or the soda? I vote for the soda!

The researchers were very clear to warn readers that this study could not prove cause and effect, yet they went on to say, paradoxically, that we should reduce red meat and processed meat to reduce type 2 diabetes. What they really should have been saying is that if you eat red meat and have an otherwise crappy diet, don't exercise, smoke and drink too much, and eat lots of sugar, your risk of diabetes goes up 1.4 percent. Not too convincing, in my opinion.

Other studies using a higher intake of meat without the accompanying sugar or starch, like grains or beans (a caveman-like diet), found that blood sugar was even better controlled than in the Mediterranean diet, which is well known to help improve blood sugar levels.[20] Another study found that the Paleolithic diet far outperformed a traditional diabetes diet in controlling blood sugar and cardiovascular risk factors.[21] And in a two-year study on obese postmenopausal women, the women following the Paleolithic diet lost twice as much weight after two years and reduced their belly fat by twice as much as the women following recommendations for weight loss according to the Nordic Nutrition Recommendations.[22] These recommendations are what the Nordic scientists and countries deem a healthy dietary pattern and include plenty of vegetables, fruits and berries, beans, regular intake of fish, vegetable oils, whole grains, low-fat versions of dairy and meat, and limited intake of red and processed meat, sugar, salt, and alcohol.

DOES RED MEAT CAUSE CANCER?

This is a big, scary question, I know ... so let's tackle it.

Most of the data we have is about colon cancer. In a review of more than thirty-five prospective studies on colon cancer and meat consumption, there was little risk found.[23] In fact, in some studies, those with the highest meat intake had lower risk than those with the lowest intake. What they did find, of course, was that meat eating was also associated with other dietary and lifestyle habits that promote cancer, including high intake of refined sugar and alcohol and low intake of fruits, vegetables, and fiber. The meat eaters also generally didn't exercise, smoked more than non–meat eaters, and were more overweight, all of which are associated with an increased risk of cancer.

As I've mentioned, some studies do link processed red meat, such as hot dogs, bacon, and luncheon meats, to cancer.[24] A 2015 World Health Organization (WHO) report on meat and cancer found that processed meats did increase cancer risk. The effects of red meat were not conclusive. Let me translate what that increased risk actually means. The WHO found that processed meat increased cancer risk by about 20 percent; that is what we call *relative risk*. It is quite different than the *absolute risk,* or the true change in risk. If your absolute risk goes from 1 to 2 percent, the relative risk increase is 100 percent. Sounds impressive. But the absolute risk increase was only 1 percent. Not too impressive. So in the WHO study, the absolute risk of getting cancer would be an increase from a 2.6 percent to a 3.2 percent chance of getting cancer—or about a 0.6 absolute increase in risk. In other words, about three extra appearances of colon cancer in every 100,000 people, for the bacon eaters. This is not too impressive. Cancer is also linked to compounds that form when you cook meat;[25] we've all heard the dire warnings about charred meat being carcinogenic. What's the real story?

Indeed, some things happen when you cook meat that may be harmful. High-temperature cooking, grilling, frying, smoking, or charring meat, including fish and chicken, all lead to the production of compounds call polycyclic aromatic hydrocarbons (PAH) and heterocyclic amines (HCA).[26] HCAs and PAHs have been shown to cause cancer in animal models, and it is a good idea to reduce your exposure to these toxic compounds.[27] But meat is not the only source of PAHs. Surprisingly, other than meat charred over an open flame, the most common source is vegetables and grains.[28] So much for grilled vegetables!

The take-home message is to focus on low-temperature cooking of meat (and veggies), including baking, roasting, poaching, and stewing. Think crockpots and a method of low-temperature poaching that is gaining popularity called sous vide, where food is cooked in water in airtight plastic bags. I don't like to cook in plastic, but some may choose to do this. Just be sure to get BPA-free and heat-stable plastic so toxins don't leach into the food.

Cooking meat can also produce compounds called AGEs, which result from protein interacting with sugars in food. These are what make things crispy—the crust that forms on a loaf of bread, crispy chicken skin, or the crunchy sugar top on crème brûlée. AGEs damage arteries and the brain, and they can cause cancer. Your best bet is to reduce high-heat cooking and grilling. Another tip to reduce AGEs, HCAs, and PAHs is to soak your meat in an acidic marinade with lemon juice or vinegar; this makes it taste better and cuts AGEs in half and HCAs by 90 percent.[29]

Most important to say here is that red meat contains compounds that *prevent* cancer, including omega-3 fats, CLA (conjugated linoleic acid), and nutrients such as selenium, vitamins B_6 and B_{12}, and vitamin D. Eating a healthy diet full of cancer-fighting plant foods, rich in phytochemicals and spices, and including lots of fiber to feed good gut bacteria can help you ward off cancer.

DOES MEAT CAUSE INFLAMMATION?

By now, you can probably answer this yourself! If you eat meat in the context of the average Western diet full of sugar and processed food and low in fruits and vegetables, nuts, and seeds, then yes. But if you eat a whole-foods, high-quality, grass-fed, organic, low-glycemic, high-fiber diet like the one laid out in Part III of *Eat Fat, Get Thin*, then the answer is no. In fact, in studies that replaced meat with carbohydrates, levels of inflammation went up.[30]

The omega-6 fat arachidonic acid is found in meat. It is in every one of your cell membranes and helps your body control inflammation, grow, and repair. Grass-fed meat actually increases levels of both omega-3s and the right omega-6s—it helps keep the fats in balance. In large population studies, those with the highest levels of both omega-3s and arachidonic acid had the lowest levels of inflammation[31] and heart disease. Population studies, as I have said, are imperfect, but they are often the best we have.

IS EATING MEAT IMMORAL OR UNETHICAL?

The ethical concerns about eating meat inspire many vegetarians, including millions of Buddhists around the world. I spent two weeks in a Tibetan monastery with a Bon abbot. (Bon is the pre-Buddhist indigenous religion of Tibet.) His beliefs dictated that he not harm any living creature, because you never know which being (human, animal, or insect) was your mother in your last life, or who will be your mother in your next life. That surely engenders loving kindness to all beings. There was only one problem: Because he followed his traditional diet, the abbot was overweight and a poorly controlled diabetic.

One morning in his private quarters, he and I shared a breakfast of tsampa, a traditional Tibetan roasted barley flour, *dri* cheese (from a female yak), and hot salted tea. I suggested that he might not want to eat flour for breakfast since he had type 2 diabetes. He protested, saying that was his traditional breakfast. I said yes, that may be so, but that diet would make sense only if he were herding yaks all day at an elevation of 17,000 feet, not sitting on a meditation cushion all day. We checked his blood sugar after eating it. It was over 300 mg/dl (normal is less than 90 mg/dl).

While I didn't convince him to start eating meat, I did get him on a high-protein, high-fat, lower-sugar, and lower-carb diet of nuts, seeds, beans, and vegetables and had him walk around the monastery every day for an hour. He lost thirty-five pounds and reversed his diabetes. Now I have 1.5 million Bon people praying for me!

I honor those who want to be vegetarians for moral or religious reasons, and I do believe you can construct a healthy vegan or vegetarian diet if it follows the basic principles of good-quality fats and low-sugar, high-fiber, and unprocessed foods. It may be harder to eat that way, but with a good plan and discipline, it can work for many people. In full disclosure, I was a vegetarian for nine years and did pretty well, although my health is much better now, with less inflammation, baggy eyes, and allergies, fewer rashes and digestive problems, and more muscle mass, even though I am 25 years older.

Vegans quote studies of large populations who are vegetarian that show they live longer and are healthier. This is true, but the question is, Why? Is it the absence of meat, or is it their other lifestyle habits? Vegetarians on the whole are more health conscious and more likely to exercise and to avoid junk, sugar, processed foods, and smoking; they even floss their teeth more.[32] Remember, this is called the healthy user effect. On the other hand, as we've discussed, meat eaters tend to have worse habits. So is it the meat or is it the bad habits that cause more deaths? Studies that compare health-conscious meat eaters with vegetarians show no difference in health outcomes.

One of the most eye-opening discussions of the ethical issues surrounding vegetarianism is *The Vegetarian Myth* by Lierre Keith. While you may not agree with all of her arguments, she points out that in the plowing of fields, clearing of forests, and growing of plants, there is wholesale destruction of natural ecosystems, including the death of birds, rodents, bugs, worms, and trillions of microbes in the soil. She says, "The truth is that agriculture is the most destructive thing humans have done to the planet, and more of the same won't save us. The truth is that agriculture requires the wholesale destruction of entire ecosystems. The truth is also that life isn't possible without death, that no matter what you eat, someone has to die to feed you."

What most vegetarians don't realize is that many organic agriculture practices require animal products to build up the soil. I recently visited the largest rooftop organic farm in America, the Brooklyn Grange, on top of an old navy shipyard. It was a marvel to behold, and as we toured the farm, I asked about the soil, and how they cared for it. It turns out it is fortified with bone meal and oyster shells. Who knew that your vegetables were carnivores!

It is well known that vegans are more likely to have nutritional deficiencies of B_{12}, omega-3 fats, fat-soluble vitamins like A and D, iron, calcium, vitamin K_2, and zinc.[33] I have treated tens of thousands of patients and have seen serious nutritional deficiencies and health problems in vegans and vegetarians. It can be a healthful choice, but you need to make sure you are getting the right nutrients: focus on eating seaweed and DHA supplements from algae, and high-fat plant foods such as nuts and seeds, avocados, and coconut oil; and minimize starchy foods, sticking instead with high-fiber, low-glycemic grains like black rice and quinoa. Eat non-GMO soy foods such as tempeh or tofu, which have been consumed safely for thousands of years in Asian countries. Eat more mushrooms, which contain minerals and vitamin D. Avoid sugar and refined vegetable oils, except extra virgin olive oil.

I support my friends who choose to be vegetarian or vegan for moral, health, or environmental reasons. The key is making it a high-fat vegan diet. But as I've said, each of us is genetically and biochemically different and may do better on different diets. Find out what is best for *you* by monitoring yourself. How do you feel? What does the scale say? What are your numbers: your blood pressure, waist size, blood sugar, levels of inflammation, HDL, and triglycerides, and the size of your LDL particles? Monitor your levels of nutrients such as vitamin D, zinc, B_{12}, and iron. Find out what's optimal for *you*.

IS GRASS-FED MEAT BETTER?

From an environmental perspective, factory farming puts more pressure on the environment through degradation of the topsoil, depletion of our aquifers and global freshwater supplies (because 70 percent of the world's freshwater is used to grow animals for human consumption), negative effects on climate change, use of fossil fuels for fertilizers and agricultural chemicals, overuse of antibiotics in animal feed, and the need for extensive food transportation because of centralized food production. Those considerations alone should move us all toward more sustainably raised, local animal products (and vegetables). From a moral perspective, the intensive, crowded, and harsh conditions for animals on factory farms should also inspire us to boycott those foods. If you haven't seen the movie *Food, Inc.* yet, it might convince you.

Grass-fed meat is better not just for the planet, but for our bodies as well. It would be hard for anyone to argue that the higher amounts of antibiotics, hormones, and pesticides in factory-farmed meat are good for you, and there is much evidence to show they are harmful. The main reason that grass-fed meat is better for you is that you are not what you eat—you are what your food eats! The difference in diets of grass-fed vs. grain-fed cows has a big impact on the health effects of the meat. Let me break this down.

Cows are ruminants that have special stomachs designed to eat grass. When they are fed grains, the levels of the inflammatory omega-6 fats in their bodies—and thus in the meat we eat—increase. Cows also have to be given antibiotics to prevent their stomachs from exploding from the bloat caused by their gut bacteria fermenting the corn feed (isn't that a lovely image?). Grass-fed cows, on the other hand, don't need antibiotics. We use about 24 million pounds of antibiotics per year in America; about 19 million of those are used in animal feed. This causes serious antibiotic resistance in animals and humans and has led to the growth of superbugs that don't respond to antibiotics.

Grass-fed meat has a healthier fat profile than conventionally raised meat, with two to five times more omega-3 fats.[34] It also has lower levels of omega-6 fats. The ratio of omega-6 to omega-3 fats in grass-fed beef is about 1.5 to 1. In grain-fed beef it is about 7.5 to 1. Grass-fed beef has more stearic acid, the saturated fat that has no impact on cholesterol. It also has two to three times as much conjugated linoleic acid (CLA) as grain-fed beef, a potent antioxidant that is protective against heart disease,[35] diabetes,[36] and cancer and even helps with weight loss and metabolism.[37]

In addition to having a better fat profile, grass-fed meat has more vitamin E, beta-carotene, vitamin A, zinc, iron, phosphorous, sodium, and potassium.[38] It also has higher levels of antioxidants, including glutathione, catalase, and superoxide dismutase.[39]

Yes, it is more expensive to eat grass-fed meat. But I believe it is worth the price, given its health and environmental benefits. You can find cheaper sources online. You can even buy a cow or a lamb with friends and share it. Some call it "cowpooling." Check out the website Mark's Daily Apple (www.marksdailyapple.com) for sources of grass-fed meat and cowpooling, or the website US Wellness Meats (www .grasslandbeef.com) for more grass-fed beef options. Eating smaller amounts of good-quality animal products is better for you, your wallet, and the planet. Save on quantity, splurge on quality!

8

Controversial Foods — What's Good, What's Bad?

I know you're reading this book because you want to know the truth about what's good for you and what isn't, so let's clear up any confusion you might have about the fat in some of your favorite foods.

EGGS: FRIEND OR FOE?

How many of us have begrudgingly eaten dry, tasteless egg-white omelets because we thought we were "supposed to"? Well, no more!

In a large analysis of sixteen major studies, each of which had anywhere from 1,600 to more than 90,000 participants, eggs were found *not* to be linked to heart disease.[1] In one detailed case report in the *New England Journal of Medicine,* one man had been eating twenty-five eggs every day for more than 15 years, and it had no impact at all on his cholesterol or his heart.[2] He might have been crazy, but he had no heart disease!

In the Physicians' Health Study, no link could be found between eggs and heart disease.[3] Other experimental studies have found protein- and fat-rich eggs aid weight loss by suppressing your appetite, speeding up your metabolism, and reducing your overall food intake during the day.[4]

Eggs have been *eggs*onerated!

In fact, eggs might be the cheapest and best new health food. But stick to pasture-raised or omega-3 eggs, which are much higher in nutrients and antioxidants. Avoid eggs with pale yellow yolks (the ones from commercial, industrial operations) and go for the ones with dark, deeply colored orange-yellow yolks. It turns out that the yolks are a treasure trove of nutrients (after all, they must supply the ingredients for creating new life). While the whites have vitamins B_2 (riboflavin) and B_3 (niacin), the yolks contain B_6 and B_{12}, folic acid (B_9), pantothenic acid (B_5), and thiamin (B_1). The yolks are also rich sources of vitamins A, E, K, and D. In fact, egg yolks are one of the few foods that naturally contain vitamin D.

Eggs are one of the best sources of choline (needed for brain health, cell membrane formation, and detoxification; it also protects against Alzheimer's disease). Egg yolks contain lutein and zeaxanthin (which gives them their yellow color), antioxidants that help prevent macular degeneration or premature blindness. The yolk contains more calcium, copper, iron, manganese, phosphorus, potassium, selenium, and zinc than the white. Eggs also prevent LDL oxidation and increase LDL and HDL particle size, so they protect against heart disease.[5] Not bad for a food that has been on the "do not eat" list for decades. It just might be nature's most perfect and complete food. After all, it contains all the nutrients needed to create a new life!

One important tip about eggs: Don't heat them in hot oil. The fats can oxidize and become harmful. Poach or soft-boil your eggs or cook them at low temperature.

BETTER OFF WITH (OR WITHOUT) BUTTER?

Butter has been indicted but not convicted in the court of science. The truth is there is no good evidence proving its link to heart disease.[6] In fact, the opposite may be true; butter may be good for heart disease prevention.[7] There may be reasons to avoid dairy, but the saturated fat content is not one of them. In fact, some studies measuring blood levels of the saturated fats that are in dairy have found them to be associated with a lower risk of heart attacks.[8]

We have seen a reduction in butter consumption from about eighteen pounds per person per year in 1900 to about four pounds in 2009.

All the while, obesity, heart disease, diabetes, and cancer are on the rise. This is only a correlation and doesn't prove cause and effect. But there is more to the story.

If I had to choose between butter and a bagel, I would choose the butter. Its potential for harm has been exaggerated, and there may be many benefits. Would I eat sticks of butter every day? Probably not. But in the context of a diet low in refined carbs and sugars and high in fiber, I don't worry about butter.

The problem with butter has been thought to be its high content of saturated fats (60 percent of the fat is saturated fat). But look at breast milk—50 percent of its fat is saturated fat,[9] and it has been linked to reduced diseases of all sorts in kids who breastfed.[10] In fact breastfed kids seem to have a lower risk later in life of obesity, type 2 diabetes, and heart disease, despite having higher cholesterol levels.[11]

Butter is essentially pure animal fat with only minor traces of dairy proteins and sugars remaining. The nutritional content of the animal's flesh depends on the content of its diet. This applies especially to butter. Whether it's grass-fed or grain-fed, butter is rich in saturated fat (about 60 percent) and monounsaturated fat (about 20 percent). The rest is polyunsaturated, but this is where grass-fed and grain-fed really differ. Cows raised on pasture produce milk fat with an omega-6 to omega-3 ratio of 1:1, which is ideal.[12] Grain-fed cows, on the other hand, produce a ratio tilted heavily toward omega-6. In grass-fed beef the ratio of omega-6 to omega-3 is 1.5:1, and in grain-fed beef it jumps way up to 7.6:1.

Personally I would never eat conventionally raised butter because, apart from the excess omega-6s, it stores pesticides and environmental toxins. But there are other reasons. An equivalent serving of grass-fed butter has the same nutrition facts as conventional butter, but it is three to five times higher in CLA (conjugated linoleic acid).[13] Grass-fed butter is deep yellow because it has more carotene and vitamin A.[14]

Cow stomach fermentation turns vitamin K_1 (found in leafy greens, like kale, chard, spinach, and, yes, grass) into K_2, which then shows up in the dairy fat.[15] K_2 is important for bone and heart health, among many other things. Grass-fed butter also contains a fatty acid called that promotes intestinal health and fights inflammation ....but the body, especially in the cardiovascular system.[16]

It's best to purchase organic butter from grass-fed cows. Kerrygold, an Irish dairy whose cows are all pasture raised, can be found fairly easily in local grocery and health food stores and even Costco. Anchor and Organic Valley are also good brands of grass-fed butter.

And then there is ghee, a form of Indian butter that is processed by melting and allowing it to simmer on low until most of the water evaporates off, leaving the fat and the milk solids. Ghee is used in Indian, Middle Eastern, and western Asian cooking in place of butter and is preferred for its higher smoking point. Butter smokes between 325°F and 375°F (163°C and 191°C) and ghee smokes at 400°F to 500°F (204°C to 260°C). Since it is best to cook below the smoking point for any oil, ghee can be used with high-heat cooking, searing, and even frying. (The smoking point is the temperature when the oil starts to smoke in the pan. It's different for different oils.) All of the same nutrients found in grass-fed butter are found in grass-fed ghee. It is high in vitamins D and A, omega-3 fats, CLA, and butyrate.

Clarified butter has had the water and milk solids removed, so it can be used by those allergic to dairy. You can purchase ghee or clarified butter from several excellent sources online. You can also make ghee from grass-fed butter by heating it, which separates out the fat from the milk solids, and then straining out the milk solids with cheesecloth.

COCONUT OIL: HEALTHY OR HARMFUL?

Coconut oil and coconut butter seem to be the latest fad, but what's the real story behind these creamy, yummy delights? They are mostly saturated fat and have been maligned along with butter. But again, being indicted is not the same as being convicted. Far from it!

Countries such as those in the South Pacific with the highest intake of coconut oil eat up to 40 percent of their calories from saturated fat (the coconut oil is almost 90 percent saturated fat, while butter is only 60 percent saturated fat). Yet surprisingly they have some of the lowest rates of heart disease in the world.[17] In fact, there is a surprising amount of research[18] showing that even though coconut oil has the highest amount of saturated fat found in any food, and it increases total cholesterol (actually it increases HDL, or good cholesterol, the most, so even though the total cholesterol goes up, the ratio is better), it is not correlated with increased risk of heart attack or stroke. Studies of Pacific Islanders[19] who ate up to 63 percent of their calories from coconut fat found them to be lean and free of heart disease or stroke.[20] Their total cholesterol was higher, but so was their good cholesterol, or HDL. Other studies have found that lipid profiles improve on high-fat diets containing coconut oil—good cholesterol is higher and triglycerides and the number of the small LDL cholesterol particles are lower.[21] Coconut fat is also associated with lower insulin levels.[22]

Just to clarify: There is coconut oil and there is coconut butter. Coconut butter is made from whole coconut flesh, with all its delicious fat and solids. It is essentially pureed or pulverized coconut meat and has a thick, creamy, smooth texture. It is about 60 percent oil. The fiber content of coconut butter differentiates it from coconut oil: One tablespoon of coconut butter has 3 grams of fiber.

Coconut oil is extracted from the dried flesh of the coconut. Coconut oil is made up of 86 percent saturated fat, 6 percent monounsaturated fat, and 1.4 percent polyunsaturated fat. About half of the saturated fat in coconut oil is a rare, special type of saturated fat called lauric acid. It is known as a medium-chain triglyceride or MCT (and there are other MCTs in coconut oil as well). In the body, lauric acid converts to monolaurin, one of the compounds found in breast milk that boost a baby's immune system (as do antibodies and colostrum). It is like superfuel for your cells, your metabolism, your bones, and your brain. It is now being studied for its antifungal, antiviral, and antibacterial health-protecting properties. It also can boost sports performance. Not bad for a fat that has been shunned for years.

Medium-Chain Triglycerides (MCT): The Superfat

The saturated fat in coconut oil is a very rare, very beneficial type called medium-chain triglycerides (MCT). These saturated fats actually reduce the ratio of total cholesterol to HDL (a good thing) and promote weight loss, and can even heal fatty liver caused by obesity. MCTs are a unique form of saturated fat that have been shown to possess antioxidant and antimicrobial properties, which help support the immune system. In the body, MCTs convert easily into energy; therefore, very little MCT oil is stored as fat, because it is used for energy. This is how MCTs help you burn fat and lose weight.

In a study published in the journal *Obesity Research* in 2003, scientists at McGill University carried out a randomized controlled trial to compare the effects of medium-chain triglycerides and long-chain triglycerides on body fat, energy expenditure, appetite, and other aspects of weight loss in overweight men.[23] They recruited twenty-four overweight men and put them on different diets for twenty-eight days. They switched the diets after a period of time so they could analyze the differences in the same people—this is called a crossover design. One group ate a diet rich in medium-chain triglycerides, like coconut oil. The other group ate a diet rich in long-chain triglycerides, like olive oil. Then the participants switched diets midway through the study. When the study was over, the researchers found that men on the MCT diet lost more body fat (especially belly fat). The MCT oil boosted energy expenditure and fat oxidation, or burning—in other words, their metabolism was faster. They were also less hungry than those who ate the olive oil diet.

Another small study carried out at the University of Rochester Medical Center and published in the *American Journal of Clinical Nutrition* looked at what happened when a group of men consumed meals with either MCTs or LCTs.[24] The test meals contained either 45 grams of MCT or 45 grams of LCT in the form of corn oil, and the scientists measured the subjects' metabolic rates both before the meals and up to six hours after. They measured oxygen consumption (which is an indirect measurement of metabolism—the more oxygen you can burn per minute, the more calories you can burn and the faster your metabolism) and found that oxygen consumption after the meal rich in MCTs increased by 12 percent—about triple the increase seen after the LCT meal. They also found that blood levels of triglycerides soared by 68 percent after the LCT meal with corn oil, but there was no increase in triglycerides after the MCT meal. The authors state, "This study also raises the possibility that replacing LCT with MCT over long periods of time could produce weight loss in the absence of reduced energy intake." Eat more, weigh less. Sounds good to me!

Lots of other studies support the benefits of MCT oils. MCT oils are good for many reasons. They get absorbed directly from the gut to the liver and burned quickly, while omega-6 fats from seed, bean, or grain oils — like corn, soy, sunflower, and canola — are transported into the lymphatic system, not the blood, which allows them to be taken up in your fat tissues. That is why MCT oils boost your metabolism and help you burn more calories, reduce fat storage, and cut your appetite. They are like superfuel for your cells. Studies show they cause you to burn about 460 extra calories a day for men and about 190 extra calories for women (sorry, ladies). They also affect your hormones differently than other fats do, helping you feel full.

In another study, consumption of MCTs reduced body fat and triglycerides more than omega-6 vegetable oils. After eight weeks, the experiment showed that the group having the MCT had greater reductions in their weight, body fat percentage, and levels of subcutaneous fat and a 15 percent drop in triglycerides and LDL, or bad cholesterol (even though the MCT is a saturated fat), despite no differences in exercise levels or daily consumption of total calories, protein, fat, and carbs. That's right: no fewer calories, but more weight loss. The researchers attributed this to increased metabolism and fat burning.

In the 1940s, when farmers wanted to fatten up their livestock, they gave them coconut oil. This plan backfired. The animals lost weight and had more energy!

In a randomized, placebo-controlled, double-blind study from Brazil,[25] researchers tested the effects of coconut oil on forty women between the ages of twenty and forty with abdominal obesity (waist circumference of more than 88 centimeters, or about 35 inches). They split the women into two groups. One was given soybean oil and the other coconut oil for twelve weeks. They were both told to eat a healthy, balanced diet and walk for fifty minutes a day. The coconut oil group lost more belly fat than the soybean group. Those taking the coconut oil also had higher levels of the good cholesterol, HDL. Their ratio of LDL to HDL went down (a good thing!). So, spoonful for spoonful, the coconut oil group did better with weight loss and their cholesterol profiles.

This is why I love coconut oil so much. I use it every morning to speed up my metabolism and keep me feeling focused and clear and satisfied longer.

Other Benefits of Coconut Oil

Researchers have also discovered significant antifungal effects of coconut oil. When compared to the standard drug treatment for Candida, called fluconazole or Diflucan, the coconut oil won out! It worked better and at a lower dose than the drug.[26]

Coconut oil is also an antibacterial. Virgin coconut oil can even help treat skin infections.[27] It also fights dry skin, and scientists have found that it works against bacteria, fungi, and viruses.

Coconut oil also has benefits for the heart! In one study, scientists followed about 2,500 people from the Polynesian islands of Tokelau and Pukapuka. They ate a very high-fat diet, mostly from coconuts. They basically ate some form of coconut at every meal.[28] The study found that the islanders' health was good and that heart disease was almost unknown. They also did not suffer from most chronic diseases, including colon cancer and digestive problems. The lead researcher, Dr. Ian Prior, suggested that there was no evidence that high saturated fat intake from coconut oil had adverse health consequences.

Tips for Using Coconut Oil

- Look for coconut oil that is virgin, organic, cold-pressed, unrefined, and never deodorized or bleached.
- You can use expeller-pressed, unrefined coconut oil for cooking at up to 400°F, so this is a go-to oil for high-heat stir-fries, medium-high heat sautéing, and most baking.

Like coconut oil, coconut butter is highly stable because of its high content of saturated fats. It will last quite a while in your cabinet. But don't use it for any high-heat cooking, as the bits of coconut flesh will burn. Spoon coconut butter straight from the jar and eat it. Melt it and pour it over a sweet potato or winter squash, or make a sweet potato sandwich using coconut butter and almond butter (if you slightly undercook the sweet potatoes, they form "resistant starch," which doesn't spike blood sugar). Use it in curry dishes and stir-fries for an extra burst of flavor. Add it to smoothies or soups, or stir it into hot beverages. Enjoy your coconut!

WHAT ABOUT PALM OIL?

Palm oil is a vegetable oil derived from the fruit of the oil palm tree. It has also gotten a bad rap because of its saturated fat content. It has been shunned by people and denigrated by advisory groups despite research showing it's not harmful and has no connection to heart disease. In fact, it has been shown to be protective of blood vessels[29] and to reduce blood pressure and heart disease risk.[30] It even seems to improve cholesterol profile.[31]

The confusion about palm oil stems from the fact that it contains palmitic acid, a saturated fat that is considered to be bad if it is in high levels in your bloodstream. However, as you now know, dietary saturated fats don't raise blood saturated fats except in the context of a high-carb and high-sugar diet. In fact, through lipogenesis, palmitic acid in the blood is produced in the liver from eating carbs and sugar, not from eating palmitic acid in the palm oil or other fats.

Palm oil is grown commercially in several tropical countries but mainly in Indonesia and Malaysia. In its highly processed form it is a common ingredient in margarines, biscuits, breads, breakfast cereals, instant noodles, shampoos, lipsticks, candles, detergents, chocolates, and ice creams (and should be avoided in these products). Palm oil has a light, buttery flavor. But there are different kinds of palm oil and they are not all good for your health or the environment.

Red palm oil is the virgin, unrefined stuff that comes from the flesh or fruit. Palm oil is naturally reddish, and it comes chock full of vitamins and antioxidants, including vitamin E, beta-carotene (much more than carrots or tomatoes), and coenzyme Q10 (key for cellular respiration). While the vitamin E in most foods is mainly tocopherol, the vitamin E in red palm oil is made up of both tocopherols and tocotrienols, which are especially effective antioxidants. If you want to use palm oil, this is the one to use.

Refined palm oil is about 50 percent saturated fat, 39 percent monounsaturated fat, and only around 11 percent polyunsaturated fat. While it is stable for cooking (and storage), you shouldn't use it. When palm oil is highly refined, it loses its color and taste right along with the inarguably beneficial effects.

Palm kernel oil comes from the same tree, but instead of coming from the fruit, it comes from the seeds of the plant—the kernels. Palm kernel oil is highly saturated (around 80 percent SFA, 15 percent MUFA, and 2.5 percent PUFA). Be careful not to confuse fresh palm fruit oil (or red palm oil from the fleshy fruit part of the plant), which is the good stuff full of antioxidants such as tocotrienols and carotenoids, with palm kernel oil or refined palm oil, the bad stuff, which is found in roughly half of the packaged goods in American grocery stores. The bad palm oil goes by many names, including palm kernel oil, palmitate, and glyceryl stearate, and can be hidden in processed foods.

The Dark Side of Palm Oil

Palm oil is now the most widely used vegetable oil on the planet (though corn and soybean oil are the most common in the United States), accounting for 65 percent of all vegetable oil traded internationally. By 2020, the use of palm oil is expected to double, as the world's population increases and as people—especially in countries like China and India—become more affluent and consume more processed foods containing palm oil.

Clearing land for oil palm plantations has led to widespread deforestation in Indonesia and Malaysia as well as other regions. This has pushed many animal species to the brink of extinction, including rhinos, elephants, orangutans, and tigers. The clear cutting of forests has also forced indigenous peoples off their land, depriving them of their livelihoods and damaging the ecosystem, depleting clean water and fertile soil. Globally, the destruction of tropical forests is a major contributor to climate change. The annual carbon emissions that result from the deforestation of much of Indonesia's rainforests (which are then turned into palm oil plantations) exceed emissions from all the cars, trucks, planes, and ships in the United States combined.

Indonesia and Malaysia produce more than 85 percent of the palm oil in America's processed foods. In 2014 *Business Week* published an investigation by the Schuster Institute of Investigative Journalism on the extensive use of child labor on palm oil plantations. Most of the palm oil found in America's food supply, dubbed conflict palm oil, is produced in ways that cause large-scale rain forest destruction and human rights abuses.

The FDA has declared trans fats a nonsafe food additive that must be eliminated from the food supply. This has forced the junk food industry to frantically search for alternatives. Unfortunately, conflict palm oil is the main substitute for trans fats. Since 2006, when the FDA first required labeling of foods with trans fats, manufacturers started swapping palm oil for trans fats and its use has increased 500 percent in the last ten years and is found in over half of all packaged goods.

Practical Tips for Purchasing Palm Oil

Ensure you buy products that contain sustainable palm oil. Look for the CSPO (certified sustainable palm oil) label. You can recognize products made from sustainable palm oil because they carry the CSPO trademark. This mark assures you that the palm oil was produced using sustainable practices that address both social and environmental concerns. Around 15 percent of the world's palm oil production was certified sustainable in 2013, up from 10 percent in 2011.

Nutiva's Red Palm Oil is sustainably grown in Ecuador and doesn't contribute to deforestation or habitat destruction. You can purchase vegan shortening from Spectrum or Nutiva, which use sustainably farmed palm and coconut oil in a blend that works well for baking.

OLIVE OIL: LIQUID GOLD

A trove of studies has shown that the Mediterranean diet prevents heart disease, cancer, and diabetes, and even reduces risk of death. Many of the protective benefits seem to come from olive oil. And that's a good thing because olive oil makes your food taste amazing and is a health-promoting fat that is easy to find and use.

Olive oil is produced by crushing olives and then putting them through a press to squeeze out the oil. The crushed olives can be pressed many times. The first pressing creates what is known as extra virgin olive oil, and it is the only type you should consume because it has the most benefits. It also has the best flavor.

Olive oil is made up of a blend of fats. Most of this (about 75 percent) is a monounsaturated fat called oleic acid. About another 20 percent are saturated fats, and olive oil also contains vitamin E, beta carotene, and squalene, an important antioxidant that is great for your skin.

But the unique feature of olive oil is the powerful antioxidant and anti-inflammatory phytonutrients it contains, called polyphenols. As you know by now, most chronic diseases, including obesity, type 2 diabetes, heart disease, dementia, and cancer, all have roots in inflammation. You don't have to consume large quantities of olive oil to get these benefits. Just 1 to 2 tablespoons of extra virgin olive oil per day has significant anti-inflammatory effects.[32]

Olive Oil and Your Heart

Olive oil has powerful antioxidant properties that are good for your heart and protect your blood vessels. Remember, free radical damage or oxidative stress is the main way that your cholesterol becomes damaged and is the actual cause of heart disease (only rancid fat or cholesterol damages arteries). Fat-containing molecules, including LDL (bad cholesterol), need to be protected from oxygen damage. One of the common mechanisms of aging and chronic diseases—especially atherosclerosis, or hardening of the arteries—is damage from free radicals and oxidative stress, which is why we need to consume a diet rich in antioxidants.[33]

Olive oil also helps prevent platelets from clumping together excessively, therefore protecting against blood clots. There are lots of poly-phenols in olive oil—including hydroxytyrosol, oleuropein, and luteolin. These help keep your blood thin and prevent your platelets from form-ing the blood clots that cause heart attacks.[34]

The oleic acid content of olive oil helps to improve your cholesterol profile, raising the HDL, lowering the LDL, and improving the particle size and the overall LDL to HDL ratio. When other vegetable oils were exchanged for olive oil, the cholesterol profile for research participants improved.[35]

Recent research also shows that the oleic acid found in olive oil can help lower blood pressure. The olive oil works its way into your cell membranes and changes the ways your cells communicate, leading to lower blood pressure.[36]

Olive oil and its polyphenols lower blood levels of C-reactive pro-tein (CRP), therefore lowering inflammation, a risk factor in heart dis-ease. Polyphenols also improve endothelial function (the health of blood vessels) in young women.[37]

Olive Oil and Your Gut

Not only is olive oil good for your heart, it is also good for your gut. Studies on cancer of the stomach and small intestine found lower rates of cancer in people who used olive oil on a regular basis. The anti-cancer benefits likely come from the antioxidant and anti-inflammatory properties of the polyphenols in olive oil.[38]

We have learned that some fats, like the refined omega-6 oils, can harm the gut bacteria. But the polyphenols in olive oil can help balance your gut flora and prevent the growth of bad bugs like *Helicobacter pylori,* the bacteria responsible for ulcers and reflux.[39]

Olive Oil and Your Brain

Olive oil is also good for your brain. A large French study found that older adults who used a lot of olive oil in cooking and in sauces and dressings improved their visual memory and verbal fluency.[40] In studies of animals deprived of oxygen, which caused brain injury, olive oil helped their brains heal and recover.

Olive Oil and Cancer

Olive oil also seems to have anti-cancer properties. As little as one to two tablespoons a day lowers the risk of many cancers, including stomach, colon, breast, and lung cancer.[41]

Much of the research showing olive oil's relationship to cancer focused on the polyphenols in olive oil and their antioxidant and anti-inflammatory properties. But other studies have found that olive oil improves the function of your cell membranes, reducing the risk of cancer and boosting your body's own antioxidant system by turning on antioxidant genes. The myriad of antioxidants in olive oil protect your DNA from free radical damage. Your cells function better and the risk of cancer goes down.[42]

Olive Oil: Practical Considerations

Olive oil is good but it is easily damaged by exposure to light, air, and too much heat. If you buy a bottle of dark extra virgin olive oil and leave it on the counter, over time it will turn pale. That means it has oxidized or turned rancid. Buying better quality extra virgin olive oil and keeping in a dark place inside the cupboard will prevent this from happening.

You might be tempted to buy the cheap olive oil, and not get the extra virgin type. But studies have shown that the anti-inflammatory properties of the polyphenols found in extra virgin olive oil are far greater than those from later pressings or non-virgin olive oil.[43] Don't be duped by health claims like "pure olive oil" on the label either. Only buy what says "extra virgin olive oil." If a label says "pure," it usually means that it is a combination of refined and unrefined olive oils.

Another term that you may see is "cold-pressed." This means that very minimal heating (less than 81°F [27°C]) was used to extract the oil from the olives. This allows for more of the powerful nutrients to be preserved.

Buyers beware: Much of the extra virgin olive oil sold in the United States is adulterated with other oils like soybean, rapeseed, or canola oil.[44] In an expert taste and smell test, one study found that 69 percent of imported olive oil labeled "extra virgin" did not meet the standard for that label. Thankfully, olive oil expert Tom Mueller has compiled a list of extra virgin olive oils you can buy at your local grocery store (including at chains like Costco, Trader Joe's, and Whole Foods); see his website, Truth in Olive Oil: http://www.truthinoliveoil.com/2012/09/toms-supermarket-picks-quality-oils-good-prices. If you'd like to learn more about this issue, read Mueller's book, *Extra Virginity: The Sublime and Scandalous World of Olive Oil.*

Look for extra virgin olive oils sold in dark-tinted glass bottles, as the packaging will help protect the oil from oxidation caused by exposure to light. If you purchase large tins of olive oil, pour out what you'll need for a few weeks into a dark bottle so that you can avoid opening the tin often and exposing the oil to oxygen.

Once you've got your hands on a quality extra virgin olive oil, be sure to store it properly: store in a cool, dark place, out of direct sunlight and away from a heat source (do not store near the stove). Olive oil should be used within one to two months to ensure its healthy phytonutrient profile remains intact.

The take-home message is clear: Enjoy fresh extra virgin olive oil as part of your diet. It helps improve your heart health, helps you lose weight, reduces the risk of heart attacks and death, prevents cancer, and is good for your gut and your brain. Best of all, it makes your food taste delicious!

THE GOOD NEWS ON NUTS AND SEEDS

Cutting out nuts and seeds entirely from your diet because they are fattening is one of the worst pieces of advice ever offered to the American public. Study after study[45] has shown that increased nut consumption is associated with a lower risk of heart disease,[46] type 2 diabetes,[47] obesity, cancer, and death.[48] In fact, in one of the largest randomized trials ever done on heart disease, the PREDIMED study, those who ate nuts every day reduced their risk of getting heart attacks by 30 percent—equal to or better than taking statin drugs. In another study on weight loss, researchers compared a low-fat vegan diet with a high-fat vegan diet, including nuts, avocados, and olive oil. The high-fat diet led to more weight loss and better cholesterol.[49]

The results of a review of the evidence linking nuts and lower risk of coronary heart disease were published in the *British Journal of Nutrition*.[50] In this review, researchers looked at four large prospective epidemiological studies—the Adventist Health Study, Iowa Women's Study, Nurses' Health Study, and Physicians' Health Study. When evidence from all four studies was combined, subjects consuming nuts at least four times a week showed a 37 percent reduced risk of coronary heart disease compared to those who never or seldom ate nuts. Each additional serving of nuts per week was associated with an average 8.3 percent reduced risk of coronary heart disease.[51]

A study published in the journal *Obesity* showed that people who ate nuts at least twice a week were much less likely to gain weight than those who almost never ate nuts. The twenty-eight-month study, involving 8,865 adult men and women in Spain, found that participants who ate nuts at least twice per week were 31 percent less likely to gain weight than participants who never or almost never ate nuts.[52]

Nuts are high in protein, fiber, vitamins, and minerals. Packed with healthy fats, they help reduce appetite. The key is to eat them in moderation. You want them as part of a healthy diet. But just like you wouldn't binge on three bags of broccoli, you shouldn't binge on three bags of nuts. You can overdo it and end up eating just too much food. A handful or two a day is all it takes to reap their potent benefits—and to satisfy your crunch desires!

How to Buy and Prepare Nuts and Seeds

I recommend purchasing certified organic raw nuts and seeds; that way, you will protect yourself from exposure to potential contaminants. Avoid roasted or salted nuts, as the high temperature used by commercial roasters damages the many delicate fats found in nuts and seeds. If you like, you can lightly roast them yourself at a very low oven temperatures (250°F).

It's a good idea to soak your nuts and seeds to reduce lectins, phytates, and enzyme inhibitors. These are considered "anti-nutrients" that can block nutrient absorption, cause digestive distress, and inhibit enzymes. While raw nuts and seeds are extremely nutritious foods, preparation is key in order to unlock maximum nutrient potential and deactivate any substances that could be irritating to the gut. The soaking process germinates nuts and seeds, allowing increased enzyme activity.[53] Soaking also enhances the flavor.

Simply soak raw nuts or seeds in warm salt water overnight or up to twenty-four hours. Make sure there is enough warm water in the bowl to cover the nuts or seeds by an inch. Add 1 tablespoon of sea salt to 4 cups (150g) of nuts or seeds. When they're done soaking, rinse them thoroughly so that the rinsing water runs clear. Then it's crucial to thoroughly dry them. The best way to ensure they'll dry all the way through is to spread them out in a single layer in a warm oven at the lowest possible setting—ideally not more than 120°F.

9

The Bonus Benefits — Fat Makes You Smart, Sexy, and Happy

Weight loss from eating good fats? Check.

Heart disease prevention? Check.

Revved metabolism? Check.

But the health benefits from eating more of the right fats don't end there! Here's a look at all the other good things healthy fats can do for your body, your brain, your mood, and more.

EATING FAT REVERSES TYPE 2 DIABETES (AND IMPROVES BLOOD SUGAR CONTROL FOR TYPE 1)

Of all of my patients, those with diabetes and pre-diabetes do the best on a high-fat, low-carb diet. One patient with type 2 diabetes recently told me she got off 56 units of insulin in four days on the *Eat Fat, Get Thin* program, and she went on to lose thirty-six pounds. Another patient with type 2 diabetes got off 48 units of insulin and all his diabetes medication and lost fifty pounds. Still another patient with type 2 diabetes got off her insulin in three days and lost eighteen pounds in the first ten days (she had been eating a lot of refined carbs and sugar).

> I was taking 200 units of Lantus insulin daily and my hemoglobin A1c (average blood sugar) was still over the top. I came off insulin the third day on the program, lost thirty-five pounds so far, and my last hemoglobin A1c was down to 6.9 from over 11.
>
> — Kerry Otteso

Type 2 diabetes and pre-diabetes together now affect 1 in 2 Americans and 1 in 4 kids. Eighty percent of the world's type 2 diabetics are in the developing world. We now know how to prevent and reverse this global epidemic. Although the ADA and our government dietary guidelines still recommend high-carb diets for diabetics, the world leader in diabetes treatment and care, Harvard's Joslin Diabetes Center, is moving toward a high-fat diet. It is my hope that the tide will continue to turn.

Comprehensive reviews of all the research in 2008[1] and 2015[2] both came to the conclusion that a low-carb, high-fat diet was the best prevention and treatment for type 2 diabetes and pre-diabetes. In these reviews, scientists document twelve reasons why high-fat, lower-carb diets are the way to go, even for better management of type 1 diabetes:

1. Restricting dietary carbs and increasing fat have the greatest impact on lowering blood sugar levels.
2. During the obesity and type 2 diabetes epidemics, the increase in the number of calories consumed has been due almost entirely to refined carbs and sugar, while fat consumption as a percentage of our total calories has decreased.
3. You don't need to lose weight to reap the benefits of lower-carb, higher-fat diets.
4. Even though weight loss is not necessary, no dietary intervention is more effective for weight loss.
5. People are much more likely to adhere to lower-carb, higher-fat diets because they reduce cravings and are more satisfying.
6. Replacing some of the carbs with protein is helpful.
7. Total and saturated fat intake do not correlate with risk for cardiovascular disease.
8. Blood levels of saturated fat are controlled by dietary carbohydrates far more than dietary fats.
9. The best predictor of small blood vessel damage (the type that causes amputations) is the average level of blood sugar (hemoglobin A1c), which is better controlled on a high-fat, low-carb diet.
10. Dietary carb restriction and higher fat intake are the most effective way to reduce blood levels of triglycerides and raise HDL.

11. The best way to reduce or eliminate medication and insulin in type 2 diabetes is a low-carb, high-fat diet. And people with type 1 diabetes can use less insulin and get more steady blood sugars.
12. The diet has no side effects, as opposed to medications and insulin, which increase risks of heart attacks and death.[3]

Just a reminder: This approach of a higher-fat, lower-carb diet is so powerful that you should be sure to be careful as you eat better. You will need less medication and insulin and your blood sugars could bottom out when you dramatically change your diet, so be cautious. Be sure to work with your doctor before reducing any medication.

EATING FAT PREVENTS BRAIN AGING AND DEMENTIA

Low-fat diets have been associated with dementia and higher-fat diets shown to prevent it. In fact, leading Alzheimer's researchers are promoting a very high-fat (or ketogenic) diet for the treatment of dementia. In his paper "Reversal of Cognitive Decline: A Novel Therapeutic Program,"[4] Dr. Dale Bredesen, of the Buck Institute for Research on Aging, reviews ten case studies where dementia was actually reversed in patients on a very low-carb, low-glycemic, low-grain, high-fat diet. This is groundbreaking. After $2 billion of research and 243 studies over the last few decades on the treatment of dementia with medication, none have shown this level of success. In fact, none of those studies worked except for one, and that one only very slightly.

In Dr. David Perlmutter's groundbreaking book *Grain Brain*, he also documents the role of fat in the brain. There is an abundance of research showing that carbs cause brain aging and fat prevents it. In fact, some now call Alzheimer's type 3 diabetes because insulin resistance causes brain damage. A study from the Mayo Clinic found that people who eat a ton of carbs quadruple their risk of getting pre-dementia, known as mild cognitive impairment. The same study showed that people who ate the healthiest fats had a 44 percent lower risk of early dementia, and those who ate more good-quality protein from chicken, meat, and fish had a 21 percent lower risk of early dementia.[5]

Another study of more than 8,000 people over the age of sixty-five found that 280 of them got dementia over the span of four years. The researchers looked at the participants' diets and found that those who ate the least brain-healthy omega-3 fats had a 37 percent increased risk of dementia.[6] Those who ate the most fish had a 44 percent reduction in the risk of getting dementia. Those who ate the most olive oil, walnuts, and flaxseeds had a 60 percent reduction in the risk of getting dementia. But they also found that those who ate the most omega-6 oils had twice the risk of dementia.

EATING FAT HELPS WITH SEIZURES, DEPRESSION, ADD, AUTISM, TRAUMA, AND MORE

Your brain is 60 percent fat, and much of it is made of omega-3 fats and cholesterol. When you eat a low-fat diet, you are starving your brain.

Fat is critical for your brain. Lack of fat in the diet has been linked to neurodegenerative diseases; mental disorders such as depression,[7] suicide, and aggressive behavior;[8] ADD[9] and autism;[10] stroke; and trauma.[11] On the other hand, supplementing the diet with omega-3 and other good fats has been linked to improvement in all these conditions. Omega-3 fatty acids stimulate beneficial gene expression and boost the activity of your brain cells, increase connections between brain cells, and even help the formation of new brain cells (neurogenesis). They help reduce brain inflammation and improve cognitive function. They can aid depression and even recovery from brain injury.[12] Very high-fat ketogenic diets are used to control epilepsy[13] and are now being used for ALS (amyotrophic lateral sclerosis)[14] and other neurologic disorders, including brain cancer.[15]

Bottom line: Fat is good for your brain!

EATING FAT REDUCES INFLAMMATION AND AUTOIMMUNE DISEASE

Bad fats such as the omega-6 refined vegetable oils cause inflammation, but good fats reduce inflammation. Omega-3 fats have been extensively studied as a way of treating inflammatory and autoimmune disease. They modulate inflammatory pathways and help improve expression of anti-inflammatory genes.

There have been many studies assessing the benefits of supplementation with fish oil in inflammatory and autoimmune diseases in humans, including rheumatoid arthritis, Crohn's disease, ulcerative colitis, psoriasis, lupus erythematosus, multiple sclerosis, and migraine headaches. These studies show great benefits, including decreased disease activity and less of a need for anti-inflammatory drugs.[16] I have found that fish oil supplementation along with a low-glycemic, anti-inflammatory, higher-fat diet that is also gluten- and dairy-free can dramatically help my patients with autoimmune disease.

Gamma linolenic acid (GLA) has been well researched in autoimmune disease and shown to be effective.[17] It is found in evening primrose oil or borage oil and can be synthesized by the body, but often not very well, especially under conditions of illness. I have used it effectively in combination with diet and other therapies in many of my autoimmune patients.

EATING FAT BOOSTS YOUR SPORTS PERFORMANCE

We have all been trained to believe that if you want to enhance your sports performance, you need to carb-load. Eat that big bowl of pasta before a race to make sure you top up your muscle carbohydrate stores (glycogen) so you don't hit the wall…that sort of thing. You can store up to 2,000 calories of carbs as glycogen in your muscles, but the average lean athlete has about 40,000 calories of energy stored as fat. Wouldn't it be great if you could switch from carb burning to fat burning?

Many scientists have studied high-fat, low-carb diets for athletes. Two in particular have led the way: Dr. Jeff Volek and Dr. Stephen Phinney. They have authored hundreds of papers untangling the biology of high-fat, low-carb diets on every aspect of physiology—even in extreme athletes who are insulin sensitive and not carbohydrate intolerant. In their books *The Art and Science of Low Carbohydrate Living* and *The Art and Science of Low Carbohydrate Performance*, they go into great detail on how your body can switch from burning mostly carbs to burning mostly fat. This is called keto-adaptation. The key is to keep insulin levels very low. Higher levels of insulin inhibit or block fat burning, making it impossible to mobilize fat stored in your tissues. Drs. Volek and Phinney explain the benefits of switching from carb burning to fat burning for exercise:

- Low-carb (high-fat) diets are anti-inflammatory and so reduce oxidative stress during exercise, reduce lactic acid buildup, and help the body recover faster between exercise sessions.
- Once you adapt to a low-carb diet (which takes about two weeks), your body relies primarily on burning body fat during and between exercise sessions, so you don't have to load up on carbs to restore glycogen levels. You can eat a lot of fat without risk.
- Endurance and power- or strength-training athletes can use carb-restricted high-fat diets and even get better body composition and strength.

I know eating a low-carb, high-fat diet has made me stronger, fitter, and faster even as I've aged. And when I load up on coconut oil, which contains medium-chain triglycerides,[18] which boost performance, increase fat burning, and help build muscle, before a long bike ride, I can go and go without pooping out.

EATING FAT GIVES YOU BEAUTIFUL SKIN, HAIR, AND NAILS

Ever wonder how trainers get horses to have beautiful, shiny coats? They give them flaxseeds, which are a rich source of omega-3 fats. Lack of omega-3 fat in your diet from fish or plant sources can cause significant health problems. Most people slather creams, lotions, and potions on dry skin, put on all sorts of hair products to bring their hair back to life, and use nail products to strengthen their nails, but most of our outside problems come from inside. Omega-3 deficiency can cause dry, itchy, flaky, even discolored skin. It can also cause rough, bumpy chicken skin on the backs of your arms. I know you are checking that now! Your fingertips may crack and peel. Your hair may be dry, stiff, and tangled; you may have dandruff and hair loss. Your fingernails might grow slowly or become brittle and chipped. Omega-3 fats can relieve all of these problems. For some people with really problematic skin, applying a combination of flax and borage oil can have amazing results.

EATING FAT ENHANCES YOUR SEX LIFE

You might be surprised to learn that your sex hormones are produced from cholesterol in the body. We eat an average of 146 pounds of flour and 152 pounds of sugar per person per year in America, which spikes insulin, driving the storage of belly fat, increasing estrogen in men (belly fat cells produce more estrogen) and sending their testosterone levels plummeting. This leads to low sex drive, sexual dysfunction, muscle loss, loss of body hair, and man boobs! For most men, cutting out the carbs and boosting fats fixes the problem without having to resort to testosterone replacement.

Low-fat diets can cause women to stop menstruating or to experience irregular, heavy periods and infertility. They can increase belly fat, raise testosterone levels, and trigger acne, facial hair, and hair loss on the head, whereas high-fat, low-carb diets can reverse all that.

FAT AND CANCER: SHOULD WE BE WORRIED?

Let's take a look at whether we should be worried about fat and cancer. This probably won't surprise you by this point, but there is conflicting evidence. Some studies show that fat and cancer are not connected, others show they might be, yet others show fat might be protective, and even others are using very high-fat ketogenic diets to starve cancer cells because they can run only on sugar, not on fat. So how do we make sense of this?

Truthfully it is hard. The problem, as I have described, is the poor state of nutrition research. In large population studies where diets are assessed by food frequency questionnaires (which are not super accurate because who really remembers what they ate from week to week?) and where many other factors can explain associations, it is hard to draw clear conclusions. It is why population studies can't prove cause and effect. For example, in some studies it was found that people who had more saturated fat might be at higher risk for more cancer. But was it the saturated fat or the overall dietary and lifestyle pattern of the saturated-fat eaters (less exercise, more smoking, more refined and processed foods, more fried foods, fewer fruits and vegetables, heavier weight of the saturated-fat eaters)? It may not be the saturated fat at all. Many large population studies found, for example, that increased fat intake was linked to breast cancer, but then when large randomized controlled experiments were done to assess true cause and effect, no link between dietary fat and breast cancer could be found.[19]

Population studies also show contradictory results. Some show that more fat or certain fats cause cancer, while other studies show exactly the opposite.[20] Large reviews have trouble finding consistent links between fat and cancer.[21] That is why I rely more on basic science and experiments combined with an understanding of basic biology and, in this case, cancer biology. The data is still coming in and we don't have all the answers, which is why I advocate a sensible approach based on whole foods and good fats.

Here's what we do know about cancer. It is a complex disease that results from environmental insults (like toxins, smoking, etc.), diet, and stress. We also know certain things for sure. Insulin resistance or prediabetes or type 2 diabetes dramatically increases the risk of most common cancers (prostate, breast, colon, pancreas, liver, etc.). We also know that inflammation increases cancer risk. Everyone agrees that vegetables and fruits contain powerful anticancer compounds. One study in China measured metabolites of broccoli and cruciferous vegetables in the urine and found that those with the highest amounts of these compounds had the lowest risk of cancer.[22] Other studies link certain foods strongly with certain cancers, for example, dairy with prostate cancer.[23]

Some fats, however—the essential omega-3 fatty acids such as EPA and DHA—do seem helpful and are good for almost every other health problem because they are critical components of our biology. Many studies show that omega-3 fats have anticancer properties.[24] They reduce inflammation, improve insulin resistance, and work through other cellular mechanisms to inhibit cancer pathways in colon cancer,[25] breast cancer,[26] and prostate cancer.[27] Many studies show that in the face of a diet high in omega-6 PUFAs from vegetable oils, omega-3 fats don't work that well. Other studies have shown that saturated fats are harmful only in the face of a high-carb diet or a diet low in omega-3 fats. In fact, much research is being done now on using ketogenic or very high-fat diets (60 to 70 percent fat) for treating cancer,[28] including brain cancer and colon cancer.[29] It seems that high-fat ketogenic diets are toxic to cancer cells, while helping the patient thrive.

I don't believe there is one diet that is good for your heart, and another that prevents cancer, another that prevents dementia, and even another that prevents diabetes. I believe we were much more intelligently designed than that, that nature and our biology are more elegantly constructed. There must be one set of principles that makes sense for humans. Unfortunately, because of the sad state of nutrition science, we have to piece together the story.

Part of the problem with nutrition science is it tries to draw conclusions by teasing apart individual nutrients and separating them from the overall dietary pattern. But this just doesn't make sense. We evolved eating whole real food, not individual ingredients or types of fat that we dialed up or down based on the latest research. While there might be risks, I think that a whole-foods, evolutionary approach to eating, informed by science and our current understanding of molecular biology and physiology, makes the most sense. This perspective is the foundation of the *Eat Fat, Get Thin* Plan outlined in Part III.

So there you have it: all the research, facts, and figures on fat. I hope by now you're as convinced as I am that the low-fat era must finally be put to an end, and that eating healthy fat is the key to losing weight, preventing disease, restoring vitality, and—most of all—enjoying many of the foods you love!

THE *EAT FAT, GET THIN* PLAN

And Pharaoh said unto Joseph, Say unto thy brethren,
This do ye: lade your beasts, and go, get you unto the land
of Canaan; And take your father and your households, and
come unto me: and I will give you the good of the land of
Egypt, and ye shall eat the fat of the land.

—Genesis 45:17–18

10

What Should I Eat?

Now that you know the whole story about how we got into this big, fat mess, and why you need to change how you think about food and fat, let's get to what you really want to know:

How can I lose weight and improve my health?
What foods should I avoid?
How do I increase the fat in my diet — and which ones should I choose?
What carbs should I eat?
How much protein do I really need?
How can I combat cravings?

The *Eat Fat, Get Thin* Plan will answer these questions and more. I'm going to share with you the program I designed that will revolutionize everything from your mind-set to your pantry, and from your waistline to your overall health. In just twenty-one days, you'll know not only what to eat but how to fuel your body on every level so you can look and feel fantastic.

The *Eat Fat, Get Thin* Plan will jump-start you on the path to losing weight, rebooting your metabolism, and getting healthy. After the twenty-one days, as you'll read about in Chapter 14, you'll have the option to stay on the *Eat Fat, Get Thin* Plan to continue your weight loss and healing, or transition to what I call the Pegan Diet (my vetted combination of Paleo and vegan), which includes whole grains, beans, and — in the secondary stage — the reintroduction of some gluten, dairy, and the occasional treat. I focus specifically on the cross-section of vegan and Paleo because the middle ground between these two approaches is the most doable, sensible, sustainable, delicious, healthful, and science-based way of eating. It incorporates elements from other diets that have been found to be healthful, such as the Mediterranean diet. This long-term approach to eating is the result of decades of research and personal experience working one on one with thousands of patients.

COMPARING VEGAN AND PALEO DIETS

You'd think the research would clarify the answer to the question of what we should eat, but it just makes for more confusion. Vegan diet studies show they help with weight loss, reverse diabetes, and lower cholesterol. Paleo diets seem to do the same thing. So should you be shunning animal foods and eating only beans, grains, and veggies, or should you eat meat and fat without guilt and give up all grains and beans? There are great aspects to both perspectives, but they are incomplete by themselves. Essentially, the members of each camp adhere to their diet with near religious fervor, pointing only to studies that validate their point of view. We call this cherry picking.

Typically these studies compare high-quality versions of Paleo or vegan diets with the standard American diet, which is high in processed foods, sugar, refined carbs, poor-quality industrial animal products, and refined oils. A study of any diet of whole foods — vegan or Paleo — will do far better than the awful processed industrial diet. But what happens when you compare two whole-food, good-quality vegan diets — one low-fat and one high-fat? This has been done, and the high-fat, high-protein, low-carb, low-glycemic vegan diet (Eco-Atkins) performed better for weight loss and lowering cholesterol than the low-fat vegan diet that avoided nuts, seeds, and avocados.[1]

Comparing a vegan diet of chips, Coke, bagels, and pasta to a Paleo diet of healthy veggies and grass-fed meat wouldn't be very helpful either; nor would comparing a Paleo diet of feedlot meat, bologna, and few fresh veggies to a whole-foods, low-glycemic vegan diet. But no one has yet done the study that compares the ideal healthy Paleo diet with the ideal healthy high-fat vegan one. My guess is that both can be healthful and that some people might do better on the higher-fat animal-food diets and others better on the plant-based higher-fat diets. LeBron James, considered one of the greatest basketball players of our time, follows a Paleo diet. The number one tennis player in the world, Novak Djokovic, cut out gluten and dairy and ate a higher-fat diet and went from losing match after match to winning every major tennis tournament in a year. Rich Roll completed five Ironman triathlons in seven days on a high-fat vegan diet. Humans are amazingly adaptable. But the only important question is, What is the right diet for the human that matters most—you?!

You should base your food and lifestyle choices on how *your* body responds. Listen to your body. It will tell you what it likes. It takes observation and time to figure it out. But your body is the smartest doctor in the room.

BEST OF VEGAN + BEST OF PALEO = PEGAN

The Pegan Diet combines the best of the Paleo and vegan diets.

These are general principles that I live by because I want to live a long, healthy life. I also am in good shape and at my ideal body weight and body composition so I can enjoy a bit more varied diet. However, if you are trying to reverse diabetes, lose a lot of weight, reverse chronic health problems, and do a total body reset, then the jump-start metabolism reset *Eat Fat, Get Thin* Plan is the place to start. Think of it as a twenty-one-day program to reboot your body and mind and turn your body back to its original factory settings.

Once you have achieved your goals, you can begin to expand your way of eating to the full Pegan Diet approach. It is more of a philosophy with guidelines than a rigid way of eating; it incorporates the latest science and insights about nutrition and supports your body to thrive for the long term. So what is the Pegan Diet?

Let's focus first on what Paleo and healthy vegan have in common. They are both based on real, whole, fresh food that is sustainably raised;

rich in vitamins, minerals, and phytonutrients; and low in sugar, refined carbs, and processed foods of all kinds. An apple doesn't have a bar code, an egg doesn't have a nutrition facts label, and an almond doesn't have an ingredient list. They are all real foods.

Here are the characteristics of a healthy diet almost everyone agrees on:

1. **Ideally organic, local, fresh, whole foods.**
2. **Very low glycemic load**—low in sugar, flour, and refined carbohydrates.
3. **Very high in vegetables and fruits**—the deeper the colors, the more variety, the better (although the Paleo camp recommends sticking to lower-glycemic fruit, such as berries).
4. **Low or no pesticides, antibiotics, or hormones** and no GMO foods.
5. **Very few to no chemicals,** additives, preservatives, dyes, MSG, artificial sweeteners, and other "Frankenchemicals."
6. **Higher in good-quality fats** from olive oil, nuts, seeds, and avocados. Omega-3 fats for all! If you are a vegan and don't want to eat anything with a mother, that's perfectly okay. But it's critical to get omega-3 fats, and not just ALA found in plants. You need DHA directly from food, rather than hoping your body converts the ALA to DHA. The good news is that you can get DHA from algae.
7. **Low in refined, processed vegetable oils.** Extra virgin olive oil is a delicious, healthy alternative.
8. **Moderate protein** for appetite control and muscle synthesis, especially in the elderly (though, obviously, there's debate as to whether this should come from vegetable or animal protein sources).
9. **Animal food.** While of course vegetarians and vegans don't agree that eating animal products is okay, those who do approve are in agreement that meats should be sustainably and humanely raised, grass-fed, and antibiotic- and hormone-free.
10. **Fish.** Ditto for fish when it comes to vegans, but if you fall into the camp that eats fish, the consensus is that you should choose low-mercury and low-toxin fish such as sardines, herring, anchovies,

wild salmon, and other small fish and avoid tuna, swordfish, and Chilean sea bass because of the high mercury load. Fish should also either be from sustainable "organic" fisheries, or sustainably caught in ways that do not deplete natural fisheries.

THE AREAS OF CONTROVERSY

Here's where things start to get a little hairy. These are the areas of controversy in the nutrition world that many are still debating:

1. **Dairy.** Both the Paleo and vegan camps (and yours truly) shun dairy, for good reason. While some can tolerate it, for most it contributes to obesity, diabetes, heart disease, dementia, and cancer and may increase (not decrease) the risk of osteoporosis, not to mention allergies, asthma, eczema, postnasal drip, acne, and irritable bowel syndrome.[2] While some data suggest that it can be helpful in weight management and diabetes prevention, it is not clear if that is because milk drinkers have less soda or sugar-sweetened beverages, because of the dairy itself, or because the Dairy Council funded the studies! We'll go into more detail about dairy in Chapter 13, and why, with the exception of grass-fed butter or ghee, it's excluded from the *Eat Fat, Get Thin* Plan.

2. **Grains.** For millions of Americans (and millions in the rest of humanity!), gluten contributes to inflammation, autoimmunity, digestive disorders, mental illness,[3] autism,[4] depression, schizophrenia,[5] obesity, heart disease, dementia,[6] and cancer.[7] Celiac disease affects 1 percent of all people, but gluten sensitivity might affect up to 10 percent, or more than 30 million Americans. Less than 1 percent are diagnosed.[8] Gluten is in refined, high-glycemic foods like bread or baked goods and contributes to weight gain and insulin resistance. Even whole wheat bread spikes your blood sugar more than table sugar; any grains can increase your blood sugar, for that matter. But grains *can* be part of a healthy diet, just not in unlimited amounts, especially if you have diabesity or are carbohydrate intolerant. For type 2 diabetics wanting to get off insulin and reverse

their diabetes, those with autoimmune disease, or those with a lot of weight to lose, a grain-free diet is a good experiment.

3. **Beans.** Beans are a great source of fiber, protein, and minerals. But they do cause digestive problems for some, and if you are diabetic, a mostly bean diet can trigger spikes in blood sugar. Again, moderate amounts are okay—meaning up to 1 cup (250g) a day. Some are concerned that beans contain lectins,[9] which can create inflammation, and phytates, which impair mineral absorption.[10] In *Eat Fat, Get Thin*, we avoid beans during the initial twenty-one days, much for the same reason as we do grains.

4. **Meat.** No shocker here: Meat is a sticking point for many. I cover meat in detail in Chapter 7. But the upshot is that research on meat is fuzzy, because most studies don't look at the quality of the meat. Some studies show that red meat increases heart disease and death rates,[11] but other studies show the opposite. In truth it depends on how the study was done, but the evidence in my mind is trending toward meat not being linked to disease. On the other hand, there are many ethical and environmental reasons to downsize your meat consumption. Focus on quality, not quantity.

5. **Eggs.** I've already shared with you all the reasons why eggs have been unfairly maligned, and why they have finally been exonerated. The bottom line is that eggs, especially organic and omega-3 eggs, are a great nutrient-rich, low-cost source of protein, and they have no impact on cholesterol or heart disease risk.

So what's an eater to do?

First and foremost, don't worry about focusing on how much you eat. If you focus on *what* you eat, and choose the right foods in the right balance, your body's natural appetite control and healing systems kick into gear. I vote for resetting your body completely with the *Eat Fat, Get Thin* Plan, and then transitioning to the Pegan Diet as your long-term maintenance plan. A Pegan diet is a sensible and balanced way of eating without a ton of restrictions; it is satisfying, easy to follow, and based on the best science to date.

Here are the Pegan principles I follow, which you'll learn much more about in Chapter 14:

- Unlimited amounts of nonstarchy veggies (greens and crunchy veggies), which should make up about 50 to 70 percent of your diet by volume (how much room it takes up on your plate). See page 224 for a list.
- Moderate amounts of nuts and seeds, including almonds, walnuts, pecans, macadamia nuts, pumpkin seeds, sesame seeds, and hemp and chia seeds
- Moderate amounts of low-glycemic fruit
- Sustainably farmed and low-mercury wild fish (sardines, mackerel, herring, wild salmon)
- Grass-fed beef, bison, lamb, organic poultry
- Pasture-raised or organic eggs
- Small quantities of gluten-free grains (brown or black rice, quinoa, buckwheat)
- Small quantities of beans, if tolerated
- No dairy (except organic goat or sheep cheese or yogurt if tolerated and ghee or grass-fed butter)
- Plenty of good fats, including avocados, extra virgin olive oil, coconut oil
- Occasional treats of real sugar, maple syrup, or honey
- Moderate alcohol intake: maximum 1 glass of wine at night or 1 ounce (25m) of hard liquor, or ideally fewer than five drinks a week. Beer is a problem because of the sugar and gluten. Think "beer belly."
- Coffee or tea (1 to 2 cups a day maximum)
- Minimal amounts of gluten (but only in the form of whole grains such as steel-cut oats, whole-kernel rye bread, barley) and dairy (ideally goat or sheep and always organic), only if tolerated (but my vote is to avoid or significantly limit dairy). These are optional and only if you find you have no reaction when you reintroduce them. They do not need to be part of a healthful diet, and for most people they cause inflammation and chronic symptoms.
- What it doesn't include: processed foods, artificial anything (especially sweeteners), liquid sugar calories, and juices except green juices

That said, I have created the *Eat Fat, Get Thin* Plan as a way to jump-start health and weight loss. It takes three weeks (twenty-one days) to change habits, to learn new patterns, and to allow your biology to completely reset, cool off the inflammation, renew your gut, and adapt to a higher-fat way of eating. Think of it as the "pre-Pegan" diet to reset your brain chemistry, hormones, and metabolism.

The *Eat Fat, Get Thin* Plan starts you off by removing the grains, beans, sweets, dairy, and gluten (however minimal), and includes lots of healthy fats and clean, sustainable animal products and seafood. This helps most people hit the biological reset button. Think of it as returning your body to its original factory settings. Then, as you'll learn in Chapter 14, after twenty-one days you get to add back beans and grains in moderation—and, a few weeks later, if you want, small amounts of gluten, dairy, and treats like dark chocolate and wine—so you can see how your body responds. Pay attention. Notice how you feel. Good? Or bloated? Do you gain weight or lose weight? Does your brain fog or achiness come back or do you feel awesome? Let your body tell you. We all need a personalized approach, a way of eating that works best for us.

PERSONALIZING YOUR DIET

Even if you understand all the distinctions between the different types of fat and their effects on the body, you can't know for sure the effects these foods will have on *your* body. We are all unique and each of us requires a different, individualized approach to our health. One-size-fits-all medicine is a thing of the past.

There is no single prescription for what to eat that works for everyone. The truth is that some people do better with more fat, even up to 70 or 80 percent fat, while others do better with more starch and carbohydrates such as whole grains or beans or sweet potatoes (although no one does well with large amounts of sugars and refined carbs). The best doctor is your own body. Listen to it. Pay attention. What makes it feel good or feel bad? Learn the medicine that works. As I've said many times, food is medicine, not just calories. It contains information or instructions that regulate your genes, your metabolism, your immune system, and even your gut flora.

There are some emerging tests that can help you find out what pattern of eating might work best for you. High-fat, low-carb or lower-fat, higher-carb? Even what type of exercise you might benefit from most. This is the study of *nutrigenomics*, which we use in Functional Medicine to personalize our approach.

A few companies are now offering genetic tests that you can do on your own to help you make more personalized decisions. Much of the information you need is contained right in your own body—what I like to call the smartest doctor in the room. Your own body will give you direct and often immediate feedback about what works and what doesn't, if you need more or less fat, more or less carbs, more or less protein. It can even tell you what type of exercise works best for you. Throughout the twenty-one days on the *Eat Fat, Get Thin* Plan, it's up to you to monitor how your body is responding. In Chapter 13, I give you clues on what to look for to know if you need more or less fat, carbs, or protein.

Your own blood work and your own story and family history all are amazing guides to personalizing treatment. People who are more carbohydrate intolerant (see carbohydrate intolerance/diabesity quiz, pages 20 to 21) typically do better on a higher-fat, lower-carb diet. That's an easy way to tell what makes the most sense. Almost everyone does better on a higher-fat, lower-carb diet compared to the average American diet, but some may be able to tolerate a bit more healthy carbs, including whole grains and starchy veggies and beans (which, again, you'll test for yourself in the transition-to-Pegan stage in Chapter 14).

Checking your blood work also can be very helpful in identifying carbohydrate intolerance. Ideally you need a special cholesterol test called NMR done by LabCorp or the Cardio IQ test done by Quest Diagnostics to check particle number and size. All other cholesterol tests are inadequate and provide incomplete information. Here's what to look for to determine if you are carbohydrate intolerant:

- High triglycerides (over 100 mg/dl)
- Low HDL (less than 50 mg/dl for a man and less than 60 mg/dl for a woman)
- High triglyceride to HDL ratio (over 1:1 or 2:1)
- Many LDL particles (over 1,000)
- Many small LDL particles (over 400)
- High insulin (over 5 fasting)
- High blood sugar levels (over 90 mg/dl)
- Elevated hemoglobin A1c (over 5.5 percent; measures average blood sugar)
- Abnormal insulin tolerance test: fasting blood sugar and insulin levels at thirty minutes and one and two hours after a 75-gram drink of glucose
  - Fasting blood sugar should be less than 80 mg/dl. Thirty-minute, one-hour, and two-hour glucose should not rise above 110 mg/dl; some say 120 mg/dl
  - Fasting insulin should be between 2 and 5 µIU/dl; anything greater than 10 µIU/dl is significantly elevated. Thirty-minute, one-hour, and two-hour insulin levels should be less than 25 µIU/dl to 30 µIU/dl; anything higher than 30 µIU/dl indicates some degree of insulin resistance

If you have abnormal values on these tests you will tend to do better on a higher-fat, lower-carb diet. If they are totally normal, you may be able to include more healthy starchy veggies, whole grains, and beans once you transition to the Pegan Diet. You can monitor those numbers and see how different approaches to eating affect you.

TESTING YOUR GENES

Many of us would like to blame our parents or our genes for our weight or health problems. It would be easy to say that you have the genes for obesity or diabetes, that your parents and grandparents were overweight or had diabetes or heart disease, so you do, too. But the world of genetics is much more complicated than that.

Each of us has about 20,000 genes. Approximately 99 percent of those genes are identical to every other human on the planet; the other 1 percent is what makes us unique. You have about 112 million variations on those genes, called single nucleotide polymorphisms (SNPs for short), which influence every function of your body, including your need for vitamins, your ability to detoxify, and your tendency toward inflammation, heart disease, cancer, and much more. These SNPs also influence your weight and metabolism and your ability to process or manage fat in your diet.

Every day we are learning more about these SNPs and how they influence our health. We know enough today to start using genetic tests to help personalize our approach to health and nutrition. Soon we will be able to take a swab of our cheek, send it in, and for a few hundred dollars know our whole genome and match our food, supplement, and exercise needs to our own genes, optimizing function and metabolism. Up to 40 to 50 percent of the variance in body weight among people may be due to genetic factors, which is why different people respond differently to different diets.[12]

For some of my patients, I order genetic testing to help guide me in personalizing recommendations. There are some genes that help me tailor my approach for each person. These specific genes are linked to obesity and the tendency to gain weight, and how cholesterol profiles may respond to a high- or low-fat diet,[13] metabolic rate, absorption of dietary fat, mobilization of fat from cells, and the ability to burn fat for energy. There are genes that regulate dopamine receptors in the brain, which control your likelihood of craving carbs and sugar, and genes that can predict levels of insulin resistance, inflammation, cholesterol metabolism, and even how your body responds to different types of exercise.

I've listed below some of the genes I test for (and that you can easily test for with a home test kit—see www.eatfatgetthin.com for details):

- FABP2: influences your absorption and metabolism of fat
- PPARG: affects your insulin function, fat burning, and cholesterol levels

- ADRB2: affects how your body mobilizes fat from fat cells for energy
- ADRB3: affects how your body breaks down fat
- APOA5: regulates your triglycerides
- APOA2: affects the risk of obesity, cholesterol metabolism, risk of heart disease, and risk of diabetes
- MC4R: affects your energy intake and expenditure and appetite control
- FTO: regulates appetite, temperature, and nervous and hormonal systems
- TCF7L2: regulates blood sugar, including insulin secretion and action
- ADBR3: affects your responsiveness to exercise and fat burning
- PLIN: affects fat storage related to obesity
- TNF-A: affects inflammation, which can affect blood sugar control and cholesterol abnormalities
- LDL: removes cholesterol from circulation
- CETP: regulates metabolism of HDL and the levels of blood cholesterol
- APOA1: regulates the production of HDL (good cholesterol)
- APOC3: plays a key role in cholesterol and triglyceride metabolism
- APOE: plays an important role in the breakdown of triglycerides and cholesterol
- DRD2: affects the dopamine receptors in your brain and your risk of addiction to sugar and refined carbs

Since I am interested in this area, and because I have a strong family history of heart disease and tend to have higher cholesterol, I wanted to see what my tests showed. Let's go through my own results so you can see how this can play a practical role in personalizing your own approach to health.

On the whole, I discovered I was genetically very lucky. I had only one highly impactful gene that put me at risk of being carbohydrate intolerant, called PLIN. This didn't surprise me, since I notice that if I eat refined carbs or sugar, I gain a bit of belly fat! I also have the MC4R gene variation, which makes me likely to overeat. I do in fact have to watch myself.

My triglycerides are a bit higher than I would have expected, given how clean my everyday diet is. It was enlightening to learn that I have the APOA5 and APOA3 genes; it helps me know that I should have more olive oil or MUFAs and fewer carbs in my diet.

As you progress through the program, don't forget to listen to your body. How do you feel? Are you losing weight? Is your energy dramatically increased? Are your aches and pains better? Is your brain fog gone? Remember, your own body is the best barometer of what works and what doesn't.

11

About the Program

Welcome to twenty-one days that not only will change how you think and feel about eating fat—but will forever alter how you think and feel about your body and how you care for your health and well-being. You'll no longer have to wonder what to eat or how much. You'll learn the secrets that will give you the life-changing confidence that comes from knowing you're in command of the most potent medicine there is: what you put on the end of your fork.

The *Eat Fat, Get Thin* program is divided into three stages:

Stage 1: Lay the Foundation
Stage 2: The *Eat Fat, Get Thin* Plan
Stage 3: Your Transition Plan

Stage 1 is the preparation stage, to be done in the two days prior to beginning the program. Stage 2 covers the *Eat Fat, Get Thin* Plan and includes everything that you'll eat, drink, and do. Stage 3 lays out three options for transition plans, all of which give you a blueprint to follow for the rest of your life.

STAGE 1: LAY THE FOUNDATION

You wouldn't construct a building without first laying a solid foundation, and that's precisely what you'll do in the two days prior to beginning the *Eat Fat, Get Thin* Plan. During these two days, you'll do the following:

- **Make Over Your Kitchen.** Out with the bad, in with the good! I'll walk you through the steps to set yourself up for cooking and eating success.
- **Tackle Your Fear of Fat.** It's a challenge for us as human beings to give up deeply held beliefs—especially ones that are as deeply ingrained as our collective fear of fat. But give them up we must if we're going to succeed, and I know you're up for the challenge now that you've learned the truth about fat. I'll give you questions to answer to help you root out any mental blocks that may be standing in your way.
- **Stock Your Toolbox.** Besides the groceries you'll get as part of the kitchen makeover, there are several supplies you will need to get, including a pair of sneakers (for, you guessed it, exercise) and supplements. I'll give you a checklist to ensure you have everything you need to succeed.

STAGE 2: THE *EAT FAT, GET THIN* PLAN

For each of the twenty-one days on this program, you'll incorporate the following components into your daily routine. I'll give you specific guidelines to make each super simple and easy to follow.

Here are the three components of your daily plan:

- **Nourish.** Each day, you'll enjoy three delicious meals and two optional snacks (you may not need the snacks because fat cuts your hunger). Whether you're a novice in the kitchen or a gourmet chef, you'll find lots of recipes in Chapter 16 to satisfy your belly and delight your taste buds. I'll also give you easy guidelines for preparing ultra-simple meals, as well as for eating out successfully. To round out this aspect of the program, you'll also take the daily supplements I recommend getting in Stage 1.

- **Energize.** The best way to create energy, paradoxically, is to spend it. Moving your body, no matter your fitness level, is good for your mind, body, and soul. On pages 225 to 226, I'll give you specific advice and guidelines for exercise on this program to optimize your results.

- **Rejuvenate.** Two things can quickly sabotage your efforts at getting healthy and losing weight: stress without a way of discharging or releasing it, and inadequate sleep. The cornerstones of a life full of energy, joy, health, and pleasure are good food, movement, relaxation (de-stressing), and sleep. The last two can't be neglected. Stress literally programs you to gain weight and get sick. It causes your body to produce the hormone cortisol, which drives belly fat storage, sugar cravings, and emotional eating. And lack of sleep, or poor-quality sleep, drives the hormones that make you hungry and make you store fat. In Chapter 13, I'll give you strategies for keeping the stress in check and getting good sleep.

STAGE 3: YOUR TRANSITION PLAN

After the twenty-one days, I'll lay out three paths for you to choose from, so you can sustain your lifelong journey of health, happiness, and freedom from fat fear.

Depending on the state of your health, you can continue on the *Eat Fat, Get Thin* Plan until you reach your goals (weight loss, health, etc.). You may want to lose a hundred pounds or reverse diabetes; if so, you'll want to stay on this plan. Or you may be feeling great and have reached your ideal weight, and can transition to a way of eating for life that includes a wider variety of foods—the Pegan Diet. Some may find that the *Eat Fat, Get Thin* Plan works for them long term; others might discover they can include some grains, beans, or organic dairy.

In Chapter 14, I'll give you guidelines to help you determine the best transition plan for you. But most important, you will have to continue listening carefully to your body. Do you still feel good, or is the Feel Like Crap syndrome creeping back in? Is your weight where you want it to be (or moving in the right direction), or are you starting to gain weight or put on belly fat? Listen closely.

WHAT YOU CAN EXPECT

You don't have to believe me that this program will work. You don't even have to believe the 1,000 trial participants who dropped pounds quickly and saw astonishing improvements in their health. Just try it for twenty-one days and you'll see and feel the results for yourself. Your body has a tremendous capacity to repair itself when you know how to clear out the wrong foods and feed it the right ones.

Let's get started!

12

Stage 1: Lay the Foundation

Set aside two days before you begin the *Eat Fat, Get Thin* Plan to lay your foundation. During these two days, you'll get your supplies and—most important—your mind ready, so you can begin the program with confidence, knowing you're set up to succeed.

If you think back to the story I told you in Part I about how we got into this big, fat mess, you'll remember it came down to these two missteps: first, we were spooked into taking out dietary fat, and second, we replaced it with high amounts of sugar, refined carbs, and fake, toxic, "non-food." (There is no such thing as junk food. There is junk, and there is food. Period.) But with the *Eat Fat, Get Thin* Plan, we're going to undo those two steps so that you can reclaim your health, easily shed pounds, and revitalize how you look and feel on every level.

MAKE OVER YOUR KITCHEN

The standard American kitchen is a scary place that has been hijacked by the food industry. Unfortunately most Americans don't eat food anymore. They eat factory-made, industrially produced food-like substances (Frankenfoods), which are full of disease-causing trans fats, high-fructose corn syrup, MSG (monosodium glutamate), artificial sweeteners, colors, additives, preservatives, pesticides, antibiotics, and novel food proteins and allergens from genetic breeding and genetic engineering. We call these "anti-nutrients" because they literally rob our bodies of the nutrients we need to survive and thrive.

The Ingredients Game

All industrial food contains all the same processed ingredients — high-fructose corn syrup, flour, salt, hydrogenated fats, MSG, colors, additives, and preservatives — all squeezed into injected molded inventions of different colors, shapes, and textures, but all containing nearly the same ingredient list. If you covered the front of packages of factory-made foods and just looked at the labels, you would have a hard time telling what they were — you couldn't tell if they were Pop-Tarts or Pizza Stuffers. This should make you stop and think!

Should we really be putting this in our bodies? The National Institutes of Health spends $800 million a year trying to discover the cause of obesity. Hmm. Could it be that the average American every year consumes 29 pounds of French fries, 23 pounds of pizza, 24 pounds of ice cream, 57 gallons of soda, 24 pounds of artificial sweeteners, 2.7 pounds of salt, 90,000 milligrams of caffeine, or 2,700 calories every day? We consume about 152 pounds of sugar, 146 pounds of white flour, and 600 pounds of dairy per person each year in the US. Doesn't seem like any great mystery to me why we're in an obesity crisis!

We think of these of foods as "convenience" foods. But how convenient is it to be depressed, overweight, and tired, or to have to take multiple medications for lifestyle diseases like heart disease, depression, and reflux? How convenient is it to lose between seven and fourteen years off your life span simply because of what you're eating?

I've got to hand it to the food industry: They're clever. They artfully and intentionally muscled their way into our homes by encouraging us to "outsource" our food and cooking. That sounds like a tempting way to save time and energy, but that approach has led to a cascade of problems. When food is cooked in a factory, it is generally devoid of nutrients, fiber, or real taste, and full of sugar, fat, salt, and calories. We have now raised at least two generations of children who don't know how to cook a meal from scratch from real ingredients and who spend more time watching cooking on television than actually cooking.

These foods have hijacked our taste buds and brain chemistry. Did you know that sugar and processed foods have been shown to be eight times more addictive than cocaine? They have taken over our bodies, minds, and souls.

The good news is that a life of abundance and vitality is right around the corner—in fact, it is right in your own kitchen. Health is the most basic human right, and it has been taken from us. It's time to take it back, and *Eat Fat, Get Thin* will show you how. We have been convinced that it is time-consuming, expensive, and difficult to eat well. But I'm here to tell you that enjoying real, fresh, whole food is easy, inexpensive, and delicious and will put you on the path to health and happiness.

The *Eat Fat, Get Thin* Plan is not a diet. It is a way of living and eating that celebrates real, whole foods. It's about fun, pleasure, deliciousness, and joy, not deprivation or suffering. We want to wake up every morning feeling good and enjoying life. The *Eat Fat, Get Thin* Plan will give you that, and more.

Cooking Our Way to Health

Time and money are the biggest perceived obstacles to eating well. Neither is real. We have bought into insidious marketing messages like "You deserve a break today." Give us a break!!

Americans spend eight hours a day in front of a screen. We each spend an average of two hours a day on the Internet—something we've somehow found time for that didn't even exist in common usage 20 years ago. What's missing isn't the time to cook, but the education, basic skills, knowledge, and confidence. When you don't know what to buy, or how to cook a vegetable, how can you feed yourself or your family? One family I met, whom you'll read about in a moment, taught me that it is not lack of desire, but the prison of food addiction, food terrorism, and lack of knowledge that holds them hostage. But there is a way out.

We have to cook our way out of our health care, environmental, and financial crisis. We have abdicated one of the essential acts that makes us human—cooking—to the food industry. Making our own food is essentially a political act that allows us to take back our power. We have become food consumers, not food producers or makers, and in so doing we have lost our connection to our world and ourselves. Michael Pollan in his book *Cooked* says, "The decline of everyday home cooking doesn't only damage the health of our bodies and our land but also our families, our communities and our sense of how our eating connects us to the world."

Cooking is fun, freeing, and the most real activity we can do every day. It is a revolutionary act—one that each one of us has the ability to be a part of. As a physician I am deeply concerned about our fat and sick nation, and about our children's and your children's future. The best medicine for this ailment is something so simple, so easy, so healing, so affordable and accessible to almost everyone: cooking *real food,* in your home, with family and friends. And that's a big part of what you'll learn to do in *Eat Fat, Get Thin*.

In Part IV, I'll share the basic, easy tips for learning how to prepare healthful meals at home, as well as a myriad of delicious recipes that anyone—yes, *anyone*—can make.

Your Kitchen Makeover

The first few days of this program are key as you allow your body to detox from all the processed foods, gluten, dairy, sweeteners, and other food-like substances that contribute to insulin resistance, weight gain, poor health, and just generally feeling crappy. You'll be able to break the addiction cycle and halt your cravings. Why not stack the odds in your favor by removing the items that have kept you trapped, sick, and miserable? Or, to put that a better way: Why not set yourself up for optimal success by making your kitchen a happy, hopeful place filled only with vibrant, real, whole foods that will nourish your body and genuinely feed your soul?

Set aside a few hours during this stage to detox your kitchen of the items in the list below. Don't just tuck these away—toss them in the garbage! If you have a moment of panic, rest assured: we're going to quickly and easily replace them with delicious, healthy alternatives that will leave you more than satisfied. These are the absolute "must-go" non-foods for now (you will be able to add back some sugar from this list after the twenty-one days, but all the rest should really not be eaten by humans or other living things):

- **All fake foods.** By "fake food," I mean anything that is not whole, real, and fresh. This includes anything that comes in a bag or a box (with the exception of real food like canned whole foods such as sardines or tomatoes with only water or salt). Get rid of anything that contains preservatives, additives, or dyes or that is otherwise processed in any way. Ditch the processed snack foods, frozen dinners, and, most important, anything labeled "fat-free" or "low-fat." Anything with "natural flavors" may sound good but could contain gluten (more specifics on why we avoid gluten in the *Eat Fat, Get Thin* Plan in a moment) or even the secretion from beavers' anal glands, which is commonly used as vanilla flavor. That's right, not kidding. Look it up! If your great-great-grandmother wouldn't have it in her kitchen, then you shouldn't either. Throw it out.

- **All foods that contain sugar.** That means sugar in any form, including high-fructose corn syrup or "natural" sweeteners like honey, molasses, agave, maple syrup, coconut sugar, or organic cane juice. If you have to ask, "Is it okay?" the answer is no. If you start negotiating about sweet things you can have, whether it is stevia or raw organic coconut sugar gathered by an indigenous shaman and blessed by the pope, the answer is still no!

- **Any drinks that contain sugar.** This includes fruit juice (even if unsweetened), sweetened teas, coffees, sports drinks, and energy drinks. Juice boxes are presented as healthy kids' drinks, and orange juice is considered healthy, but fruit juice is very high in sugar and doesn't have the fiber that makes eating whole fruit fine. You wouldn't eat five apples at once, but you can easily drink them. It's a lot of sugar. Stick to water with lemon juice. After twenty-one days, you can add back in whole-food, low-sugar drinks such as green juices (without a lot of fruit), coconut water, or cold-pressed watermelon water with no added sugar.

- **Anything containing artificial sweeteners.** This includes aspartame, saccharin, sorbitol, xylitol, and basically any other chemical sweetener. If it comes in a blue, pink, or yellow packet—or any packet at all, for that matter—toss it. Artificial sweeteners have been linked to obesity and diabetes and even shown to alter your gut bacteria. Even stevia or other "natural" low- or no-calorie sweeteners need to go. These can all trigger cravings for more sugar and carbs, and we are trying to shut off that cycle. Eventually you can add a bit of stevia if you tolerate it, but not for the first twenty-one days.
- **Anything containing hydrogenated oils or refined vegetable oils** (like corn or soybean oil). As you now know, these oils contain inflammatory omega-6 fats, which we want to avoid. You will be getting plenty of omega-6 fats in nuts and seeds, animal foods, and even olive oil, but you want to avoid all those oils made in a factory. Olive oil, extra virgin coconut oil, ghee, or grass-fed butter will be your healthy oils of choice during this program, as they contain the good fats that promote weight loss and optimal health.

While it may be tempting to say, "Oh, I'll be fine...I'll just avoid those things that aren't part of this program," I strongly encourage you not to skip this very important step!

Other Foods to Avoid

For the next twenty-one days, to facilitate the detox and healing process and maximize the benefits of the good fats you'll be eating, you'll also be refraining from all gluten products, dairy products (except grass-fed butter or ghee), grains, and beans. Dairy (except grass-fed or clarified butter), gluten, and grains (such as rice, quinoa, millet, etc.) most commonly cause food sensitivities and the resulting inflammation. Inflammation is the root cause of almost all chronic ailments and diseases, from asthma and allergies to heart disease, type 2 diabetes, and even cancer, depression, and autism. Beans also contain inflammatory compounds and are not ideal for blood sugar issues because they are high in starch. As you'll read about in Chapter 14, after the twenty-one days you can reintroduce these foods if you wish, after you've given your gut a chance to heal.

If you would prefer not to completely remove these from your kitchen, simply put them out of sight during the plan. One exception: If you have nonorganic dairy, chuck it! It is full of hormones, antibiotics, and inflammatory compounds. If you have refined flours like wheat flour or rice flour, you probably don't want to keep those either. You may choose to reintroduce some of these in Stage 3, which we'll talk more about in Chapter 14.

If you're reading this list of items and feeling a little panicky, you're not alone. I've met and worked with thousands of people just like you who were convinced they could never give up sweets, processed snacks, soda, and the like. But I promise you: It's far easier than you imagine.

> EFGT is an awesome program! I never imagined how big a difference I would see in a mere three weeks and how much better I feel. Yesterday I even passed up dessert easily and without regret! Thank you for giving me the tools to make the changes I needed in life and for my health!
>
> — Pamela Barrett

I've scientifically designed this program to ensure your success. Remember, dietary fat is the ultimate cravings killer. It keeps your blood sugar balanced longer and prevents spikes and swings, and more recent research maps its effect on the brain's craving, addiction, and habit-forming centers. While sugar stimulates cravings and addiction, fat stops them. Cold!

Can I Drink Coffee?

Java lovers rejoice: coffee is allowed on the *Eat Fat, Get Thin* Plan. You can have up to two cups a day (about 150 milligrams of caffeine). In some studies, coffee has been shown to improve blood sugar, most likely because of all the antioxidants it contains. If you like milk in your coffee, don't despair; you're going to discover the magic of coffee blended with grass-fed butter or coconut oil on this program, and you'll never look back. You'll also find recipes for delicious homemade nut milks in Part IV. You don't *have to* drink coffee or caffeine on this program; in fact, some people are slow metabolizers of caffeine, which makes them intolerant of coffee. There are genetics tests to find out, but if it makes you anxious or disrupts your sleep, then best avoid it. But if not, consider it a treat.

One Family's Kitchen Revolution

If you're feeling nervous or unsure about whether you can tackle your kitchen (and cooking...and eating...) overhaul, let me put your mind at ease and share a story with you. I promise, if this family can take back their kitchen, their health, and their waistlines, so can you!

I had the remarkable opportunity to visit a very sick, overweight family in South Carolina (one of the worst food deserts in America) as part of the filming of the movie *Fed Up,* the movie the food industry doesn't want you to see. (If you haven't seen it, watch it on Netflix or iTunes!) It helped me understand the sad state of the standard American kitchen and how a simple makeover and easy cooking lessons could make a crucial difference between health and the real risk of death.

When I met this family in 2013, they were a family in crisis. Their list of difficulties was a long one: morbid obesity, pre-diabetes, renal failure, disability, financial stress, and hopelessness about how they could dig themselves out of their scary downward spiral—a spiral that is affecting more than 150 million Americans (including tens of millions of children) who struggle with the physical, social, and financial burden of obesity and its complications.

The costs of obesity and its related diseases are staggering. By the year 2040, 100 percent of our federal budget will be needed to pay for Medicare and Medicaid. Our poor diet makes our kids sicker (more obesity, ADHD, asthma, etc.), and this contributes to an "achievement gap" (they are too fat and sick to learn)[1] that limits our capacity to compete in the global marketplace.[2] Seventy percent of our kids are too fat or unfit to serve in the military, threatening our national security. These are not small problems. They greatly threaten our future.

The mother, the father, and their sixteen-year-old son were all morbidly obese. Their three other sons were "skinny fat," not overweight; even though the junk food didn't make them fat, it made them sick. The eldest was 47 percent body fat and his belly was 58 percent fat (normal for a man is 10 to 20 percent body fat). His insulin levels were sky-high, and these drove his relentless sugar cravings and food addiction and promoted storage of more and more belly fat. His life expectancy was 13 years less than kids of normal weight, and he was twice as likely to die by the age of fifty-five years old as his thin friends.

His parents were no better off. At forty-two, his father had renal failure from complications of obesity. He couldn't get the kidney transplant he needed to save his life until he lost forty pounds, and he had no clue how to lose the weight. His mother was more than 100 pounds overweight and on medication for high blood pressure. The whole family was at serious risk.

They desperately wanted to find a way out but didn't have the knowledge or skills to escape from the food industry. They were trapped in a cycle of food addiction. They blamed themselves for their failure, but it was clear they were the victims, not the perpetrators.

When I asked them what motivated them to change, the tears started to flow and the father said he didn't want to die and leave his wife and four boys. His youngest son was only seven years old. A powerful motivator if I've ever heard one.

We started in the easiest place possible to dig this family out of the mess they were in: their kitchen.

Not one member of this knew how to cook real food. They didn't know how to navigate a grocery aisle, shop for food, or read a label. Like so many Americans, they had been hoodwinked by the "health claims" on packaged, processed foods that made them fat and sick, including "low-fat," "diet," "zero trans fats," and "whole grain." Whole-grain Pop-Tarts? Zero trans fats in Cool Whip? All the fat is trans fat, but since the serving size is small, and the food lobby forced Congress to permit them to label the "food" as having zero trans fat if it has less than 0.5 grams per serving, *they can legally state such nonsense.* The family didn't know that chicken nuggets have twenty-five or more ingredients, and only one of them is chicken.

They grew up in homes where food was either fried or eaten out of a box or can. Everything was premade in a factory. They only knew about two vegetables: boiled cabbage and canned green beans. Their kitchen didn't have basic cooking implements, such as a sharp knife or even a cutting board. They existed on food stamps and disability; about half of the

$1,000 they spent per month on food went to eating out in fast-food places.

The grandmother had a garden, but the mother never learned how to grow food, even though they live in a beautiful, temperate rural area. When I met her, she didn't know how to chop a vegetable or sauté it. I realized that the best way to help them was not to shame or judge them, not to prescribe more medication or tell them to eat less and exercise more (a subtle way of blaming them), but to teach them to cook real food from scratch, good food on a tight budget, to show them they could eat well for less.

We got the whole family washing, peeling, chopping, and cooking real food—onions, garlic, carrots, sweet potatoes, cucumbers, tomatoes, salad greens. To my surprise, the mother pulled a bunch of fresh asparagus from her fridge (which I suspect she got when she found out I was coming to their home), remarking that she hated asparagus. "Once I had asparagus out of can; it was nasty," she said. "But then a friend told me to try one off the grill, and even though I didn't want to, I tried it and it was good."

I showed her and her kids how to snap asparagus to get rid of the chewy parts and how to sauté it in olive oil and garlic. They learned how to roast sweet potatoes with fennel and olive oil, and how to make turkey chili from scratch. They even made fresh salad dressing from olive oil, vinegar, mustard, salt, and pepper, instead of using gummy bottled dressings laden with high-fructose corn syrup, refined oil, and MSG.

As we were cooking, the boys came running into the kitchen, lured away from their Xbox by the sweet, warm smells of chili and roasted sweet potatoes, smells they had never had in their kitchen. They all happily ate the food and were surprised at how delicious and filling it was.

After a happy, satisfying, healing meal of real food, cooked in less time and for less money than it would take for them to drive to Denny's and order deep-fried chicken nuggets, biscuits, gravy, and canned green beans, the son, who struggled to get healthy against all odds, who wanted to go to medical school, who wanted to help his family, said in disbelief, "Dr. Hyman, do you eat real food like this with your family *every night*?" I assured him I did.

I left to go home amidst tears of relief, of hope for a different future for this family. Five days later, the mother texted me that the family had lost eighteen pounds all together and was making chili again from scratch. She went on to lose a hundred pounds and got off her blood pressure medication. The father lost forty-five pounds and was able to get a new kidney, and the eldest son lost fifty pounds. (Sadly, he gained those pounds back, and more, when he went to work at Bojangles'. As he said, it was like putting an alcoholic to work in a bar. But he soon got back on track.)

So you see: We can end this mess one kitchen, one meal at a time.

TACKLE YOUR FEAR OF FAT

Recently, we had a guest at our house. She came into the kitchen to say hello just as I was about to make myself a Bulletproof Coffee, a special drink created by my friend Dave Asprey that contains coffee blended with grass-fed butter and MCT oil (see page 267). I offered to make her one and she looked at me a bit horrified and said, "Isn't that fattening?"

Chances are, before reading this book you might have said (or thought) the exact same thing. And even now, after learning the truth about dietary fat, you may still be skeptical about eating "fattening" things like butter, nuts, coconut or olive oil, and generous helpings of avocado after so many decades of having the fat-free mantra drilled into you. I know that once you make the leap and try this program, you'll be convinced, but for now, we want to root out any of the mental obstacles that could potentially stand in the way of your success.

Set aside some time during the two days of the foundation stage to journal your responses to the following questions. It's important to actually write down your responses, rather than just answering mentally. The act of writing holds you accountable and will also allow you to look back at the end of the program to see how far you've come.

- What do I believe to be true about eating fat?
- How did I feel reading the story about how we, as a culture, came to shun fat and embrace processed foods?

- What is my history or current relationship with "fat-free" foods?
- How has eating these foods made me feel in the past?
- What worries or fears do I have about including fat in my diet?
- How can I address those worries or fears?
- Why am I doing this program?
- What three goals do I have for myself over the next twenty-one days?

STOCK YOUR TOOLBOX

Here are the supplies you'll want to gather before beginning the program:

The Right Foods

Now that you've rid your kitchen of toxic, inflammatory foods, let's restock it with the good stuff! The following is a list of basic staples you'll want to get so that you can make the recipes included in the plan and prepare basic meals according to the guidelines in Part IV:

- Extra virgin olive oil
- Extra virgin coconut oil
- Sea salt
- Black pepper
- Detoxifying and anti-inflammatory herbs and spices (ginger, turmeric, cinnamon, cayenne pepper, thyme, rosemary, cumin, sage, oregano, coriander, cilantro, paprika, and parsley)
- Nuts (walnuts, pecans, almonds, macadamia nuts, cashews, etc.; no peanuts)
- Seeds (hemp, chia, flax, pumpkin, sesame)
- Unsweetened almond or hemp milk, or homemade coconut milk (see pages 273 to 274 for recipes for homemade milks)
- Grass-fed butter or ghee
- High-quality coffee (if you drink coffee)

You'll be choosing breakfast, lunch, dinner, and snack options from the recipes in Part IV. I strongly encourage you to plan out your meals in advance, so you don't get caught hungry and scrambling to get what you need. Map out one week's worth of meals at a time and shop in advance for those meals. The worst thing that can happen to you is to find yourself in a food emergency. Planning what you are going to have or where you will be for breakfast, lunch, and dinner is key to your success.

You'll notice that I did not create a day-by-day meal plan for this program, and that was intentional. My goal is not only to help you reset your metabolism and reprogram your genes for weight loss and health, but also to give you guidelines for how you can continue to do that on your own for the rest of your life. I want to empower you to know how to choose the right foods to fuel your body, beginning with these twenty-one days. But don't worry—I'll be giving you lots of clear direction, guidelines, and tips to help you do that. I'm here to help you succeed!

Supplements

Though you will be fueling your body with real food packed with vitamins and minerals, you'll still need additional nutrients to help your body burn calories efficiently, regulate appetite, cool inflammation, optimize your gut flora, and help your cells become more insulin-sensitive.

If you eat only wild food that you hunt and gather, drink pure clean water, breathe clean air, have no chronic stress, are exposed to no environmental toxins, and sleep nine hours a night, you don't need vitamins, but the rest of us do. Ninety percent of Americans are deficient in one or more nutrients, even if we eat a healthy diet. Our soils are depleted; whole foods are hybridized (which reduces their nutrient density) and grown with artificial fertilizers, then transported over long distances and stored for long periods of time. Or they are highly processed, which further depletes their nutritional value. Everyone needs at the very least a good multivitamin and mineral, fish oil, vitamin D supplements, and ideally probiotics. Many also need magnesium, the relaxation mineral.

That is why I recommend the following basic supplements to optimize your body's fat-burning and repair mechanisms. You can purchase these as a simple twice-a-day packet for ease and convenience at www.eatfatgetthin.com (if you choose to order these, make sure to do so one week before beginning the program, to allow for shipping time), or purchase them at your local health food store. But be cautious about which brands and products you pick. You can also find sources for the hard-to-get components of this program such as MCT oil or electrolytes at www.eatfatgetthin.com. You want to use brands that are free from contaminants, fillers, and allergens like gluten, which was recently found in many probiotics.

Your daily supplements should include:

- A high-quality **multivitamin and multimineral** supplement. This contains all the B vitamins, antioxidants, and minerals you need to optimize your metabolism, blood sugar, and insulin functioning.
- 2 grams of purified **fish oil** (EPA/DHA), an anti-inflammatory, insulin-sensitizing, blood-sugar-balancing, heart-disease-preventing, brain-boosting supplement.
- 2,000 units of **vitamin D_3**, which helps insulin function. Up to 80 percent of the population is deficient in this important vitamin (take this is in addition to what's in your multivitamin).
- 300 to 400 milligrams of **L-carnitine** twice a day. Carnitine helps transport fat into your cells so you can burn fat more effectively, and boosts your metabolism.
- 30 milligrams of **coenzyme Q10** twice a day. Coenzyme Q10 is a critical nutrient for turning food into energy inside your cells.
- 100 to 150 milligrams of **magnesium glycinate** (1 capsule twice a day). Magnesium is also the relaxation mineral and helps reduce anxiety, improve sleep, improve blood sugar control, and even cure muscle cramps. If you have constipation you may need to add magnesium citrate (see optional supplements list that follows). Also, if you have kidney problems, check with your doctor before starting magnesium.
- **PGX** (in powder or capsule form)—a superfiber that slows blood sugar and insulin spikes and can also cut cravings and promote weight loss. Take 2 to 5 grams just before every meal with a large

glass of water. This can be taken in powder form (½ to 1 scoop) or in 3 to 6 capsules; the powder form tends to work better. If you have night cravings or night eating, you can also take a dose after dinner.

- **Probiotics:** 10 to 20 billion CFU (colony forming units). Probiotics help normalize your gut flora; tending your inner garden is one of the best ways to reduce inflammation, improve digestion, and even reverse diabesity and carbohydrate intolerance.

- **MCT oil:** 1 to 2 tablespoons. You can have it in coffee or a shake or put it on salad. This is a superfat from coconut oil that speeds up your metabolism and fuels your brain.

- **Electrolytes:** 1 to 2 capfuls of E-lyte (a liquid electrolyte solution). Put 1 capful in a glass of water and drink, twice a day (so 2 glasses and 2 capfuls). This combination of electrolytes and salt helps with proper tissue hydration and will make you feel amazing. If you cut out carbs you will lose a lot of fluid and need more salt and electrolytes to keep you balanced.

- **Potato starch:** Build up to 1 to 2 tablespoons in 8 ounces (200ml) of water twice a day to help balance your blood sugar and feed the good gut bugs. Use Bob's Red Mill Unmodified Potato Starch, which is easy to find in health food stores, at Whole Foods, or online. While potato starch is technically optional on this program, I strongly recommend it.

Why Potato Starch?

You might be wondering why I would recommend potato starch when I have been railing against the evils of refined carbs. White powdery starch! Deadly, right? Well, there is a special type of starch called *resistant starch* that has some unique properties, including improving your metabolism, insulin sensitivity, and blood sugar; increasing fat burning and reducing fat storage in your cells; and even optimizing your gut flora[3] in a way that helps promote weight loss.[4]

Resistant starch is not digested in the small intestine — at least not by you. It is digested only by the bacteria in your gut. When you eat resistant starch, it "resists" digestion and doesn't spike blood sugar or insulin.

Resistant starch is a *prebiotic*. Think of it as compost or fertilizer for your healthy gut bacteria. This sea of bacteria — more than ten times the number of your own cells and about three pounds' worth — is not just waste. It is profoundly connected to almost every part of your health. Imbalances in your gut flora have been linked to a whole host of diseases, including obesity,[5] diabetes, heart disease, autoimmune disease, inflammatory bowel diseases, cancer, depression,[6] anxiety, and autism.[7]

One of the best ways to get your gut back in balance is to give the bugs good food in the form of prebiotics. This food can come in many forms, including inulin (not insulin) from chicory or Jerusalem artichokes, soluble fiber from psyllium, or starch from high-amylose plants such as potatoes, green bananas, and plantains. Cooking then cooling starches like potatoes or rice and not reheating them all the way can also transform regular starch in rice or potatoes to resistant starch.

When resistant starch gets to your gut, it stimulates the growth of beneficial bugs that crowd out the bad bugs. They produce short-chain fatty acids that are fuel for colon cells — one in particular called butyrate can prevent cancer, speed up your metabolism, and reduce inflammation.[8]

Resistant starch can also improve insulin sensitivity[9] and help reduce your blood sugar after meals.[10] In other words, it helps reverse diabesity.[11] In fact, in one study, 15 to 30 grams (about 2 to 4 tablespoons) of potato starch improved insulin sensitivity in obese men as much as losing 10 percent of their body weight would![12]

It has other benefits as well: helping with weight loss, reducing insulin spikes after eating, increasing fat burning, and reducing fat storage in your cells.[13] It changes the gut bacteria in ways that promote health and weight loss. We know that you can reverse diabetes by taking the fecal matter of a thin healthy person and putting it in a diabetic. I would say that eating potato starch is more appealing to most of us than getting a fecal transplant![14]

(Continued)

The best way to add in resistant starch if you are on a low-carbohydrate diet like the *Eat Fat, Get Thin* Plan is to use Bob's Red Mill Unmodified Potato Starch (not potato flour). It has about 8 grams of resistant starch per tablespoon. You can also use plantain flour and banana flour. Potato starch is well tolerated and mixes well with water and tastes just a little like potatoes. Not so bad. It can help you sleep at night. It can also be included in smoothies or mixed in almond milk (but it should not be heated).

Resistant starch can initially cause gas because the good and bad bugs are duking it out. Start small — with ¼ teaspoon at night — and slowly increase to give your body a chance to get used to it. If you have a *lot* of gas or gut discomfort, it probably means you have small intestinal bacterial overgrowth (SIBO) or yeast overgrowth and need treatment by a Functional Medicine doctor to fix your gut. If you want to know more about how to tend your inner garden and fix your digestive symptoms, please download the special free e-book called *Beyond Food: Other Causes of Obesity and Damaged Metabolism* at www.eatfatgetthin.com.

Here is a list of optional supplements to help relieve symptoms:

- **Digestive enzymes:** 1 to 2 capsules with each meal. Good digestion is critical to good health. As you transition your diet, you may need help digesting a higher-fat diet and a higher-fiber diet. They also can reduce inflammation.
- **Magnesium citrate:** 150-milligram capsules or tablets, 2 to 3 twice a day. This is essential if you have constipation, which can be caused by extra fiber such as PGX. If you don't have a bowel movement once or twice a day, you may feel ill on this program, so be sure to pay attention to how often you are eliminating and do what's needed to enable you to go every day (see page 232 for troubleshooting if constipation becomes a problem).
- **LaxaBlend** (an herbal laxative): 2 to 3 capsules at night if you haven't had a bowel movement in a day or feel constipated.

■ **Buffered ascorbic acid:** 500 mg capsules, 2 to 4 capsules twice a
  day to help with detoxification and constipation (see pages 230 to
  231 for more tips on easing detox symptoms)

For an easy-reference chart of all the daily supplements and dos-
ages, please see pages 347 to 348 in the Resources section as well as
www.eatfatgetthin.com.

PGX: The Wonder Fiber

Most Americans don't eat enough fiber. We have gone from eating almost
100 grams a day as hunter-gatherers to eating 8 to 15 grams a day or less on
a processed-food diet. Fiber helps fertilize the good bacteria in your gut,
improve your bowel movements, and prevent cancer and heart disease.
But it also helps you lose weight. A special superfiber called PGX (polygly-
coplex) has been extensively researched over the past few years.[15, 16, 17] A
combination of konjac root (glucomannan) and seaweed fibers, it slows the
rate at which sugar (and fat) is absorbed into the bloodstream, and it has
the overall effect of balancing blood sugar and insulin, reducing appetite,
and helping with weight loss.

One of my diabetic patients got off 100 units of insulin just by using this
special fiber, and another lost forty pounds. That is why I recommend taking PGX before every meal during the program. If you choose to use only
one supplement, PGX is the most important for the program.

Please note: To ensure that the fiber moves through your system the
way it's meant to, it is essential to drink the recommended eight glasses of
water each day. Otherwise, you can get constipated. If you tend toward
constipation, please see page 232 to learn how to safely clean out your
bowels and stay ahead of this problem.

Fitness Gear

If you've read any of my other books or my blog or seen me on television, you've likely heard me say, "You can't exercise your way out of a
bad diet." It's really true. No amount of exercise can undo the harmful

effects of a fat-deficient, processed, and otherwise bad diet. You'd have to walk four and a half miles to burn off one can of soda. But that doesn't mean that exercise is not critical to a healthy, well-functioning metabolism and long-term health and well-being. On this program, you'll be eating the optimal diet to repair your health and reset your metabolism, and exercise can go a long way toward enhancing that.

One of the biggest deterrents to exercise isn't a lack of motivation— it's a lack of organization. When you make it easy for yourself to get up and out the door to exercise, you're far more likely to do it. Scrambling around trying to find the right shoes, the right clothes, or even the right time of day to fit it in throws up unnecessary roadblocks where they don't need to be. Use these two days of the foundation stage to organize what you need to get going. For instance, a good pair of sneakers, hand weights, comfortable workout clothes, motivating music downloaded onto your smartphone, and so on.

Equally important, schedule exercise into your days. For the next twenty-one days, carve out a minimum of thirty minutes each day to exercise. (Yes, every day!) Plan for it, the same as you would plan for anything else important in your life. Create an appointment with yourself in your calendar. It is as important as any meeting or deadline. I work with very busy and successful people, and they always make time to work out. Personally I don't watch TV because there are too many other fun things to do. I mean, how much time do you spend on Facebook or social media? We somehow spend seven to eight hours a day on our screens; I have to imagine we could find thirty minutes somewhere in there to move our bodies. Because, really, what's more important than your health?

Water Filter and Bottle

It is essential to drink at least eight glasses of clean, pure water each day to aid the detox process and keep your bowels functioning well. Having the right tools on hand will make daily hydration an easy habit. I recommend getting a simple carbon filter, like Brita, and pouring filtered water into a stainless steel or glass bottle to carry with you at all times. You can purchase a filter and bottle at most home supplies stores or the supermarket.

Eat Fat, Get Thin *Journal*

Your journal will be your constant companion throughout the twenty-one days. Purchase a blank notebook or journal that appeals to you so that you can record your results, thoughts, and experiences. Or you can use the online journal at www.eatfatgetthin.com.

CHECK YOUR NUMBERS

It's important to take measurements and get your numbers checked before you begin and when you've completed the program. I want you to be able to see the hard numbers and facts of your transformation!

Take Your Measurements

Take the following measurements the day before you start the program and record them in your journal (or go to www.eatfatgetthin.com to find our online health-tracking tools):

- Your weight. Weigh yourself first thing in the morning without clothes and after going to the bathroom.
- Your height. Measure it in feet and inches.
- Your waist size. Using a tape measure, find the widest point around your belly button, not where your belt is.
- Your hip size. Again using a tape measure, find the widest point around your hips.
- Your thigh circumference. Measure the widest point around each of your thighs.
- Blood pressure. This can be done by your doctor or at the drugstore, or buy a home blood pressure cuff (go to www.eatfatgetthin.com).

Also, be sure to fill out the FLC Quiz on pages 22 to 24. And if you are planning to have your cholesterol profile or basic lab testing done (which I strongly encourage you to do), now is the time. See below for the specific tests you should have done. Seeing your test results before and after you do the program can be a powerful motivator.

Test Your Blood Sugar

Many people think you need to check your blood sugar only if you are diabetic. Not so. While it's optional, I think measuring your blood sugar before, during, and after this program is a simple, great way for you to see how your body responds to what you eat. It will give you immediate and direct feedback about how dramatically and quickly your body responds to the right information in diet and lifestyle.

Some of you may already have a glucose meter and know how to test your blood sugar. Others may want to get a meter at their local drugstore. The newer ones are easy to use, and you can always ask your pharmacist to show you how. I like the ACCU-CHEK Aviva blood glucose meter with strips (this comes with a few test strips; you may need extra) or the FreeStyle Freedom Lite (you will also need extra test strips).

Here is the protocol I recommend for testing:

Measure your fasting blood sugar daily, first thing in the morning before breakfast. Ideally, your fasting blood sugar should be between 70 and 80 mg/dl.

Measure your blood sugar two hours after breakfast and two hours after dinner. Ideally, your two-hour sugars should never go over 120 mg/dl. If they go over 140 mg/dl, you have pre-diabetes. If they go over 200 mg/dl, you have type 2 diabetes. Technically, these measures are the ones we use after a 75-gram glucose load, but if your sugars go this high on the plan, you definitely have a problem. Pay attention to how they change depending on what you eat.

Get Tested by Your Doctor

Again, this is optional, but I encourage you to consider getting basic lab tests done before and after the program. These lab tests can be done through your doctor or at most hospitals or laboratories, or you can order them through personal testing companies such as SaveOnLabs (www .saveonlabs.com). For more information and detailed explanations for each of these tests, go to www.eatfatgetthin.com. There you can find my free e-book *How to Work with Your Doctor to Get What You Need*.

The tests I recommend include:

- **Insulin response test,** which is like a two-hour glucose tolerance test but measures insulin as well. It is done by measuring both insulin and glucose after fasting and one and two hours after a 75-gram glucose drink.
- **Hemoglobin A1c,** which measures your average blood sugar over the past six weeks. Anything 5.5 percent or above is considered elevated; over 6.0 percent is diabetes.
- **NMR lipid or the Cardio IQ test** (cholesterol) profile, which measures LDL, HDL, and triglycerides, and the particle number and particle size of each type of cholesterol and triglycerides (which is also important because big, large triglycerides are bad—the opposite of the HDL and LDL particles, which are better when large). This is a newer test, but I would demand it from your doctor, because the typical cholesterol tests done by most labs and doctors are out of date. These tests can be obtained only through LabCorp or Quest Diagnostics.
  - Total cholesterol—ideally under 200 mg/dl, but this matters less than the overall profile. If your total cholesterol is 300 mg/dl and your HDL is 100 mg/dl, that is much better than a total cholesterol of 150 mg/dl and an HDL of 30 mg/dl.
  - LDL cholesterol—ideally under 100 mg/dl but more important is the total particle number, which should be under 1,000, and the small LDL particle number, which should be less than 400 (or even lower).
  - HDL cholesterol—ideally over 50 mg/dl for men and over 60 mg/dl for women (although I think both men and women should be over 60 mg/dl).
  - Triglycerides—ideally less than 100 mg/dl or even under 70 mg/dl. And you want the small, not the large version of the triglycerides.
  - Total cholesterol to HDL ratio less than 3:1.
  - Triglyceride to HDL ratio less than 2:1, or ideally 1:1 (if it is over 3:1 you almost certainly have carbohydrate intolerance).

DNA Diet Testing

This exclusive panel of tests helps you identify genetic tendencies that may affect your ability to lose weight and get healthy. Depending on the results, you can create a customized approach to optimizing your metabolism. You might do better on a higher- or lower-fat diet, or you might have a tendency toward insulin resistance or sugar addiction. You can order a simple saliva test at www.eatfatgetthin.com, and also find a customized guide of recommendations to turn on your unique disease-preventing and weight loss genes and turn off your unique disease-promoting and weight gain genes.

Part of what you're doing over these twenty-one days is becoming an active partner in your health and weight loss, and that includes having a full understanding of your numbers and following them over time. I believe everyone should become empowered to learn about their bodies, interpret their test results, and use that information to track their progress.

JOIN THE *EAT FAT, GET THIN* ONLINE COMMUNITY

Losing weight and getting healthy are social activities. You *can* do the program alone, but if you find a buddy, join or create a group, or join our online community at www.eatfatgetthin.com, you will not only find support for your journey and friends on the path to help if you have questions or get discouraged; you will get twice the results.

I encourage you to join the *Eat Fat, Get Thin* Online Course at www.eatfatgetthin.com to get all the tools you need and connect with a community online to get daily support.

I am also a strong proponent of life coaching to help you get out of your own way. I have used it successfully for many years to help me grow and change behaviors that prevented me from thriving. My favorite life-coaching group is the Handel Group (www.handel group.com). You can access all these resources at www.eatfatgetthin .com.

BE SURE TO CHECK IN WITH YOUR DOCTOR

One note of caution for you before you get started: The program works so well that your blood sugar and blood pressure can drop dramatically in just a day or two. If you are on medication or insulin, you must carefully monitor your blood pressure and blood sugar and reduce your dose of medication in partnership with your doctor to make sure you don't get into trouble. Having your blood sugar or blood pressure run a little high for a week poses almost no danger (if your sugars are under 300 mg/dl and your blood pressure is under 150/100), but rapid drops in blood sugar or blood pressure can be life threatening. If you are taking insulin or oral hypoglycemic medication, you need to be especially careful, as your blood sugar can drop dramatically. So please be sure to talk with your health care provider before embarking on this journey.

> I still cannot believe how quickly I could stop taking my drugs; my blood sugar and pressure numbers were actually lower than when I was taking them. It was just like a miracle for me....I have my health back with NO drugs!
>
> —Joanne Schwien

CHECKLIST FOR STAGE 1:

- Do your kitchen makeover and throw out the bad stuff.
- Stock your pantry and fridge with the essentials listed on page 199.
- Write your answers to the journal questions on pages 198 to 199 to tackle your fear of fat.
- Read Chapter 15 and choose your meals for Days 1 to 7 to shop accordingly.
- Purchase your supplements.
- Organize your fitness apparel and any needed gear.
- Purchase a water filter and water bottle.
- Take all your body measurements and write them down in your journal (weight, height, waist size, hip size, blood pressure, and ideally blood sugar).
- Do any of the optional testing mentioned on pages 209 to 210.
- Check with your doctor before beginning the program.

13

Stage 2: The *Eat Fat, Get Thin* Plan

The *Eat Fat, Get Thin* Plan is simple and easy to follow. I designed it to give you a working template so you can learn the essentials of how and what to eat and what to do to maximize weight loss and optimize your health.

Each day includes the three core elements I introduced in Chapter 11:

- **Nourish:** This encompasses what you'll eat and drink and what you'll avoid, as well as which daily supplements to take.
- **Energize:** I'll talk about how much, when, and the ideal exercises to do on this program.
- **Rejuvenate:** I'll give you simple strategies to make sure you're relaxing and sleeping as well as you should.

NOURISH

You won't be counting calories, or weighing your food, or anything else that makes eating a chore. And most important, you won't feel deprived or hungry!

Here are the basic guidelines of what you should eat each day and what to avoid. Beginning on page 218, you'll find more detail about which foods in particular are optimal on this program.

What to Eat

- **Fat.** Use only good, healthy fats and clean (grass-fed or sustainably raised) animal foods (see pages 218 to 219 for a complete list). You should include at least one serving of fat at each meal. The best sources are avocados; extra virgin olive oil; nuts and seeds; extra virgin coconut oil; organic coconut milk; whole organic eggs; fatty fish such as sardines, wild salmon, mackerel, and herring; grass–fed lamb, bison, and beef; and organic poultry. You can also add MCT oil to salad dressings or smoothies. MCT oil is flavorless, so it can be used where you might not want the coconut taste from coconut oil, like on salads. A typical serving of fat is 1 tablespoon of oil, a handful of nuts or seeds, or 4 ounces (~100g) of fish or animal protein. You want to have four to five servings of fat a day. See pages 218 to 219 for a full list of your best fat options.

- **Protein.** Eat 4 to 6 (100 to 175g) ounces of protein at each meal. (See pages 220 to 221 for a complete list of the best proteins.) The average person needs about 0.68 gram per pound of body weight per day (or 1.5 grams per kilogram of body weight per day); you may need to adjust that up if you exercise vigorously or are recovering from an illness. Pay attention to how your body feels and you'll know. You can learn by experimenting and recording your observations each day. Check your hunger, energy level, cravings, and amount and quality of sleep to see how they change according to more or less protein. If you feel fatigued or sluggish, it may be a signal that you require more protein.

- **Carbohydrates.** Most of your diet should be carbohydrates. Shocking, right? I'm not talking about bagels, rice, potatoes, or cookies; I'm talking about the carbs in whole plant foods. All vegetables are carbs. Broccoli, asparagus, and green beans are all carbs. In fact, nonstarchy veggies full of vitamins, minerals, phytochemicals, and fiber should make up about 50 to 75 percent of your plate at every meal. You get unlimited refills, so fill up on these foods! Nuts and seeds contain carbs (as well as protein and fat), as does fruit.

- **Snacks (optional).** You can have up to two snacks a day, as needed. Easy snack options are a handful of raw nuts; raw veggies with almond or cashew butter, olive tapenade, or tahini; or half an avocado sprinkled with sea salt, pepper, and lime or lemon juice. In Part IV, you'll find other tasty snack recipes.

- **Salt.** When you cut down on carbs, your body needs more salt. You will lose water and salt initially and can feel tired, weak, and unable to exercise if you don't consume enough salt (1 to 2 teaspoons a day of sea salt). If you have salt-sensitive high blood pressure, simply watch your blood pressure daily and adjust the salt to help keep your blood pressure normal. This is why I suggest supplementing with electrolytes in the form of E-lyte.

- **Fruit.** You can include ½ to 1 cup (75–150g) per day of the following (but only these) fruits: berries, pomegranate seeds, watermelon (which has a very low glycemic load because it is mostly water), lemon, lime, or kiwi.

- **Bone broth.** Enjoy Dr. Hyman's Veggie-Bone Broth (1 to 2 cups a day; see the recipe, page 321) to help heal leaky gut, which results from food sensitivities, overgrowth of bad bugs, or overuse of antibiotics. Having a leaky gut allows bacterial toxins and food proteins to "leak" into your bloodstream, causing inflammation and weight gain. Bone broth also reduces inflammation and provides a rich source of minerals (calcium, magnesium, potassium, silicon, sulfur, and phosphorous) and body-building collagen and nutrients. Make enough for a week and store it in the fridge or freezer.

- **Coffee (optional).** If you enjoy coffee, 1 cup daily made from the highest-quality beans is fine. Try the Bulletproof Coffee on page 267, or simply blend 1 tablespoon of extra virgin coconut oil or ghee and 1 tablespoon of MCT oil into your coffee instead of milk or cream. This can be your breakfast, if you like, as it is high in healthy fats and will keep you satisfied for several hours. No sugar or other sweetener, please!

- **Water.** Drink a minimum of 8 glasses of pure, clean water throughout the day.

Additionally, take your daily supplements, detailed on pages 201 to 202. For a quick, easy reference guide of what to take and when, see the Resources section on pages 347 to 348 as well as www.eatfatgetthin.com.

What Is a Leaky Gut and Why Does It Matter in Weight Loss and Health?

Unfortunately, we modern humans have done many things to damage our inner gardens and promote the growth of bad bugs that cause weight gain, diabetes, cancer, heart disease, depression, and even autism.[1] First, we dramatically changed our diet from whole, unprocessed, high-fiber, low-sugar foods to a high-sugar, low-fiber diet high in processed foods and in omega-6 fat (soybean oil)[2] that harms our gut bacteria. Some evidence indicates that certain GMOs (genetically modified foods) damage our gut bacteria. We have also had a rise in Cesarean sections, which prevent the normal colonization of a baby's gut as it passes through the mother's birth canal.[3] And we have had a decrease in breastfeeding, necessary for the normal development of the gut and the gut immune system.[4] .The overuse of gut-busting drugs such as antibiotics, acid blockers, anti-inflammatories, birth control pills, hormones, and steroids has led to changes in our gut flora and damaged the lining of our guts.

This results in a leaky gut, in which bacterial products, toxins, and food proteins "leak" into your bloodstream and interact with your immune system, creating inflammation and causing insulin resistance and weight gain and even heart disease, diabetes, cancer, allergies, and autoimmune disease. Some even hypothesize that our overly hygienic, highly sanitized world (constant hand washing, avoiding dirt, and so on) negatively affects the normal immune function that results when we live more closely with bugs. Case in point: People who grow up on farms or live in developing countries have less asthma, allergies, and autoimmune disease than people who don't.[5]

Here are some tips to keep in mind for meals:

- **Breakfast.** For best results, eat only fat, protein, and/or veggies for breakfast. Toss some spinach in with your eggs, or try the Triple Green Smoothie, Bulletproof Coffee, or any of the other breakfast recipes in Part IV.
- **Lunch.** Lunch should consist of 75 percent nonstarchy veggies and 25 percent protein by volume on your plate, with fat included in dressings, olive oil, and coconut oil, and found naturally in proteins such as fatty fish, meat, or nuts and seeds (see pages 224 and 220 to 221 for veggie and protein sources).
- **Dinner.** Dinner is the same as lunch. If you like, include ½ to 1 cup (60–125g) of starchy veggies such as sweet potato, winter squash, or parsnips at dinner (see page 224 for starchy veggie sources).

What to Avoid

1. **Gluten.** In anything. It is hidden everywhere, so be sure to read labels carefully to look for hidden gluten or wheat products (see www.celiac .org to learn these hidden names and discover sources of gluten in our food). Gluten is found in wheat, rye, barley, oats, Kamut, spelt, and triticale or anything made from those products, as well as soy sauce. Even gluten-free oats are suspect because of potential contamination and cross-reactions! The best way to avoid it is to eat only whole, fresh foods and nothing made in a factory unless you are 100 percent sure it is gluten-free. Also be vigilant when you go to restaurants. There is a lot of cross-contamination in restaurant kitchens. If you are gluten sensitive, even a thimbleful of gluten can cause problems.

2. **All grains.** Avoid rice, quinoa, buckwheat, millet, and all other grains. Whole grains can be part of a healthy diet, but they are still starch and can spike blood sugar and insulin. They can also create gut problems and inflammation for some people. This isn't a forever thing—you may choose to reintroduce these after the twenty-one days—but for now, we're looking to reboot your system, and removing these grains will help heal your gut and lower insulin spikes that drive weight gain. Taking a break for twenty-one days and then reintroducing grains can help you identify how they affect you.

3. **All dairy products.** The only exceptions to this are grass-fed butter, clarified butter, and ghee, all of which are allowed in the program. If you know you have a dairy allergy or sensitivity, you may tolerate clarified butter because all the milk proteins are removed. Grass-fed butter and ghee have many antioxidants and good fats, including CLA, which boosts metabolism. Dairy is one of the most common allergens and causes significant inflammation for many. It's not the fat that causes problems; it's the proteins that trigger your immune system. That's why clarified butter and ghee are fine for most dairy-sensitive people.

4. **Beans.** Beans contain a fair amount of starch, and they aren't ideal for blood sugar balance. They also contain inflammatory compounds called lectins, and since you want to cool off inflammation, you should stop them for twenty-one days. And they aren't that easy to digest. The only exceptions to the no-bean rule are organic

non-GMO tofu or tempeh (soybeans that are broken down or fermented and easier to digest), green beans, snap peas, and snow peas.

5. **All fruit.** This is with the exception of the ones listed in the previous section, "What to Eat." Fruit is full of antioxidants and beneficial fiber and nutrients. But it can also be a source of sugar, and for those who are insulin resistant or trying to lose weight or kick sugar addiction and reset their metabolism, it can be a trigger. I have seen many people binge on fruit as a sugar substitute. Once you reset your body, you can add fruit back in moderation.

6. **Refined vegetable oils.** This includes corn, canola, soy, sunflower, safflower, and the like. These contain a lot of inflammatory omega-6 fats and toxic contaminants. Stay away forever. Extra virgin olive oil is good!

7. **Processed foods of any kind.** Nothing that contains additives, preservatives, dyes, or MSG. This includes processed meats like conventional bacon, salami, canned meats, hot dogs, and so forth. They are the only meats that have been linked to increased risk of disease. No more Spam sushi for you Hawaiians. These are out forever.

8. **Artificial sweeteners.** These have been linked to obesity, diabetes, and neurological problems. Run away from these and don't ever look back.

9. **Natural sweeteners.** Sweetness is one of life's great pleasures. But in order to reset your metabolism and unhook your brain from sugar addiction, we're going to take a short twenty-one-day break from honey, maple syrup, raw sugar, and so on. This will allow you to get into the right relationship with sweetness in your life, and then a little bit can go a long way.

> I thought giving up wine would be hard, but because my inflammation went down, it turned out I didn't need to drink to reduce pain. I canceled the physical therapy I had scheduled to resolve knee pain, because I no longer needed it! That was just as thrilling as losing 4 inches of belly fat in 3 weeks. I've known for a while that wheat and dairy are not good for me, but I didn't realize how closely related my inflammation was to consumption of these products. Now I'm more motivated to avoid these foods.
>
> —Polly Stecyk

10. **Carrageenan.** This is a "natural thickener" in nut and other plant milks, which can cause leaky gut and inflammation in the body.
11. **Alcohol.** It's really just another form of sugar.

Good Sources of Fat

Include the following healthy fats in your daily diet. Be sure to include 4 to 5 servings of fat per day. Serving sizes for each are in parentheses.

- Extra virgin coconut oil (1 tablespoon)
- Extra virgin olive oil, avocado oil, macadamia oil, walnut oil, almond oil (1 tablespoon); use these in salads or stews—they should not be used for high-heat cooking; for high-heat cooking, use coconut oil or ghee
- MCT oil (1 to 2 tablespoons a day); I like MCT oil from NuMedica
- Organic coconut milk (¼ cup/50g); Native Forest brand is my favorite—the cans are BPA-free
- Avocado (½ to 1 avocado)
- Fatty fish like sardines, mackerel, herring, black cod, and wild salmon (4 to 6 ounces (100g to 175g)); aim to include these 3 to 4 times per week
- Nuts and seeds (2 to 3 handfuls); all are okay except peanuts
- Olives (¼ cup/50g)
- Grass-fed butter, clarified butter, or ghee (1 tablespoon); if you are allergic to dairy, just use ghee

YOUR GUIDE TO THE BEST FAT-CONTAINING FOODS

Animal Protein

Beef, grass-fed	Ostrich, grass-fed
Bison, grass-fed	Venison or elk, grass-fed
Lamb, grass-fed	

Poultry

Organic only with no hormones or antibiotics	Duck
	Eggs—farm, omega-3, or organic
Chicken—with or without skin	Turkey

Seafood

Fish — Sustainable and Low in Toxins (Mercury)

Check out the Environmental Working Group (ewg.org), Seafood Watch (seafoodwatch.org), or Natural Resources Defense Council (nrdc.org) for more information about fish choices. Check out CleanFish (cleanfish.com) to find the best brands of clean, sustainably farmed fish or sustainably caught fish. If the fish are not on this list, they are high in toxins or not sustainably farmed or harvested.

Anchovies
Catfish
Herring
Mackerel
Sardines
Sole (Pacific)
Squid (calamari)
Tilapia
Trout (freshwater)
Wild salmon (canned)
Wild salmon (fresh) or organic salmon

Shellfish

Clams
Crab
Mussels

Oysters
Scallops
Shrimp

Dairy

Clarified grass-fed butter
Grass-fed butter

Grass-fed ghee

Nondairy Milks

Be sure they have no carrageenan or sweeteners. Homemade is best.

Almond
Cashew
Coconut
Hemp

Nuts

Almonds
Brazil nuts
Cashews
Chestnuts

Hazelnuts
Macadamias
Pecans

Seeds

Chia
Black sesame
Flax
Hemp

Pumpkin
Sesame
Sunflower
Walnuts

Nut and Seed Butters

Almond
Cashew
Hazelnut
Macadamia

Pecan
Sunflower seed
Walnut

Saturated Plant Fats

Coconut milk (canned, not boxed or packaged stuff with weird ingredients)
Extra virgin organic coconut butter (don't
use for cooking)

Extra virgin organic coconut oil (best for
high-heat cooking)
Palm oil (sustainable only; check for the
CSPO label or buy Nutiva red palm oil or
Spectrum palm oil)

Healthy Oils

Almond oil (for salads)
Extra virgin olive oil (only for very low-heat
cooking)
Macadamia oil (for salads)

Sesame oil — expeller-pressed only for
higher-heat cooking
Walnut oil (for salads)

Other Foods with Good Fat

Avocados
Cocoa butter

Dark chocolate (as a treat at the end of the
twenty-one days)
Olives

Good Sources of Protein

Protein should be divided up throughout the day because the body can
use only about 30 to 40 grams at any one meal for muscle synthesis. A
steady intake of protein also helps increase what we call thermogenesis,
or your metabolic heat. Protein literally turns up your metabolic engine
and will increase your calorie burning.[6] By adding protein to your
breakfast, for example, you can increase your calorie burning so it adds
up to eleven pounds of weight loss in a year.

Your best choices for protein are:

- Whole free-range organic or omega-3 eggs (unlimited amount).
- Grass-fed, organic, sustainably raised lamb, beef, bison, venison, or
other game (three to four times per week maximum). Avoid pork,
which accumulates more toxins than other animals. See Meat Eater's
Guide from the Environmental Working Group to learn how to
source grass-fed or sustainably raised products (www.ewg.org/
meateatersguide).
- Fatty fish such as sardines, mackerel, herring, black cod, and wild
salmon (at least three to four times per week). As you'll recall, these
also count as good fat sources, so you hit two targets with one arrow.

Go to Vital Choice Wild Seafood & Organics (www.vitalchoice .com) to order organic frozen or canned fish.

- Shellfish, including clams, oysters, mussels, shrimp, scallops, and crab. Avoid lobster, which is higher in mercury.
- Calamari or octopus.
- Organic poultry (chicken, turkey, duck).
- Organic non-GMO tofu or tempeh.
- Seeds, including hemp, chia, pumpkin, sesame (maximum 2 to 3 handfuls daily).
- Nuts, including almonds, macadamia, walnuts, pecans, and Brazil nuts (maximum 2 to 3 handfuls daily). Avoid peanuts, which are legumes, not nuts.

What About Protein Powders?

I prefer you avoid protein powders while on this plan—both vegan and animal based—for two reasons. First, most tend to contain sweeteners and flavorings that interfere with normal metabolic function and keep you trapped in the cravings cycle. Even "healthy" sweeteners like stevia are not ideal for weight loss, blood sugar control, or normalizing addictive behavior around food and sweets.

Second, because this program uses food as medicine to reset your metabolism, your goal is to eat only real, whole foods. Protein powders by definition are processed, and so their nutrient content may be compromised. Exposing protein, fats, and phytonutrients to heat of any kind denatures the molecular structures we are depending on to fuel your body.

With that said, if supplementing your smoothies with a little protein powder feels right for you and has a positive effect on your energy and glucose levels, follow these guidelines to make the best selection:

1. Choose plant-based proteins such as hemp or chia, egg proteins, collagen protein, or a combination of these. I also sometimes recommend hydrolyzed beef protein, a low-allergy, good-quality protein. Avoid pea protein; it can be useful long term, but not for the twenty-one days.

2. Look for plain, unflavored, and unsweetened varieties. Nothing with sugar alcohols or "natural" flavors. A little stevia is fine for most people. Even though I recommend getting off sweeteners completely for the first twenty-one days, if you feel you want to use some protein powder (especially for vegans), then you can have a little stevia in the shake—but not in other foods!

3. Avoid consuming protein powder daily. Eating the same protein repeatedly in concentrated forms increases its allergenic potential. Rotate it with other, whole-food protein sources in your shakes and smoothies, like nut butters or seeds, or choose an egg- or meat-based breakfast.

Good Carbs

It's become pretty standard these days for people to be afraid of carbs. The problem isn't carbs, per se—it's the *wrong* carbs. Refined grains, processed foods, sugary cereals and snacks...absolutely, we should all be wary of those carbs, for all the reasons I've already shared. It may sound like I've been making carbs into the bad guys, but what I mean are the refined, processed carbs: flour and sugar in all their forms. The reality is that all veggies are carbs. Yes, broccoli is a carb! So the key is to eat the *right* carbs.

The carbs in the *Eat Fat, Get Thin* Plan are the good ones: vegetables and plant foods. Most of your diet should come from whole plant foods, and all plant foods (vegetables, fruit, nuts, and seeds) contain carbs. Plants contain powerful antioxidants, vitamins and minerals, and phytonutrients that have critical healing properties. For example, broccoli has glucosinolates, which help your body detoxify and prevent cancer. Tomatoes have lycopene, another anticancer compound. To learn more about the amazing compounds in whole plant foods, I encourage you to look up your favorite fruits and vegetables at the World's Healthiest Foods (www.whfoods.com).

While you won't be counting carb grams on this program (because by choosing the right foods you won't have to worry about counting anything), I think it's helpful to understand why certain carbs (like, say, broccoli or nuts) are better than others (like flour or sugar). Really, it all comes down to the fiber content, which determines what's called the *net carbs* of any given food, or the net effect of any given carbohydrate on your metabolism. Net carbs are calculated by subtracting the number of grams of fiber from the total number of carb grams. So, if you have 45 grams of carbs in a serving but 15 grams of fiber, the net carbs are 30 grams.

If you increase the fiber in your diet, you decrease the spike effect of carbohydrates on your blood sugar. And when you eat more fat, you need more fiber to keep the right balance of flora in your gut. This plan is not just about increasing the amount of fat in your diet; it's about striking the right balance. As I've said, resistant starch and PGX help to reduce the effect of carbs on your blood sugar and insulin, and therefore they help you manage your weight, metabolism, and even cholesterol.

Given all that, it's less important to worry about net carb amounts than it is to focus on the quality of the carbohydrate you are choosing. You don't need to count grams of food or calories. You just need to choose the right foods, and the rest takes care of itself. When we focus on quality, the quantity takes care of itself because your appetite is naturally regulated (I mean, you can't eat 750 calories of broccoli, which is 21 cups or nearly 2kg!). When we have poor-quality, processed, high-sugar, or refined foods, our normal mechanisms that regulate appetite and metabolism get completely derailed. The whole science behind *Eat Fat, Get Thin* is to reset our biology to its original factory settings so we can easily and naturally live in balance with our bodies and minds without having to struggle or restrict or control how much we eat. If we just focus on eating the right foods, the rest takes care of itself. Your body can shed unnecessary pounds and reach a new healthy equilibrium.

A quality carbohydrate will contain both phytonutrients and fiber. It will be whole and unprocessed and have had a very short distance from field to fork. How many "processing steps" does broccoli need to get to your plate? Hardly any—just cut it off the stalk, wash off the dirt, steam or sauté, and voilà, it's on your plate. If your food took a pit stop in a factory, you might want to reconsider eating it unless you can still recognize it, like an artichoke in a can or jar, or a nut that has been removed from its shell. A quality carb will not contain refined flours, additives, preservatives, fillers, sweeteners, dyes, or any other ingredient normally found in processed foods. Bottom line: If you can't pronounce an ingredient or recognize it as originating from nature, don't eat it!

Here are the best carbohydrates to stick to on the *Eat Fat, Get Thin* Plan:

Nonstarchy Veggies

Unlimited amounts — knock yourself out!

Artichokes
Arugula
Asparagus
Avocados
Bean sprouts (not alfalfa sprouts, which contain natural carcinogens)
Beet greens
Bell peppers
Broccoli
Brussels sprouts
Cabbage
Carrots (no juicing, because it becomes like sugar)
Cauliflower
Celery
Chives
Collard greens
Dandelion greens
Eggplant
Endive
Fennel
Fresh herbs
Garlic
Ginger
Green beans
Hearts of palm
Jalapeños
Kale
Lettuce
Mushrooms
Mustard greens
Onions
Radicchio
Radishes
Seaweeds (kelp, aramae, wakame, etc.)
Shallots
Snap peas
Snow peas
Spinach
Summer squash
Swiss chard
Tomatoes
Turnip greens
Watercress
Zucchini

Starchy Veggies

Eat only at dinner, ½ to 1 cup (60–125g) maximum, up to four times per week

Beets
Celeriac
Parsnips
Pumpkin
Rutabaga
Sweet potatoes
Turnips
Winter squash (butternut, kabocha, acorn, etc.)

Fruit

Limit to ½ cup to 1 cup (75–150g) per day

Berries (fresh or frozen blackberries, raspberries, wild blueberries, or cranberries; not strawberries, as they are higher in sugar)
Kiwi
Lemon
Lime
Pomegranate seeds
Watermelon

Note: Check out the Environmental Working Group website (www.ewg.org) to learn the list of the Dirty Dozen fruits and veggies (the ones that you should always choose organic) and the Clean Fifteen (which have very low levels of pesticides, even if not organic).

Condiments, Staples, and Spices

Almond flour or almond meal
Apple cider vinegar
Arrowroot (a natural thickener)
Balsamic vinegar
Black pepper
Cocoa powder (unsweetened)
Coconut flour
Dijon mustard
Dried or fresh herbs and spices, such as basil, cayenne pepper, chili powder, cinnamon, coriander, cardamom, ginger, cumin, onion powder, oregano, paprika, parsley, rosemary, sage, thyme, turmeric
Gluten-free tamari
Sea salt (at least 1 to 2 teaspoons per day, unless you have salt-sensitive hypertension or kidney failure)
Tahini (sesame seed paste)
Vanilla powder (unsweetened)
Vegetable or chicken stock (organic, no MSG or gluten)

What to Drink

Each day, be sure to consume a minimum of 8 glasses of filtered water. This is especially important for detoxification and to prevent constipation. Additionally, you can enjoy any of these beverages throughout the day:

- Hot lemon water (helps detoxification)
- Sparkling water or mineral water
- Herbal or green teas
- Butter coffee or tea (see Bulletproof Coffee, page 267)
- Bone broth (see Dr. Hyman's Veggie-Bone Broth, page 321)
- Organic coconut milk (1 can mixed with 3 to 4 cans of water); use mostly for smoothies or cooking

ENERGIZE

Exercise boosts your energy, revs your metabolism, increases mental clarity, and—when done in tandem with an anti-inflammatory, detoxifying, health-boosting program like *Eat Fat, Get Thin*—facilitates weight loss.

The trick is to find what you enjoy (although if you are not used to exercise, getting going might require a bit of determination). New research on exercise has shown that you don't have to spend hours on the treadmill to succeed. High-intensity shorter workouts (what is called burst training or high-intensity interval training), combined with muscle building with weights or your own body weight, lead to amazing gains in metabolism and well-being. You will find that fat fuels your workouts much better than gooey sugar-filled packets or "sports" drinks.

I have everyone start with walking, at least thirty minutes a day if they don't do any other exercise. If you already do exercise, you can continue what you are doing, or boost it up with burst or interval training and some resistance training (either with weights or using your body weight) for strength. Exercise is not a strategy for weight loss alone, but it has a thousand other benefits and will boost your metabolism. To find free workout programs and resources for how to exercise smarter, not harder, go to www.eatfatgetthin.com. To start, though, there is nothing better or simpler than taking a brisk thirty-minute walk every day. Then you can build from there. After the first few weeks you will have the energy to begin a program of movement that works for you.

> Regular distance walking wasn't easy at first, but is getting easier now that the inflammation I had in my hips and lower back is simply gone. I am now walking nature trails with my boys, and it is actually how I spent my forty-second birthday on Memorial Day.
> — Heather Barnes

As I've said in the past, you can't exercise your way out of a bad diet, but exercise combined with a high-quality diet will help build muscle and speed your metabolism, not to mention prevent almost every known disease of aging. And it's a better treatment for depression than Prozac!

REJUVENATE

The two metabolism boosters and appetite quenchers we all need are sleep and relaxation.

Let's start with sleep. If you want to get healthy and lose weight, sleep needs to be as much of a priority as eating right. Aim for seven to eight hours minimum per night. Here are my favorite tips to ensure you get good, healthy z's:

- **Get on a regular schedule.** Going to sleep and waking up at the same time each day instills a familiar rhythm.

- **Use your bed for sleep and romance only.**
- **Make your bedroom a peaceful, quiet haven.**
- **Get at least twenty minutes of sunshine every day,** preferably in the morning. This triggers your brain to release chemicals that help regulate sleep cycles.
- **Shut off bright screens before bed.** Try to avoid screens for at least one to two hours before bed. Download the app f.lux to change the light spectrum coming from your screen so it doesn't suppress melatonin and inhibit sleep.
- **Try low blue-light nights.** Low blue-spectrum light helps your brain reset for sleep and increases melatonin. Try to put on only low blue lights for three hours before bed. You can buy them at LowBlueLights.com.
- **Reset your nervous system.** Using an acupressure mat helps to increase your parasympathetic nervous system and get you into deep relaxation before sleep. Lie on it for thirty-five minutes before bed. You can find one at the Spoonk website (www.spoonkspace.com).
- **Get grounded.** Sometimes electromagnetic frequencies (EMFs) impair sleep. Turn off Wi-Fi. Keep electronic devices (like your phone or radio) away from your bed. Try an "earthing sheet," which grounds you to the earth and disconnects you from EMFs that can disrupt your sleep. Check out Earthing.com.
- **Clear your mind.** Keep a journal or notebook by your bed and write down all your to-dos or ruminations before you go to sleep so when you close your eyes your mind will be less likely to spin.
- **Do some light stretching or yoga before bedtime.** Relax your body.
- **Warm your core.** This raises your core temperature and triggers the proper chemistry for sleep. Use a hot water bottle or a heating pad.
- **Use herbal therapies.** Try 300 to 600 milligrams of passionflower or 320 to 480 milligrams of valerian root extract before bed.
- **Try other natural sleep supplements.** Try one at a time and see what works. You can start with melatonin and magnesium, which are often enough for most people. Some of these come in combination.
  - 1 to 3 milligrams of melatonin
  - 150 to 300 milligrams of magnesium

- 200 to 400 milligrams of theanine
- 500 to 1,000 milligrams of GABA
- 50 to 200 milligrams of 5 hydroxytryptophan
- 365 milligrams of magnolia
- **Use relaxation practices before bedtime to unwind.** Examples include guided imagery, meditation, deep breathing, etc.; see the next section for more information). Try the app called Headspace for simple, short, guided meditations.

You'll find product recommendations for sleep at www.eatfatgetthin .com.

Now let's talk about relaxation. And by relaxation, I don't mean sacking out on the couch and binging on Netflix! For relaxation to have the intended effect on your metabolism, it needs to be deep and active. For instance, set aside, ideally, thirty minutes a day (but at least five) for any of the following:

- Yoga
- Meditation
- Chanting
- Deep breathing (see box following)
- Guided imagery
- A steam or sauna
- A hot bath (with 2 cups of Epsom salt and 10 drops of lavender oil— what I call my Detox Bath)

The Take-Five Breathing Break

Here's the breathing exercise I often recommend: Breathe in slowly through your nose to the count of five, then out for five. Doing this five times a day — when you wake up, before each meal, and before bed — has a profound effect.

If you can't find 5 to 10 minutes a day to stop, reset, and get still, then you should rethink how you spend your time. You can access more resources for sleep and relaxation in the Resources section on page 349 and at www.eatfatgetthin.com.

YOUR DAILY SCHEDULE

Here is your daily schedule for the *Eat Fat, Get Thin* Plan:

Morning

- Begin the day with thirty minutes of brisk walking (or any other workout)
- Before breakfast, take 2 to 5 grams of PGX fiber: 1 to 2 packets or ½ to 1 scoop of the powder in 10 ounces (300ml) of water, or in 3 to 6 capsules of Ultra Matrix Softgels by WellBetX
- Make your shake or breakfast
- Take your supplements with breakfast
- Take your MCT oil
- Enjoy a midmorning snack (optional)
- Drink water (at least 8 glasses throughout the day); use at least 1 capful of E-lyte in 8 ounces (200ml) of water twice a day

Afternoon

- Before lunch, take 2 to 5 grams of PGX fiber
- Eat lunch
- Enjoy a midafternoon snack (optional)

Evening

- Take 2 to 5 grams of PGX before dinner
- Eat dinner
- Take your second dose of supplements at dinner
- Do one or more of your relaxation practices (alternatively, this can be done at any time of the day that works best for you)
- Take 1 tablespoon of potato starch in water before bed (optional)
- Get seven to eight hours of sleep

IF YOU GET STUCK: TROUBLESHOOTING

Each of us starts from a different place and has unique needs and biology. Different questions or concerns or problems can arise when changing your lifestyle or diet. But don't worry. The doctor is in! Here's how I advise my patients when problems crop up:

> **PROBLEM:** You don't feel great the first few days on the program.
>
> **LIKELY CAUSE:** Detox symptoms or not enough salt.
>
> **SOLUTIONS:** It's not uncommon for the body to have a strong reaction when you stop feeding it the processed foods and chemicals it is accustomed to, or when you get off inflammatory foods or foods to which you are addicted. We're cleaning your system of these toxic foods and drinks, and just as with any detox, that can cause some uncomfortable reactions, such as achy, flu-like feelings, irritability, nausea, headaches, and brain fog. The good news is that the discomfort usually passes within forty-eight hours. See the box following for tips on how to help alleviate detox symptoms.
>
> You may also not be getting enough salt. When you cut down on sugar and unhealthy carbs, you dump fluid and water from your kidneys, along with salt. That is because when you cut carbs, you cut insulin, and that causes your kidneys to excrete sodium, or salt. This causes a contraction of your blood volume and a general feeling of dizziness, weakness, and generally feeling crappy. So be sure you are getting at least 1 to 2 teaspoons of sea salt daily in your food. If you have salt-sensitive blood pressure or heart failure, be sure to monitor your blood pressure and symptoms. E-lyte can have profound benefits of rehydration and replenishment, so be sure to use it too.

Tips for Easing Your Detox

- Take a sauna, get a massage, or do gentle stretching or yoga to flush out your circulation and lymphatic system.
- Make sure your elimination system is running smoothly! If you are backed up, so, too, will be the toxins you're trying to flush out. See page 232 for how to combat constipation.

- Drink plenty of water to flush out the toxins.
- Get up and get going! Light exercise gets everything circulating and flushes out the lymphatic fluid that transports the toxins out of your body. Your lymph system works only through the contraction of your muscles. So get contracting!
- Take 1,000 to 2,000 milligrams of buffered vitamin C once or twice daily.
- Get plenty of rest. Even naps or ten minutes of lying down are good.
- Trust the process. These symptoms are a sign that your detox is working, and you're only days away from feeling lighter, cleaner, and more energized than ever before.
- Take E-lyte, 1 capful in 8 ounces (200ml) of water twice a day, to make sure you are fully hydrated.

PROBLEM: Digestive issues such as bloating and gas, feeling abnormally stuffed after a moderate meal, diarrhea, or constipation.

LIKELY CAUSES: Some people are not used to eating fat and it can cause loose stools. It may take a little time to adjust or you may need some digestive enzymes. Changing your diet can also sometimes cause constipation, as can not drinking enough water, especially if you increase fiber such as PGX. Without water, fiber turns to cement in your intestinal tract. If you have bacterial overgrowth and add resistant starch, it can cause bloating or gas. As your bacteria change in your gut from optimizing your diet, your body will eventually adjust.

SOLUTION: Take a comprehensive digestive enzyme to help break down fats (lipase), proteins (proteases), and carbohydrates (amylases). Plant- or animal-based enzymes are both okay; just make sure they're ones that don't contain fillers, gluten, dairy, dyes, or binders. I like Pure Encapsulations Digestive Enzymes Ultra, 2 capsules with each meal. They help you digest fats and alleviate bloating and gas. (Find out where to get it at www.eatfatgetthin. com.) If you are constipated, see page 232 for tips on how to safely and easily get your elimination system in gear.

If you are still having problems after a few weeks, see my free e-book *Beyond Food: Other Causes of Obesity and Damaged Metabolism* and follow the section titled "How to Tend Your Inner Garden." You can download it at www.eatfatgetthin.com. If your problems continue, see a Functional Medicine practitioner.

Tips to Combat Constipation

- First and foremost, be sure you are drinking enough water to clean out your bowels. The PGX fiber can cause constipation if it is not taken with enough water! Be sure to drink at least one full glass of water with each dose of PGX.

- Sprinkle ground flaxseeds into your salads or smoothies. They are high in fiber, absorb a lot of water, and help relieve constipation.

- Increase the amount of daily magnesium citrate to 600 to 1,000 milligrams until the constipation resolves. If you take too much you will get loose stools, so you may need to adjust to find the right level. If you have kidney failure check with your doctor before taking magnesium.

- Take 1,000 to 2,000 milligrams of buffered vitamin C once or twice a day. You can even increase it to 2,000 to 4,000 milligrams once or twice a day to help you go. As with magnesium, ease up on the amount if you get loose stools.

- Get up and get moving! Exercise is one of the best ways to jump-start your elimination system.

- If none of these strategies work, you can take an herbal laxative such as cascara, senna, or rhubarb at bedtime for short-term help. I like Laxa-Blend, 2 to 3 tablets at night, if you are constipated, which you can find at www.eatfatgetthin.com. If these don't work, try liquid magnesium citrate or use a glycerin or bisacodyl suppository or a Fleet enema. If still nothing, it's time to check in with your doctor, as something else is likely going on.

PROBLEM: Fatigue

LIKELY CAUSES: Inadequate sleep, or not enough carbohydrates or protein

SOLUTIONS: First, and most obviously, be sure you are getting enough sleep each night. Poor-quality or inadequate sleep will sabotage your efforts at weight loss and health. It will alter your appetite signals, making you crave carbs and sugar, and will slow your metabolism. If you're sleeping well and enough and are still fatigued, it may be a signal that your body needs additional carbohydrates or protein (especially if you are exercising often or vigorously). If you aren't already eating a starchy carbohydrate like sweet potato or winter squash with dinner (see page 224), consider adding that in now. You can also increase your protein intake throughout the day. Keep track in a journal of how you feel as you increase carbs and/or protein to help you land on the optimal amount for your body.

PROBLEM: You hit a weight loss plateau or are otherwise not getting results.

LIKELY CAUSES AND SOLUTIONS: There could be a few reasons for this that may require further evaluation for hormonal, inflammatory, gut, or toxin problems, genetics, or other issues. To learn more about why you may have hit a plateau and how to address it, check out my free e-book *Beyond Food: Other Causes of Obesity and Damaged Metabolism* at www.eatfatgetthin.com. But first, let's start with the easy and often most common causes:

- Gluten, dairy, sugar or sugar substitutes, peanuts, hidden additives, preservatives, or other chemicals are slipping into your diet. I encourage you to read labels carefully and/or just cook at home for a while, to minimize exposure to these.

- Your body may require more carbohydrates. For some people, a very low-carbohydrate diet may not be optimal. If you have hit a weight loss plateau and are not doing so already, try adding a starchy veggie at dinner.

- Your body requires even fewer carbohydrates. Some people are carbohydrate intolerant and need to cut way down on carbs in order to reset their body systems. If you are diabetic or pre-diabetic, have high triglycerides or very low HDL, and have extra belly fat, you are mostly likely very carbohydrate intolerant. Cut out the starchy veggie at dinner and all fruit, and record how you feel (energy level, mental sharpness, digestive functioning, etc.) and your weight loss over the next few days. You may need to experiment to get to the right level of carb intake, and the best way to do this is to track it closely.

- If you are drinking coffee, it may be having a negative effect on your system. Try going off coffee and continue on the program to see if this is the case. (See the following box for tips on minimizing discomfort from caffeine withdrawal.)

- Not adhering closely to the program. The meal recommendations, supplements, and practices are all scientifically designed to work in tandem, which is why I encourage you to follow the program to the letter. Record your meals, exercise, and sleep to make sure you are staying on track. If you need extra support, seek out a health coach or a life coach. I recommend you work with the Handel Group (www.handelgroup.com).

If none of this helps, it may be useful to see a Functional Medicine doctor to evaluate other causes of weight loss resistance, such as low thyroid function (or check out my e-book *The UltraThyroid Solution* at www .eatfatgetthin.com), adrenal dysfunction, intestinal bacterial overgrowth and leaky gut, overload of toxins, latent infections, mitochondrial dysfunction, or more. Go to the website for the Institute for Functional Medicine (www.functionalmedicine.org) to find a practitioner in your area. You can also come see me or another doctor on my team at The Ultra-Wellness Center, in Lenox, Massachusetts (www.ultrawellnesscenter.com) or the Cleveland Clinic Center for Functional Medicine in Cleveland, Ohio (my.clevelandclinic.org/services/center-for-functional-medicine).

Tips to Ease Caffeine Withdrawal

Kicking caffeine to the curb is easier than you might think…if you follow the right protocol. Here's how to make it as painless as possible:

- Do it slowly. Reduce your caffeine intake by half on the first day, then by another half on the second day, and then down to zero.
- To reduce headaches, drink lots of water, do gentle exercise, and take 1,000 milligrams of vitamin C twice a day. If needed, try 400 milligrams of ibuprofen. I don't believe in unnecessary suffering!
- If you're tired, nap. Ideally you can quit caffeine on a weekend to allow yourself some extra rest as needed.

With your prep days done and your *Eat Fat, Get Thin* guidelines in hand, you're now ready to embark on the twenty-one days that will change everything about how you relate to food and how you look and feel. I'm so excited for you to experience the revitalization and renewal that await you!

14

Stage 3: Your Transition Plan

So what happens now that you've gotten the toxic, health-robbing, waistline-sabotaging foods and substances out of your system and replaced them with whole, real, and fresh food with a healthy dose of good fats? Where do you go from here to continue your health and weight loss journey?

Before we get to that, I want to ask you a question: How do you feel? What's changed for you over the past twenty-one days? As I've said all the way through, you are your own best judge of what works for your body. My aim with this book is to empower you not only with knowledge about fats and free you from "fat fear," but with the tools you need to be able to answer for yourself—now and forever—the question, "What should I eat to achieve (or maintain) my healthiest, happiest, and slim self?"

YOUR PERSONAL "EXIT INTERVIEW"

Let's start with a little self-assessment, to give you a full picture of how far you've come.

Retake the Feel Like Crap Quiz

Now that you've finished the twenty-one day *Eat Fat, Get Thin* Plan, go back and complete the "after" section in the FLC Quiz on pages 22 to 24. I think you're going to be amazed by the changes! That is the power of food, and the power of the body to recover and heal.

Recheck Your Numbers

Redo your numbers. Record your weight, waist size (around your belly button), hip circumference (around the widest point), blood pressure, and fasting blood sugar, and compare them to where you started.

Recheck Your Lab Tests

If you did basic lab tests before beginning the *Eat Fat, Get Thin* Plan, it is well worth repeating those same tests to see the changes.

Review Your Journal Questions

Remember the journal questions you answered before beginning the program? Well, now is the time to look back and ask yourself the questions again. What's changed? What's improved? What areas do you still feel you want to work on?

It is important to track your progress and see where you are. That is how you'll know which transition plan you should be on. If you still have diabetes or want to lose a lot more weight and get off your medications, then continue with the *Eat Fat, Get Thin* Plan. Just because it was a jump-start doesn't mean you can't continue past the twenty-one days! If you have gotten most of the way toward your goals, you might choose to transition to the Pegan Diet, which has more flexibility and can easily be your long-term eating plan for life. To know exactly what plan you should be on, follow the guidelines in the next few sections.

> I have done other elimination-type diets in the past and as soon as they were over I was very excited to get back to "regular eating." I feel like this is the first time I've been excited to keep going and see where I will end up if I continue on the program.
>
> — Teri Dodds

TRANSITION OPTION #1: CONTINUE WITH THE *EAT FAT, GET THIN* PLAN

If you want to continue to lose weight at the same rate you have been for the past twenty-one days (or you just love how you feel), you can continue with the same protocol you've been following. You can do this for another twenty-one days, or however long you like, until you reach your goals. I suggest staying on the *Eat Fat, Get Thin* Plan if you:

- Want to lose an additional twenty-five pounds or more
- Still have diabetes and want to reverse it
- Still are on diabetes medication or insulin and want to get off them
- Still have high triglycerides and low HDL and want to get off statin medication
- Still have high blood pressure and want to get off medication
- Just feel so great and want to experience even greater levels of wellness

Review and follow the protocol on pages 239 to 242 to continue with the *Eat Fat, Get Thin* Plan.

TRANSITION OPTION #2: THE PEGAN DIET

In Chapter 10, you learned about what I call the Pegan Diet, which I believe is the optimal long-term diet for us humans. The transition to the Pegan Diet happens in two stages. First, you'll follow a basic version, as a way to keep the healing and weight loss going while reintroducing legumes (beans and lentils) and ½ cup (100g) per day of nongluten grains. Ideally, I encourage you to stay on this portion of the transition for at least three months.

After that, you can move on to the second stage, which allows for more flexibility. During this second stage, there are options to test and add back in small amounts of gluten, dairy, and treats. If, after testing, you determine you're okay with gluten, dairy, and the occasional treat, I encourage you to incorporate those options only sparingly, for all the reasons you've learned throughout this program. In the pages that follow, I'll walk you through exactly when and how to test these foods and the best ways to include them in your diet, if you choose, in a balanced, smart way. This is indeed a diet meant for life, as it allows for great flexibility and enjoyment of good food that supports your healthy new lifestyle.

The Pegan Diet: Stage 1

Transition to stage 1 of the Pegan Diet if you:

- Want to continue to get the benefits of the *Eat Fat, Get Thin* Plan and add beans and/or nongluten grains back to your diet to see how you respond to them. (Some people with diabesity can't tolerate beans and grains because they contain enough starch to spike blood sugar as well as lectins that create inflammation and weight gain.)
- You have normal blood sugars and blood pressure but want to lose more weight and/or belly fat
- You have any health conditions or inflammation or generally don't feel fabulous
- You don't have a history of heart disease or diabetes
- Your lab tests show you still have high triglycerides, low HDL, small LDL particles, high blood sugar, and insulin resistance

Here is the protocol for stage 1 of the Pegan Diet:

- Continue to eliminate all gluten- and flour-based products (including gluten-free) and dairy (except grass-fed butter or ghee).
- Continue to eliminate all forms of sugar and sweeteners.
- Continue to avoid processed foods.
- Avoid overdoing it on fruit (stick with ½ cup to 1 cup/75 to 150g per day of berries, pomegranate seeds, watermelon, kiwi, lemon, or lime).
- Avoid inflammatory beverages (alcohol, soda or sweetened drinks of any kind, and juice).
- Include up to ½ cup (100g) per day of gluten-free grains in their whole-kernel form: quinoa; black, brown, or red rice; buckwheat.
- Include as many nonstarchy vegetables as you want in all meals and snacks.
- If you like, include one serving of a starchy vegetable at dinner.
- Include 4 to 6 ounces (100g - 175g) of protein (eggs, fish, chicken, or animal protein) or ½ (125g) cup beans or legumes per meal.
- Have four to five servings of healthy fats per day (e.g., ½ to 1 avocado, or 1 tablespoon extra virgin olive oil, grass-fed butter, clarified butter,

walnut oil, sesame oil, extra virgin coconut butter or oil, or nut or seed butter such as almond or cashew). See pages 218 to 220 in Chapter 13 for a review of your good fat options.

- Continue with your daily practices: thirty minutes of exercise, supplements, relaxation, and seven to eight hours' sleep.
- Use your favorite recipes from the *Eat Fat, Get Thin* recipes, or check out *The Blood Sugar Solution Cookbook* or *The Blood Sugar Solution 10-Day Detox Diet Cookbook* for more recipe ideas. Avoid the recipes with gluten or dairy and the desserts.
- Continue to take the same supplements that you have been taking during the *Eat Fat, Get Thin* Plan. You can order them at www.eat fatgetthin.com.

As you reintroduce beans or nongluten grains, it is important to notice how you feel. How is your digestion? Are you bloated? Are you tired? Are you gaining weight or still losing weight? Do you have any other inflammatory symptoms? Your body is the best feedback mechanism. It will tell you exactly what works and what doesn't, what feels good and what doesn't. If reintroducing these foods doesn't work for you, then stay off them for three months and try again. Sometimes it takes a while to reset your body, and after a time you can broaden your diet without side effects.

The Pegan Diet: Stage 2

You've met your weight loss goals ... your health is where you want it to be ... you feel fabulous and scored well on the FLC Quiz. It's time to become a lifelong Pegan!

Stage 2 of the Pegan Diet is similar to the basic Pegan Diet but allows for more flexibility. It introduces gluten and dairy (to see if you can tolerate a little bit) and, if you wish, some treats.

Here is the protocol for the lifelong Pegan Diet:

- Avoid liquid sugar calories such as soda or juices (fresh green juices are fine).
- Continue to eliminate all artificial sweeteners — now and forever!

- Minimize all forms of sugar, but especially avoid foods with added sugars. You can always add a little bit of sugar, maple syrup, or honey to the food you cook yourself. That way you know exactly how much you are getting. Note that you should watch to see if any sweetener (sugar, maple syrup, honey, etc.) triggers an addictive pattern of eating. If so, you may have zero tolerance, and I'd encourage you to stay away from any type of sugar or sweetener and get your "sugar" exclusively from whole fresh fruit.

- Enjoy a little alcohol if you want (optional). One glass of wine or alcohol three to four times a week can eventually be well tolerated by most people. Just pay attention and notice how alcohol makes you feel. Avoid all other liquid sugar calories.

- Continue to avoid processed foods.

- Include as many nonstarchy vegetables as you want in all meals and snacks. Remember, if half to three-quarters of your plate is filled with nonstarchy vegetables, you're on the right track.

- Include up to ½ cup (100g) of gluten-free grains in their whole-kernel form: quinoa; black, brown, or red rice; buckwheat.

- Avoid all processed grains or flours (with the exception of the pasta you will use to test gluten according to the instructions provided in the section following, "Reintroducing Gluten and Dairy").

- Include nutrient-dense starchy vegetables such as sweet potatoes and winter squash, up to two servings per day (see page 224 for portion sizes).

- Include ½ to 1 cup (75–150g) of low-glycemic fruit such as apples, pears, berries, pomegranate seeds, watermelon, kiwi, lemon and lime, one to two servings per day.

- Include a moderate amount of beans and legumes, ½ to 1 cup (125–250g) cooked or canned per day.

- **Continue with your daily practices:** supplements, thirty minutes of physical exercise, relaxation, hydration, and seven to eight hours of sleep.

- **Use your favorite recipes** from *Eat Fat, Get Thin,* or experiment with some new ones from *The Blood Sugar Solution Cookbook* or *The Blood Sugar Solution 10-Day Detox Diet Cookbook.*

▪ Reintroduce gluten and dairy by following the steps detailed in the next section.

How to Dine Out Without Getting Sick and Fat!

Eating out not only costs more money; it can cost you your health, too. Food scientists and industrial food–based restaurant chains have tantalized us with addictive, salty, sugary, high-calorie, nutrient-poor foods that negatively affect our health. But you can enjoy delicious, real food when you eat out, without getting sick and fat.

I want you to succeed on your journey through *Eat Fat, Get Thin,* and I understand that business luncheons, family gatherings, and other social obligations are a part of life that you can't always escape. I also think eating out is one of life's great pleasures and can be done without jeopardizing your health or expanding your waistline. Many people have started to demand better-quality food at restaurants nationwide.

I travel a lot and have become a connoisseur at scoping out the good from the bad and knowing how to pinpoint hidden ingredients in seemingly "healthy" meals such as salads or soups. I have created a guide, *The Restaurant Rescue Guide,* which empowers you to make the best of any dining experience outside the home. You can download this free e-book at www.eatfatgetthin.com. It will show you how to choose the best restaurants and what and how to order from the menu so you can navigate your way to health and well-being while enjoying delicious food.

REINTRODUCING GLUTEN AND DAIRY

The process for reintroducing gluten and dairy is slow and systematic. This is a unique chance to really see how your body tolerates these high-sensitivity foods. We want to add these foods to your diet responsibly and without compromising all your hard work. Here are the steps I recommend:

1. Start with dairy.
2. Eat it at least two to three times a day for three days. Stick to plain milk or plain yogurt without anything added to see how you feel.

3. Track your response for the next seventy-two hours using the food log that follows.
4. If you have a reaction, stop dairy immediately.

Wait at least three days before testing gluten next. Follow these steps:

1. Eat foods containing gluten at least two to three times a day for three days. Use only plain wheat without added ingredients. The best thing to try is pasta, because most breads also contain yeast and sugar. Or you might try cream of wheat cereal for breakfast.
2. Track your response for seventy-two hours using the food log that follows.
3. If you have a reaction, stop gluten immediately.

Tracking your symptoms and reactions is pretty straightforward. You can use the following food log and monitor your progress. (You can download it at www.eatfatgetthin.com and print out as many copies as you need to keep track of all your reactions as you transition off the program.)

DATE	FOOD INTRODUCED	SYMPTOMS

(Continued)

DATE	FOOD INTRODUCED	SYMPTOMS

Each person's body is unique; everyone responds differently to food sensitivities. But to help you know what to be on the lookout for, here are some of the most common food–sensitivity reactions:

- Weight gain
- Resurgence of cravings
- Fluid retention
- Nasal congestion
- Headaches
- Brain fog
- Mood problems (depression, anxiety, anger, etc.)
- Sleep problems
- Joint aches
- Muscle aches
- Pain
- Fatigue
- Changes in your skin (acne, rashes, or eczema)
- Changes in digestion or bowel function (bloating, gas, diarrhea, constipation, reflux)

Gluten and dairy are by nature inflammatory (dairy may raise your insulin level even if you are not sensitive or allergic, so I recommend eating it only occasionally if you have diabesity). If within seventy-two hours you don't experience any reactions like the ones listed, you should be fine and can incorporate the food.

In general, if you tolerate gluten and dairy, it is okay to eat them from time to time, but don't make them staples of your diet. For dairy choices, be sure to stay away from industrial processed cheese, as it is full of chemicals, additives, and hormones. Also, modern forms of wheat have much higher starch content and more gluten proteins than more ancient forms of wheat, which make them more likely to cause inflammation. Try to find "heirloom" sources of gluten and dairy, such as locally sourced cheeses from grass-fed, heirloom cows. They may be more expensive, but they taste better and you'll need less of them to satisfy your appetite.

You can also experiment with other grains such as spelt, rye, or kamut. If you are not gluten sensitive, whole-kernel German rye bread can be a wonderful addition to your diet. Or try einkorn wheat, which was eaten by the ancient Sumerians.

If you do experience a reaction, I recommend eliminating the offending food entirely from your diet for twelve weeks. Often, one primary problem food, either gluten or dairy, can trigger a reaction to a lot of other foods. Once you remove the trigger, other allergens simply won't affect you as much. For most people, twelve weeks is enough time to allow the inflammation to cool. After that, you will likely once again be able to consume the food in small doses. I suggest limiting any problem food to once or twice a week so you don't trigger a cycle of illness.

If you still react after eliminating that food for twelve weeks, avoid that food entirely, or see a physician, dietitian, or nutritionist skilled in managing food allergies.

REINTRODUCING TREATS

Treats should be enjoyed as an occasional pleasure, not a staple of everyday life. Some good options include dark chocolate, chia seed pudding with maple syrup, berry coconut ice cream with honey (made from coconut cream and coconut milk), and chocolate chip cookies made with almond flour. You can find healthy sweets and treats in *The Blood Sugar Solution Cookbook*.

Remember to pay attention and track your responses. If you notice that cravings get triggered or you have other negative reactions, it's a sign to scale back on the treats.

THE CONTINUING JOURNEY

As with any journey, there may be times when you veer off course. You may find yourself thrown off your plan by unanticipated circumstances, distractions, or stresses. If this happens, be kind to yourself. Just acknowledge what happened and return to your plan without judgment or shame. If you've veered very far, I recommend doing the full twenty-one-day *Eat Fat, Get Thin* Plan again to hit the big reset and get yourself back on track. Then, in a very short period of time, you'll be back to feeling good again. Veering off course is easily fixable, because now you know the way back home.

PART IV

EAT FAT, GET THIN COOKING AND RECIPES

Cooking is all about connection, I've learned, between us and other species, other times, other cultures (human and microbial both), but, most important, other people. Cooking is one of the more beautiful forms that human generosity takes; that much I sort of knew. But the very best cooking, I discovered, is also a form of intimacy.

— Michael Pollan, *Cooked: A Natural History of Transformation*

15

Simple, Healthy Cooking 101

Just like you, I get busy. I really do. As rewarding as my work is, it's also pretty demanding. I founded and run The UltraWellness Center in Lenox, Massachusetts, and recently launched the Cleveland Clinic Center for Functional Medicine, which is growing and expanding daily. I travel back and forth from Massachusetts to Ohio twice a month. I have written a dozen books in as many years. I serve as the chairman of the board of the Institute for Functional Medicine, where I help teach and support the development of training for the next generation of Functional Medicine practitioners. Oh, and I'm also a single parent taking care of four kids (my two kids plus my sister's, since she died a few years ago)—and a dog!

I'm not telling you all this to give you the idea I'm superhuman, because I'm not! I am telling you this to dispel the myth that you can't take good care of yourself in the midst of a busy life. With everything I just listed above, I exercise regularly, get eight hours of sleep a night (well, most nights), and make sure I eat well even when I am on the road speaking and teaching. Believe me, if I can do it, you can, too.

But preparing healthy food is a skill, like riding a bike or driving a car. It takes a little time to learn, but it's really not that hard. All you need are a few simple techniques, some basic tools, and a plan. There is no excuse these days. You can even learn to cook by watching YouTube videos. Just type "how to sauté salmon" in your search engine and in three minutes you can learn how to cook the perfect fish.

Healthy meals can be simple and easy to prepare when there is little time and your schedule is spread thin. I don't have time to cook elaborate recipes. So I have learned how to prepare three meals in a day in thirty minutes total. Yes, that's right, three meals in thirty minutes total. Here's how:

For breakfast, I make a whole-food protein shake (you'll find some of my favorite recipes for these on pages 267 to 272). The key is to have all the ingredients ready so I can just pop them in the blender. Prep time: three to five minutes.

For lunch, I make a salad (with prewashed greens and veggies, to save time). My favorite combo is arugula, avocado, a can of wild salmon, cherry tomatoes (no cutting required!), and pumpkin seeds sprinkled on top. Dressing is a mix of extra virgin olive oil, balsamic vinegar, salt, and pepper. Prep time: five to ten minutes at most.

For dinner, I'll cook a piece of fish, a lamp chop, grass-fed beef, or organic chicken in a skillet with a little bit of coconut oil. For veggies, I'll stir-fry chopped greens like bok choy or broccoli with garlic (the prepeeled kind to save time), and have that along with a sweet potato (baked the night before and heated up) with salt and a little grass-fed butter. Super-simple, delicious, and easy—fifteen minutes total. Less time than it takes to drive to the takeout and order.

In the next few pages, I'll give you some basic ideas for simple cooking, which, along with the *Eat Fat, Get Thin* recipes, will help you turn your kitchen into your new favorite eating establishment.

PLAN YOUR EATING FOR THE WEEK

The single most important ingredient in any healthy diet is planning. If we don't plan, we might be tempted to make unhealthy choices out of sheer desperation. Think about it: How often have you found yourself at 6 p.m. without a plan for dinner or ingredients to make a healthy meal? More often than not, that leads to takeout, fast food, or packaged, prepared foods...and then lots of remorse!

The easiest way to make a healthy eating plan is to pull it together over the weekend. Make a list—in writing—of what you are going to cook each night during the coming week (or, if you know you'll be dining out at a particular restaurant, what you'll order). Start with dinner, as that is usually the most difficult meal to get on the table. Plan for one to two kinds of vegetables, a protein source, healthy fats, and maybe a tossed green salad for extra vegetables at every meal. With this basic framework, you can't go wrong.

Choose your proteins first: chicken, fish, shrimp, beef, lamb, turkey, duck, and so on. Maybe your list for a week is one to two chicken dishes, one to two seafood dishes, one beef, one lamb or turkey dish, and one vegetarian dish with tofu or tempeh, for example.

Next, choose your vegetables. Choose one or two cooked vegetables from the list of basic vegetables on pages 253 to 255, along with a salad. As a general rule, you always want to have lots of salad greens on hand. Prewashed greens save time and might cost a bit more, but you can buy heads of dark lettuce greens, wash and spin them dry, and refrigerate them in containers for quick salads.

Do the same for lunch throughout the week. Make a list of the fresh greens, veggies, nuts, and other proteins you can add to a salad to premake and store in a container to take with you on the go. Or choose from the easy recipes on pages 284 to 294 and get all the necessary ingredients.

Breakfast is also pretty easy to plan for. Choose a few of the delicious smoothie recipes on pages 267 to 272 and stock up on the ingredients you need. The Chia and Berry Breakfast Pudding is another easy option that can be made ahead and enjoyed for a few days. It's also always a good idea to keep eggs on hand, as they take only a few short minutes to prepare (eggs are also great in a pinch for dinner, if you have a night that's especially short on time).

I strongly encourage you to take the time to write out your weekly meal plans, as opposed to just having a loose idea of what you'll make. This removes the guesswork and last-minute scrambling and enables you to enjoy your meals rather than feel stressed about them.

HOW TO COOK VEGETABLES

A few simple techniques can help you get vegetables on the table in just minutes without a recipe. First, though, get veggie savvy! Here are a few essential tips:

- For best taste and maximum nutrition, don't overcook your vegetables. Many vegetables can be enjoyed raw or just lightly cooked.
- Finish your vegetables with a drizzle of olive oil, coconut oil, sesame oil, melted clarified butter, or ghee for healthy fat and flavor. Or try a dollop of one of the sauces in the recipe section.
- Chopped nuts and seeds are a great way to add healthy fat to basic vegetables, as well as a nice crunch. For more flavor and eye appeal, add chopped fresh herbs and a sprinkle of sea salt, pepper, or a specialty salt like sea salt with truffle.

Here are the basics you need to know to prepare all your veggies quickly and easily.

To Blanch (cook quickly in boiling water)

Fill a large pot three-quarters full of water and bring it to a boil. Add 1 teaspoon of salt. Drop the vegetables in and cook for 1 to 3 minutes or until crisp-tender. Serve immediately. Vegetables can also be cooked ahead. When done, plunge into a bowl of ice water to stop the cooking process, drain, dry, and refrigerate. Reheat when needed.

To Broil

Preheat the broiler on high with the oven rack one level down from the top. Arrange the vegetables on a rimmed baking sheet. Drizzle with olive oil, sea salt, and black pepper. Broil the vegetables until crisp-tender, turning once if needed. Most vegetables will take 3 to 5 minutes. Test by piercing with the tip of a sharp paring knife.

To Grill

Heat a grill pan or an outdoor gas grill with cleaned grates over high heat. Brush with a little oil to prevent sticking. Place the vegetables on the grill and cook, turning once, until browned but not limp. For an outdoor grill, a nonstick grill basket works great. Many vegetables, like zucchini, mushrooms, tomatoes, and onions, can also be skewered, then grilled.

To Roast

Preheat the oven to 425°F. Line a rimmed baking sheet with foil or parchment paper for easier cleanup. Toss the vegetables with olive oil and season with sea salt and pepper. Arrange in a flat layer on the baking sheet and roast until crisp-tender and the edges are browned. Times will vary by vegetable. Asparagus will take just 3 to 4 minutes, cauliflower or broccoli might take 20 to 30 minutes, and root vegetables 45 minutes. The smaller the pieces, the faster they cook, but don't cut them too small because they will cook too quickly and burn.

To Sauté

Heat a large (12-inch) sauté or frying pan over medium heat. Add 1 tablespoon of coconut oil, ghee, or expeller-pressed sesame oil to the pan. When the oil is hot, add the vegetables, allowing them to cook for a minute or two, and stir. Asparagus will cook in just 3 to 4 minutes for crisp-tender, and sturdier vegetables such as cauliflower will take a few minutes longer.

To Steam

Insert a steamer basket into a large (4- to 5-quart) pot. Fill the pot with several inches of water to just below the steamer rack. With a lid on, bring the water to a boil over medium-high heat. Add the vegetables to the steamer, turn the heat down to medium, and steam until crisp-tender. Most vegetables take 2 to 5 minutes.

Tips for Purchasing, Prepping, and Storing Favorite Veggies

Asparagus: One bundle or pound generally serves four. Select stalks with fresh, compact tips (not dried or frayed). Trim off the bottom of the spears and stand the bundle in a tall container with 1 inch of water. Cover the spears loosely with plastic wrap and refrigerate until ready to cook. Before cooking, snap off the tough bottom part of the spear. You can cook the spears whole or cut them into bite-size pieces for steaming.

Broccoli: 16 ounces (450g) of bagged florets or 1 large bundle serves 4. Select bright green broccoli (no brown or yellowing spots) that is firm to the touch, not limp or soft. Store in an airtight baggie for up to a week in the crisper drawer. Bags of florets are ready to cook. Or trim the florets from a head of broccoli, leaving some of the stem attached, then cut into bite-size pieces.

Broccolini: Two bundles serves 4. Select bundles that are firm to the touch, not limp or soft, and that are bright green (it's okay if they have a few yellow flowers). Store in an airtight baggie in the crisper drawer for up to 4 days. To prep, trim a little off the end and split fat stalks in half lengthwise or leave them whole (the entire stalk is edible).

Cauliflower: One large head serves 2 to 4 people, depending on how hungry they are. Heads (of any color) should not have any brown spots; if they do, they are past their nutritional peak. Choose heads surrounded by lots of green leaves. Store in an airtight baggie in the refrigerator for up to a week. To prepare, trim the florets from the heads, leaving some of the stem attached, then cut into bite-size pieces.

Green Beans: 12 to 16 ounces serves 4. Select fresh, green, plump pods without any brown spots (the thin French green beans, called haricots verts, are the most tender). Green beans will last in the refrigerator for 4 to 5 days, stored in an airtight baggie. Before cooking, snap or cut off the bottom of the stem, leaving the pigtail end (the end that was not attached to the plant).

Snap Peas: 12 to 16 ounces serves 4. Select fresh, plump, green peas that are firm — not withered. These can be stored in a bag for 3 to 4 days in the refrigerator, ideally in the crisper. To prepare for cooking (or eating raw), snap off the top tip, then pull down the side to remove the tough string.

Snow Peas: 8 to 12 ounces serves 4. Choose pea pods that look fresh and crisp. These can be stored in a bag in the refrigerator, ideally in the crisper, for 3 to 4 days. To prepare for cooking (or eating raw), snap off the top tip, then pull down the side to remove the tough string.

Zucchini (Summer Squash): 1½ pounds serves 4. Select green or yellow squash with firm, bright, smooth skin. Smaller squash are less seedy than their larger counterparts; larger squash can be bitter. Zucchini will last 4 to

5 days in the refrigerator, ideally in the crisper. To prep, trim off the stem end, quarter or halve lengthwise, and chop into pieces (or make raw zucchini noodles with a spiralizer tool).

HOW TO COOK CHICKEN, SEAFOOD, AND MEAT

When purchasing proteins, figure on 4 to 6 ounces (100g–175g) per person if the protein is boneless and skinless. When you are buying proteins such as bone-in chicken breasts, bone-in steaks, or lamb chops, you should generally buy the whole piece. If you buy too much, leftovers are a good thing and can become a quick lunch.

To Sauté

Season with sea salt, ground black pepper, and maybe garlic or other seasonings you enjoy. Heat 1 to 2 tablespoons of olive oil in a sauté or frying pan over medium heat. When the pan and oil are hot (but not smoking), place the chicken, fish, or meat in the pan and sear until you get a golden crust on one side. Turn the pieces over and cook on the other side. Don't overcook meats or fish. It makes them hard and dry. Over time, you'll get a feel when something is done, but to begin, I recommend getting a meat thermometer to measure temperatures. Just stick the thermometer into the thickest part of the meat. Chicken is done when it reaches 160°F to 165°F. Fish is ready at 145°F. Meat will depend on your preference, from 130°F to 135°F for medium-rare steak, or 140°F to 145°F for steak cooked medium. Ground meat should be cooked to 165°F. If the pieces are thick, chicken (such as bone-in breasts), steaks, and even thick fish fillets can be quickly finished in just a few minutes in a hot (400°F to 425°F) oven.

To Broil or Grill

To broil, preheat the broiler, grill pan, or outdoor gas grill on high until hot. For the broiler, place the rack one level down from the top of the oven. First drizzle the meat, chicken, or fish with olive oil, then season with sea salt, ground black pepper, and other seasonings you like. For the broiler, place on a foil-lined rimmed baking sheet and broil, turning once or twice, until the food is evenly cooked to the temperatures listed in the previous section.

To grill, turn the heat down to medium-high and place the food on the hot grill. Allow one side to get golden with nice grill marks, then flip and turn the heat down to low. The second side may not take as long.

Timing will depend on the protein and the thickness of what you are cooking. Fish should take 7 to 10 minutes, boneless chicken breast should take 12 to 15 minutes, and steaks will vary. If the outside is getting too done, move the pieces to a cooler part of the grill while they finish cooking. (Note: Small foods like shrimp cook very quickly under the broiler or on the grill. Once the first side is pink, turn them over and cook another minute or just until the second side is also pink. Don't overcook, and keep them tender.)

Whether grilling or broiling, remember not to char your food to ensure you avoid exposure to toxic compounds.

SHOPPING TIPS

Following are my favorite strategies for making grocery shopping as easy as possible. Just like healthy cooking, healthy shopping doesn't have to be a chore if you're armed with the right information (and the right lists!).

Fresh Shopping

- Buy as much organic as you can. If price or availability is an issue, use the Dirty Dozen and Clean Fifteen lists for guidance. Check out the Environmental Working Group's website at http://www.ewg .org/foodnews/ and be sure to download the smartphone app to make shopping easier.
- Shop seasonally for the best prices and availability.
- Shop at farmers' markets.
- To save money, watch for sales and use coupons.

- When properly stored, most produce will last the better part of a week in your refrigerator, so plan smart, and save time at the store.
- Produce like onions, shallots, and garlic do well in a cool pantry and are easy to keep on hand.
- Buy fresh herbs or try growing your own to save money and have instant availability.
- Packaged salad greens save time. You can also buy heads of fresh lettuce, wash and dry them, and package them for the week. If buying packaged, be sure to read labels for expiration dates and choose wisely.
- I love avocados for their healthy fat, creamy flavor, and buttery texture. You can purchase hard ones and let them ripen on the countertop for a few days, or slightly soft ones that will yield to gentle pressure and be ready to eat. Don't buy them too soft and squishy.

Pantry Shopping

With these healthy staples in your pantry, you'll be amazed at the delicious and nutritious dishes you can create.

- Oils and fats: Extra virgin olive oil, avocado oil, and extra virgin coconut oil will be your mainstays. Clarified butter or ghee can also be used, as well as sesame oil.
- Nuts: Raw almonds, cashews, walnuts, pine nuts, pecans, macadamias (not peanuts).
- Seeds: Hemp, chia, pumpkin, sunflower, sesame, and flaxseeds.
- Nut and seed butters: Pure cashew, almond, sunflower, and coconut butter.
- Flours: Blanched almond flour and coconut flour.
- Milks: Almond, coconut (unsweetened and no additives). See pages 272 to 274 for how to make your own milks, which is the best option. For canned coconut milk, my favorite brand is Native Forest.
- Broths: Low- or no-sodium frozen or boxed vegetable, beef, and chicken broth (homemade is best, but if you buy, be sure to read labels for additives).

- Dried herbs and spices:
  - Sea salt, ground black pepper, and garlic. White pepper is nice, too, when you don't want black specks, although the flavor is a bit different from that of black pepper.
  - Dried herbs such as oregano, basil, thyme, rosemary, bay leaves, Italian blends, and herbes de Provence.
  - Spices such as cumin, coriander, turmeric, allspice, ancho chili powder, chipotle, paprika, smoked paprika, cinnamon, red pepper flakes, nutmeg, ginger (fresh, dried, and organic jarred puree; refrigerate fresh and jarred puree after opening), saffron.
- Condiments:
  - Dijon mustard (look for pure mustard without sugar or chemicals)
  - Capers
  - Low-sodium tamari (gluten-free soy sauce)
  - Vinegar: Balsamic, unseasoned rice, red wine, white wine, sherry, and champagne
  - Pitted Greek olives
  - Nutritional yeast (while it sounds strange, it is very good for you and has a delicious, cheesy taste)

Freezer Items

- Frozen berries: blueberries, raspberries, blackberries, unsweetened acai berry puree
- Frozen organic vegetables (if fresh are out of season or unavailable locally)
- Frozen shrimp and other seafood
- Frozen grass-fed meats (beef, bison, lamb), organic chicken and turkey, and clean fish. See the Natural Resources Defense Council website (www.nrdc.org) for low-mercury fish, and the CleanFish website (www.cleanfish.com) for sustainably raised or harvested fish sources.

How to Eat Well for Less!

Cooking food that tastes great and nourishes your body doesn't need to break the bank. That's why I stock my pantry with food from Thrive Market. You will find all of my favorite pantry staples and more on this site, all for prices 25 to 50 percent lower than what you would find in natural foods stores. For the first time, you can buy the natural, nontoxic pantry staples you need for the same price as or less than that of their processed alternatives. To get your complimentary three-month membership, please visit www.thrivemarket.com/EFGT. There is one other great resource for eating well for less — a guide called Good Food on a Tight Budget from the Environmental Working Group (where I am on the board). You can download it for free at www.ewg.org. It tells you how to eat food that is good for you, good for the wallet, and good for the planet.

BASIC KITCHEN TOOLS

You want to invest in good kitchen tools to make cooking as easy and efficient as possible. Here are the basics I suggest everyone have in their kitchens.

Knives

Good knives will last a lifetime and are worth the investment. Choose knives that fit your hand comfortably (you can try them out at a knife or cooking store). Don't buy a set, which often has knives you won't use; buy them individually. I suggest starting with an 8- to 9-inch French or chef's knife, a paring knife, and a 7-inch Santoku (a multi-purpose Japanese-style knife that I couldn't live without!). You can also add a thin slicing knife, a fillet knife to skin fish, and a 10-inch chef's knife for bigger jobs.

To keep your knives sharp, store them in a block or a drawer with edge covers to protect the blades. Have them professionally sharpened a few times a year and never put them in the dishwasher.

Pots and Pans

The sizes you buy should depend on how many people you generally cook for; a family of two and a family of six will have different needs. Buy pans that feel heavy, as weight conducts heat. Well-cared-for, good pots and pans will last for many years. I suggest you have the following in your kitchen:

- An 11- to 12-inch stainless steel skillet with sloped sides.
- Nonstick, non-Teflon skillets such as ceramic. Small sizes like 8 to 9 inches are good for scrambling eggs, making omelets, and searing fish and delicate foods. A 10- to 11-inch skillet is useful for larger amounts of food. If you have nonstick pans that are scratched and flaking, invest in new ones.
- Stainless steel sauté pans with straight sides. A 3- to 4-quart one is a good size. For big families, add a 6-quart.
- Saucepans: 2-quart, 4-quart, and 5-quart are good basic sizes.
- Dutch ovens: enamel-coated cast iron (such as Le Creuset) in 3½- and 5½-quart sizes.
- A traditional 10½-inch cast-iron frying pan (preseasoned) is a classic, versatile, and inexpensive pan, but don't ever wash it with soap. With special care it will last a lifetime.
- A nonstick grill pan will provide nice grill marks when the weather prevents outdoor grilling or if you do not have access to a gas grill.
- An 8- to 10-quart stockpot for large batches of soups and homemade broth.
- Rimmed baking sheets—half-sheet and quarter-sheet sizes; buy heavy ones that won't warp.

Other Tools

In addition, I recommend the following useful tools.

- Good high-speed blender—they're great for making quick and healthy smoothies

- Standard-size (not mini) food processor with different blade options
- Garlic press
- Vegetable peeler
- Microplane zester
- Handheld citrus juicer
- Small handheld can opener
- Nesting set of dry measuring cups
- Liquid measuring cups in 1-, 2-, and 4-cup sizes
- Nesting set of glass or stainless steel mixing bowls
- Assorted measuring spoons, preferably stainless steel
- Box grater with sharp holes (look for the kind that fold flat)
- Large and small fine-mesh strainers
- Colander
- Steamer rack or basket to fit inside pots and pans
- Fish pliers or tweezers
- Flexible silicone spatulas
- Flat fish spatula
- Spring tongs
- Wire whisks—a French whisk and small sizes for foods like vinaigrette and eggs
- Wooden spoons
- Wood or eco-friendly wood fiber (such as Epicurean or bamboo) cutting boards, one for produce and one for raw proteins
- Digital kitchen thermometer
- Several kitchen timers

Storage and Supplies

Lastly, I suggest:

- Natural parchment paper, either rolls or precut sheets
- Heavy-duty foil
- Cloth kitchen towels
- Sealable glass containers with lids in a variety of sizes for storing prep work and leftovers

★   ★   ★

Take the time to set yourself up right in your kitchen. It truly is one of the essential keys to success for eating healthy—not just for the next twenty-one days, but also for life. While you may need to spend a little extra money and time to get the supplies you need, look at this as a long-term investment in your health and weight management. It's well worth it.

Now let's get to the recipes, which will prove to you that eating healthy is much easier—and far more delicious—than you might think!

16

The Recipes

SNACKS

Spanish Romesco Dip with Veggies

A classic sauce from the Catalonia region of Spain, romesco works beautifully over fish or chicken, and also as a snack dip with raw vegetables. For an extra layer of flavour, use smoked paprika. For a more fluid sauce, thin with almond milk. For a thick dip, leave as it is.

Yield: about 400 ml (14 fl oz)
Prep time: 5 minutes

- 20 g (3/4 oz) whole almonds
- 3 garlic cloves, peeled
- about 175 g (6 oz) roasted sweet red peppers from a jar
- 2 tomatoes (about 225 g/8 oz), quartered
- 75 g (3 oz) onion, finely chopped
- 3 tablespoons olive oil
- 1½ teaspoons paprika, regular or smoked
- 1 teaspoon sherry vinegar or red wine vinegar
- ¼ teaspoon sea salt
- ¼ teaspoon ground black pepper

Insert the steel knife into the food processor work bowl. With the motor running, drop in the almonds and garlic cloves through the feed tube. Process until ground, about 20–30 seconds.

Drain and seed the peppers, then roughly chop. Add to the food processor along with the tomatoes, onion, oil, paprika, vinegar, salt and pepper. Process until a fairly smooth sauce is achieved, about 1–2 minutes.

Serve with freshly cut non-starchy vegetables, such as celery, sugarsnap peas, cauliflower and broccoli.

Nutritional analysis per serving (50g/2oz vegetables, 50g/2oz sauce): calories 150, fat 13 g, saturated fat 2 g, cholesterol 0 mg, fibre 4 g, protein 3 g, carbohydrate 7 g, sodium 170 mg

Avocado Cream with Crudités

Creamy, luscious avocado puréed with smooth avocado mayonnaise and lime makes a great topping for burgers or chicken, as well as a dip with raw veggies for a snack.

Yield: about 250 g (8 oz)
Prep time: 5 minutes

- 1 ripe avocado, peeled and stoned
- 50g (2 oz) avocado mayonnaise
- 1 teaspoon lemon juice
- 2 pinches sea salt

Place the avocado, mayonnaise, lemon juice and salt into the bowl of a food processor with the steel knife and purée until smooth and creamy. Serve with your favourite freshly cut veggies.

Nutritional analysis per serving (50g/2oz vegetables, 50g/2oz sauce): calories 180, fat 18 g, saturated fat 3 g, cholesterol 25 mg, fibre 4 g, protein 2 g, carbohydrate 6 g, sodium 115 mg

SMOOTHIES AND MORE

DR. HYMAN'S GREEN BREAKFAST SMOOTHIE

Yield: 1 serving
Prep time: 5 minutes

- 1 lemon, quartered
- 1 avocado, peeled and stoned
- 2 celery sticks
- 65 g (21/2 oz) spinach
- 50 g (2 oz) parsley
- 50 g (2 oz) coriander
- 1 cucumber
- 1 teaspoon organic extra virgin olive oil
- pinch of sea salt
- water (as needed to achieve desired consistency)

Blend all the ingredients together until smooth.

Nutritional analysis per serving (1 smoothie):
calories 420, fat 30 g, saturated fat 5 g, cholesterol 0 mg,
fibre 23 g, protein 12 g, carbohydrate 36 g, sodium 180 mg

BULLETPROOF COFFEE

This is a version of my friend Dave Asprey's Bulletproof Coffee
Tip: For best results, make your coffee using a metal mesh filter or cafetière.

Yield: 1 serving
Prep time: 5 minutes

- 500 ml (16 fl oz) hot coffee (regular or decaff), ideally freshly brewed with organic beans
- 2 tablespoons grass-fed butter or ghee
- 2 tablespoons organic extra virgin coconut oil (Dr. Bronner's or Nutiva), or 2 tablespoons MCT oil
- optional: ½ teaspoon organic cinnamon, or 1 teaspoon organic cocoa powder

Blend all the ingredients together until creamy and frothy.

Nutritional analysis per serving (500 ml/16 fl oz or 2 mugs):
calories 500, fat 54 g, saturated fat 44 g, cholesterol 80 mg, fibre 1 g,
protein 0 g, carbohydrate 1 g, sodium 15 mg

NON-COFFEE VANILLA LATTE

For those who don't want coffee, this is a great morning drink that
provides fat without caffeine.

Yield: 1 serving
Prep time: 5 minutes

- 500 ml (16 fl oz) hot filtered water
- 2 tablespoons grass-fed butter or ghee
- 2 tablespoons Dr. Bronner's organic coconut oil or 2 tablespoons MCT oil
- 1 teaspoon unsweetened vanilla powder, or no-alcohol, gluten-free, pure
  vanilla extract
- optional: ½ teaspoon organic ground cinnamon and ¼ teaspoon organic
  ground cardamom
- optional: 1 teaspoon of organic cocoa powder

Blend all the ingredients together until creamy.

Nutritional analysis per serving (250 ml/8 fl oz):
calories 520, fat 54 g, saturated fat 44 g, cholesterol 0 mg,
fibre 1 g, protein 1 g, carbohydrate 2 g, sodium 0 mg

GREEN MACHINE SMOOTHIE

This bright green smoothie gets its creaminess from nutrient-dense
avocado, an excellent source of the nine essential amino acids our bodies
need to build muscle, as well as brain and heart-healthy omega-3 fats.
And the green tea, which is loaded with bioactive compounds, helps us
increase fat burning. For this I use Republic of Tea Organic Double
Green Matcha Tea.

Yield: 1 serving
Prep time: 5 minutes

- 250 ml (8 fl oz) unsweetened almond milk
- 60 ml (2 1/4 fl oz) full-fat coconut milk
- 50 g (2 oz) baby spinach leaves (2 big handfuls)
- 1/2 small avocado
- 2 tablespoons hemp seeds
- juice of 1 lime
- 1 teaspoon green matcha tea

Place all the ingredients in a blender and blend until smooth and creamy.

Nutritional analysis per serving (about 500 ml (16 fl oz):
calories 480, fat 39 g, saturated fat 7 g, cholesterol 0 mg,
fibre 12 g, protein 16 g, carbohydrate 22 g, sodium 65 mg

Ruby Smoothie

With nutty almond milk and creamy almond butter, this raspberry smoothie will blast off your day with healthy fat, antioxidants and phytonutrients. Those with nut allergies can use rice milk, hemp milk or organic soya milk instead.

Yield: 1 serving
Prep time: 5 minutes

- 300 ml (1/2 pint) unsweetened almond milk
- 75 g (3 oz) frozen unsweetened raspberries
- 2 tablespoons ground flaxseed
- 2 tablespoons creamy almond butter
- 1 tablespoon chia seeds
- 1 tablespoon pomegranate powder, or 3 strawberries

Place all the ingredients in a blender and start to blend at a low speed, gradually increasing to high speed. Blend until creamy and well combined.

Nutritional analysis per serving (500 ml/16 fl oz):
calories: 430, fat 31 g, saturated fat 2 g, cholesterol 0 mg,
fibre 15 g, protein 13 g, carbohydrate 31 g, sodium 320 mg

ISLAND DREAM SMOOTHIE

A creamy, light way to start the day with a touch of greens.

Yield: 1 serving
Prep time: 5 minutes

- 175 ml (6 fl oz) unsweetened almond milk
- 175 ml (6 fl oz) full-fat coconut milk
- 1 teaspoon no-alcohol, gluten-free, pure vanilla extract, or unsweetened vanilla powder
- 1 teaspoon cinnamon
- 1 handful baby spinach

Place all the ingredients in a blender and blend until smooth and creamy.

Nutritional analysis per serving (375 ml /13 fl oz):
calories 250, fat 20 g, saturated fat 10 g, cholesterol 9 mg,
fibre 5 g, protein 6 g, carbohydrate 9 g, sodium 55 mg

GINGER SPICE SMOOTHIE

This creamy, spiced, low-carb smoothie is a great way to start your day and get it into fat-burning mode. The ginger is also great for digestion.

Yield: 1 serving
Prep time: 5 minutes

- 350 ml (12 fl oz) almond or cashew milk
- 2 tablespoons raw almond butter
- 2 teaspoons grated ginger
- 1/4 teaspoon ground nutmeg
- optional: 1 handful baby spinach or greens of choice

Place all the ingredients in a blender and blend until smooth and creamy.

Nutritional analysis per serving (375 ml /13 fl oz):
calories 400, fat 31 g, saturated fat 4 g, cholesterol 0 mg,
fibre 7 g, protein 13 g, carbohydrate 19 g, sodium 30 mg

TRIPLE GREEN SMOOTHIE

Full of high-quality fat from coconut milk and avocado, this bright green smoothie helps you to burn fat and keeps you fuelled.

Yield: 1 serving
Prep time: 5 minutes

- 350 ml (12 fl oz) full-fat coconut milk
- 1/2 small avocado
- juice of 1 lime
- 1 handful baby spinach leaves

Place all the ingredients in a blender and blend until smooth and creamy.

Nutritional analysis per serving (375 ml/13 fl oz):
calories 330, fat 29 g, saturated fat 15 g, cholesterol 0 mg,
fibre 7 g, protein 4 g, carbohydrate 14 g, sodium 65 mg

COCOA BLISS SMOOTHIE

Chocolate lovers rejoice! You get to drink a chocolate shake for breakfast, and this one is power-packed with creamy, healthy fat. Cacao not only adds great flavour, but is a good source of antioxidants, vitamins and minerals.

Yield: 1 serving
Prep time: 5 minutes

- 250 ml (8 fl oz) almond or cashew milk
- 120 ml (4 fl oz) full-fat coconut milk
- 1 tablespoon raw cacao powder
- 1 teaspoon no-alcohol, gluten-free, pure vanilla extract
- 1 tablespoon coconut butter

Place all the ingredients in a blender and blend until smooth and creamy.

Nutritional analysis per serving (375 ml/13 fl oz):
calories 420, fat 33 g, saturated fat 18 g, cholesterol 0 mg,
fibre 9 g, protein 10 g, carbohydrate 17 g, sodium 40 mg

AMAZON COCOA BERRY SMOOTHIE

This vivid purple smoothie will power your morning with blueberries and Amazonian acai berries. A rich source of healthy omega fats, acai also provides vitamins and minerals. The cocoa powder, another good source of minerals, plays off the natural cocoa flavour of the acai berry.

Yield: 1 serving
Prep time: 5 minutes

- 90 g (31⁄2 oz) unsweetened frozen acai purée
- 150 ml (5 fl oz) filtered water
- 120 ml (4 fl oz) full-fat coconut milk
- 50 g (2 oz) frozen blueberries
- 1 tablespoon hemp seeds
- 1 tablespoon chia seeds
- 1 tablespoon coconut butter
- 1 tablespoon cashew butter
- 1 tablespoon raw natural cocoa powder

Hold the frozen acai packet under running cold water for a few seconds and break it up with your fingers. Cut open the top and squeeze the acai into a blender. Add all the remaining ingredients and purée until smooth and creamy.

Nutritional analysis per serving 500 ml (16 fl oz):
calories: 450, fat 37 g, saturated fat 18 g, cholesterol 0 mg,
fibre 8 g, protein 10 g, carbohydrate 24 g, sodium 25 mg

KIWI-LIME SMOOTHIE

At first sip, you would never guess that the creaminess and protein in this smoothie come from tofu and cashew butter. All you will taste is the zesty zing of lime and kiwi. The tofu is a great source of protein.

Yield: 1 serving
Prep time: 5 minutes

- 300 ml (1/2 pint) unsweetened almond milk
- 90 g (3½ oz) organic silken tofu, drained
- 2 kiwi fruits, peeled and quartered
- 2 tablespoons creamy raw cashew butter
- 2 tablespoons hemp seeds
- juice of 1 lime
- optional: 1/2 teaspoon no-alcohol, gluten-free pure vanilla extract, or unsweetened vanilla powder

Place all the ingredients in a blender and purée until smooth and creamy.

Nutritional analysis per serving (550 ml/18 fl oz):
calories 500, fat 30 g, saturated fat 4 g, cholesterol 75 mg,
fibre 8 g, protein 19 g, carbohydrate 41 g, sodium 170 mg

Speciality milks

There are many wonderful speciality milk alternatives to standard dairy milk. Here we give recipes for three easy basics that cover most needs, unless you have a nut allergy. Making homemade milks eliminates unnecessary additives, sweeteners, thickeners and preservatives that are often found in ready-made brands. Once again, homemade wins!

COCONUT MILK

Here is an easy way to whip up your own homemade coconut milk.

Yield: 1 litre (1¾ pints)
Prep time: 5 minutes

- 1 x 400 ml (14 oz) can full-fat coconut milk, well shaken
- 550 ml (18 fl oz) filtered water

Place the coconut milk and water in a glass container with a tight-fitting lid. Shake until well blended. Refrigerate and use within 4–5 days.

Nutritional analysis per serving (250 ml/8 fl oz): calories 236, fat 25.3 g, cholesterol 0 mg, fibre 0 g, protein 1 g, carbohydrate 3 g, sodium 35 mg,

ALMOND MILK

Before making the milk below, soak the almonds in water overnight to make them soft and easier to blend. Soaking also unlocks nutrients, making them easier to absorb and digest.

Yield: 650 ml (22 fl oz), unstrained
Prep time: overnight soaking, plus 2 minutes to blend

- 40 g (1½ oz) raw almonds
- 1 litre (1¾ pints) filtered water

Place the almonds in a bowl, add enough water to cover them by 5 cm (2 in) and leave to soak overnight.

Drain the almonds and place them in a blender. Add the filtered water and start blending slowly, gradually increasing to a high speed. Continue to blend at high speed for 1–1½ minutes.

The mixture can be used as it is, but for smoother, finer almond milk, strain it through a nut milk bag (available online or at healthfood stores), squeezing the bag to get as much milk as possible from the almond pulp. Cover and refrigerate the milk, and use within 3 days. Stir well or shake before using.

Nutritional analysis per serving (250 ml/8 fl oz unstrained):
calories 180, fat 15 g, saturated fat 1 g, cholesterol 0 mg,
fibre 4 g, protein 6 g, carbohydrate 6 g, sodium 5 mg

Nutritional analysis per serving (250 ml/8 fl oz strained):
calories 90, fat 8 g, saturated fat 1 g, cholesterol 0 mg,
fibre 2 g, protein 3 g, carbohydrate 3 g, sodium 5 mg

CASHEW MILK

Once the nuts are soaked and puréed, cashew milk is smooth and creamy – there is no need to strain it.

Yield: 1.25 litres (2¼ pints)
Prep time: overnight soaking, plus 2 minutes to blend

- 175 g (6 oz) raw cashews
- 1 litre (1¾ pints) filtered water

Place the cashews in a bowl, add enough water to cover them by 5 cm (2 in) and leave to soak overnight.

Drain the nuts and place them in a blender. Add the filtered water and start blending slowly, gradually increasing to a high speed. Continue to blend at high speed for 1–1½ minutes, until smooth and creamy. Cover and refrigerate the unstrained milk. Use within 3–4 days. Stir well or shake before using.

Tip: For flavoured milk, try the following ideas. Scrape the seeds of 1–2 vanilla pods into the milk, or stir in some ground cinnamon or other aromatic spice.

Nutritional analysis per serving (250 ml/8 fl oz):
calories 243, fat 18 g, saturated fat 3 g, cholesterol 0 mg,
fibre 1.5 g, protein 7.6 g, carbohydrate 13.7 g, sodium 7 mg

CHIA AND BERRY BREAKFAST PUDDING

A nice departure from smoothies and eggs, this pudding is almost like eating dessert. Make it ahead of time for a quick and delicious start to the day. Chia seeds add protein, fibre, healthy omega-3 fats and important minerals.

Yield: 4 servings
Prep time: 10 minutes

- 375 ml (13 fl oz) full-fat coconut milk
- 375 ml (13 fl oz) unsweetened almond milk
- 120 g (4½ oz) chia seeds
- 2 teaspoons no-alcohol, gluten-free pure vanilla extract
- 2 teaspoons ground cinnamon
- 250 g (9 oz) fresh berries
- 25 g (1 oz) finely chopped walnuts, for garnish
- optional: ¾ teaspoon ground nutmeg

Place all the ingredients, except the walnuts, in a large mixing bowl and stir until everything is incorporated. Pour the mixture into four 275 g (10 oz) serving bowls. Cover and refrigerate overnight to set.

To serve, top each bowl with equal amounts of the berries, chopped walnuts, and ground nutmeg, if using.

Nutritional analysis per serving (1 pudding with berries):
calories 430, fat 31 g, saturated fat 12 g, cholesterol 0 mg,
fibre 15 g, protein 9 g, carbohydrate 28 g, sodium 95 mg

EGGS AND PANCAKES

Broccoli Sausage Frittata

With a few veggies and pre-cooked chicken sausage, you can have this satisfying, savory frittata on the table in under 45 minutes, perfect for a weekend breakfast or brunch. Serve with diced avocado and fresh berries on the side.

Yield: 4 servings
Prep time: 20 minutes
Cook time: 15 minutes

- 175 g (6 oz) broccoli florets
- 2 pre-cooked, Italian-seasoned, organic, nitrate-free chicken or turkey sausages
- 1 small leek, white and pale green parts only
- 1 tablespoon clarified unsalted butter or ghee
- 8 large omega-3 eggs
- 1/4 teaspoon ground black pepper
- 1 tablespoon chopped fresh oregano or parsley leaves
- 1 avocado, peeled, stoned and diced

Preheat the oven to 200°C/400°F/Gas mark 6. Meanwhile, cook the broccoli florets in boiling water 2 minutes. Drain immediately and chop into small pieces. This step can be done in advance to make the preparation quicker.

Quarter the sausages lengthways, then chop widthways into small pieces.

Halve the trimmed leek lengthways and rinse well in cold water to dislodge any sand or dirt. Chop widthways into thin slices.

Melt the clarified butter in a medium-sized ovenproof frying pan. Add the leeks and cook over a medium heat until softened (about 2 minutes). Add the sausage pieces and brown for 3–4 minutes, mixing them with the leeks. Stir in the broccoli and spread the mixture into an even layer in the pan.

Whisk the eggs in a bowl until smooth, then pour evenly over the vegetables, spreading with a spatula if necessary. Sprinkle with the pepper.

Place the pan in the oven and bake until the frittata is set in the centre and the top is a light golden brown (about 14–16 minutes).

The frittata can be eaten immediately or at room temperature. To serve, cut it into 4 wedges and top each serving with a quarter of the avocado. Leftovers should be covered and refrigerated for up to 2 days. Reheat in a warm oven or enjoy at room temperature.

Nutritional analysis per serving (1 wedge):
calories 340, fat 25 g, saturated fat 7 g, cholesterol 495 mg,
fibre 5 g, protein 24 g, carbohydrate 13 g, sodium 570 mg

GRAIN-FREE DUTCH BABY PANCAKES WITH SAUTÉED DANDELION GREENS

When this pancake comes out of the oven it looks almost like cornbread, but don't be fooled. No grains were used, just gluten-free almond and coconut flours. Serve in wedges piled with sautéed dandelion greens, which give a nice bitter edge, or with kale, spinach or chard.

Yield: 4 servings
Prep time: 15 minutes
Cook time: 25 minutes

- 65 g (2½ oz) blanched almond flour
- 35 g (1¼ oz) coconut flour
- ½ teaspoon baking powder
- pinch of sea salt
- 6 large omega-3 eggs
- 250 ml (8 fl oz) strained unsweetened almond milk
- 2 tablespoons butter
- 175 g (6 oz) dandelion greens, washed and dried
- 1 tablespoon extra virgin olive oil
- 1 large shallot
- 3 garlic cloves, finely chopped
- ¼ teaspoon sea salt
- ¼ teaspoon ground black pepper

Place a medium-sized, ovenproof frying pan in the oven and preheat both to 220°C/425°F/Gas mark 7.

Meanwhile, put the flours, baking powder and salt in a bowl and whisk together. In another bowl or large measuring jug, whisk the eggs until smooth, then whisk in the almond milk. Gradually pour this liquid into the dry mixture and whisk until you have a smooth batter.

When the oven has reached the correct temperature, add the butter to the hot pan and wait for it to melt completely (about 45 seconds). Pour in the batter, return the pan to the oven and bake for 20 minutes. When done, the frittata will resemble cornbread, with a lightly golden, puffed top and edges that are just pulling away from the sides of the pan. Set aside to cool for a minute or so.

While the pancake is baking, prepare the greens. Chop 7.5–10 cm (3–4 in) off the bottom of the dandelion stems, then chop them widthways into small pieces. It will seem like a lot, but greens wilt down quickly. Peel the shallot, cut in half lengthways, then slice widthways into half-moons.

Heat the oil in a large sauté pan over a medium heat. When hot, add the shallots and cook until softened (about 1–2 minutes), stirring to keep them from burning, and lowering the heat, if necessary. Add the garlic and sauté for another 30–60 seconds, then add the chopped greens and cook, stirring until they are wilted and soft (about 3–4 minutes).

To serve, cut the pancake into 4 wedges and place on plates. Pile a quarter of the wilted greens onto each wedge and sprinkle with salt and pepper to taste.

Nutritional analysis per serving:
calories 350, fat 27 g, saturated fat 9 g, cholesterol 350 mg,
fibre 7 g, protein 17 g, carbohydrate 18 g, sodium 390 mg

MEXICAN-STYLE EGG AND VEGETABLE SCRAMBLE

Lots of colour and vegetables make for an out-of-the-ordinary breakfast scramble with south-of-the-border flavour. The bacon can be cooked ahead of time for faster cooking on busy mornings. Add as much chilli as you dare. Serve with a small side of fresh berries.

Yield: 4 servings
Prep time: 10 minutes
Cook time: 10–20 minutes

- 4 strips uncured turkey bacon
- 6 large omega-3 eggs
- 2 tablespoons full-fat coconut milk
- 20g (3/4 oz) clarified unsalted butter or ghee
- 1 small onion, finely chopped
- 1 red or orange pepper, seeded and finely chopped
- 1 tomato, cored, seeded and finely chopped
- 1 small jalapeño chilli, seeded and finely chopped (optional if heat sensitive)
- 1 tablespoon freshly chopped coriander leaves
- 1 avocado, peeled, stoned and sliced into eighths
- ¼ teaspoon sea salt
- ¼ teaspoon ground black pepper

Preheat the oven to 180°C/350°F/Gas mark 4. Line a rimmed baking sheet with foil, and place a wire rack on top if you wish (this will facilitate browning). When the oven is ready, place the bacon strips on the foil or rack and bake for 9–10 minutes. Turn and bake the other side for another 9–10 minutes, or until crisp and brown. Chop the bacon into small pieces and set aside.

Crack the eggs into a bowl, add the coconut milk and whisk until smooth. Set aside.

Heat the oil in a large, non-stick frying pan over a medium heat. When hot, add the onion, pepper and tomato. Stir and cook until the vegetables are softened (about 2 minutes). Add the chilli and cook until softened (about 1 more minute).

Add the whisked eggs to the pan and reduce the heat to low. Sprinkle the chopped bacon over the eggs. Cook slowly, pushing the eggs around the pan with a wooden spoon or spatula until they are creamy and scrambled.

Sprinkle the eggs with the coriander and serve with the avocado slices. Season to taste with salt and pepper.

> **Tool Tip:** If your non-stick pan is scratched and flaking, it's time for a new one. Use only wooden or heat-resistant silicone tools in non-stick pans to extend their life, and be sure to hand-wash them. Always use liquid oils or butter – not sprays – in non-stick pans.

Nutritional analysis per serving:
calories 290, fat 21 g, saturated fa: 5 g, cholesterol 360 mg, fibre 5 g, protein 17 g, carbohydrate 11 g, sodium 540 mg

QUICK HERB AND AVOCADO OMELETTE

This combo is fast enough for a quick breakfast and equally excellent for lunch along with a tossed green salad.

Yield: 1 serving
Prep time: 5 minutes
Cook time: 5 minutes

- 2 teaspoons unsalted butter
- 2 large omega-3 eggs
- 2 teaspoons filtered water
- 1 tablespoon chopped parsley or coriander leaves
- 1 spring onion, thinly chopped
- pinch of sea salt
- pinch of ground black pepper
- 1/4 avocado, sliced
- 1/2 small tomato, thinly sliced

Place a small ovenproof non-stick frying pan over a medium-low heat and add the butter. Meanwhile, whisk the eggs, water and herbs together. Add the salt and pepper and whisk again.

When the butter has melted and the frying pan is hot, pour in the eggs and allow them to sit undisturbed until the bottom has set (about 1–2 minutes). With a flexible spatula, gently lift the edges of the omelette and allow the liquid eggs to flow underneath. Cook for another minute, until set but creamy, then place the slices of tomato and avocado on one half of the omelette. Fold the other half on top and serve.

For a firmer omelette, finish cooking it under a hot grill for 15–30 seconds to set the still-creamy eggs. Place the slices of tomato and avocado on one half of the omelette. Fold the other half on top and serve.

Nutritional analysis per serving:
calories 300, fat 25 g, saturated fat 9 g, cholesterol 470 mg, fibre 4 g, protein 16 g, carbohydrate 9 g, sodium 230 mg

Sautéed Cavolo Nero and Peppers with Poached Eggs

Poached eggs seem to work for almost any meal, and this colourful, vegetable-filled dish is perfect for a weekend lunch or brunch. A mustardy sauce recipe is included, but you could also use Avocado Cream (page 266) or the No-Cheese Sauce (page 330).

Yield: 4 servings
Prep time: 25 minutes
Cook time: 20 minutes

- 400 g (14 oz) cavolo nero or kale
- 2 large red or orange peppers, cored, seeded and cut into thin strips
- 1 sweet onion
- 11/2 tablespoons extra virgin olive oil
- 4 garlic cloves, finely chopped
- 1/4 teaspoon sea salt
- 1/4 teaspoon ground black pepper, plus a little extra to serve
- 8 large omega-3 eggs, poached

FOR THE EGGS

- 100 g (4 oz) organic or homemade mayonnaise (see page 332)
- 2 tablespoons Dijon mustard
- 1 teaspoon finely chopped fresh tarragon
- optional: few drops of hot chilli sauce
- optional: 1/2 teaspoon paprika

Hold a cavolo nero stalk in one hand and run your other hand upwards to strip off the leaf. Alternatively, cut out the stem with a sharp knife.

Repeat with the remaining cavolo nero, then cut the leaves widthways into thin ribbons.

Cut the onion in half from stem to root end, then slice the halves into thin half-moons.

Heat the oil in a large sauté or frying pan over a medium heat. When hot, add the onion and peppers and cook, stirring now and then, until soft (about 4 minutes). Add the garlic and cook for another 30 seconds, stirring. Sprinkle with the salt and pepper. Add the cavolo nero and stir to combine. It will look big, but soon cooks down. It will reduce and soften in 5–7 minutes. If you like softer kale, add 1–2 tablespoons water to the pan to steam it. When done to your liking, cover the pan and turn off the heat.

To make the sauce, whisk together the mayonnaise, mustard, tarragon leaves and hot chilli sauce (if using). Set aside.

To serve, divide the vegetables between 4 shallow bowls, top with 2 poached eggs per bowl, then drizzle each serving with 2 tablespoons of the sauce. Sprinkle with the paprika and some freshly ground black pepper.

Nutritional analysis per serving:
calories 470, fat 37 g, saturated fat 7 g, cholesterol 495 mg,
fibre 4 g, protein 19 g, carbohydrate 22 g, sodium 620 mg

ALMOND PANCAKES WITH BERRIES

Golden pancakes for a weekend breakfast treat – with no wheat or grains! Top with fresh berries and a drizzle of warmed coconut oil, clarified butter or ghee.

Yield: 4 servings (about twelve 10 cm/4-in pancakes)
Prep time: 10 minutes
Cook time: 20 minutes

- 4 large omega-3 eggs
- 120 ml (4 fl oz) full-fat coconut milk
- 120 ml (4 fl oz) filtered water
- 2 tablespoons clarified butter, ghee or coconut oil
- 2 teaspoons no-alcohol, gluten-free pure vanilla or almond extract

- 120 g (4½ oz) almond flour
- 35 g (1¼ oz) coconut flour
- 1 teaspoon bicarbonate of soda
- ½ teaspoon cinnamon
- ¼ teaspoon sea salt
- 1 teaspoon coconut oil (for the griddle)

FOR THE PANCAKE TOPPING

- 40 g (1½ oz) melted coconut oil or clarified butter
- 250 g (9 oz) raspberries, blackberries, blueberries or sliced strawberries

Preheat the oven to its lowest setting and place an ovenproof plate inside.

In a medium bowl, whisk together the eggs, coconut milk, water, butter and vanilla until smooth.

In a separate bowl, whisk together the flours, bicarbonate of soda, cinnamon and salt. Gradually whisk the wet ingredients into the dry mixture until it forms a thick, slightly grainy batter.

Heat the coconut oil in a non-stick flat griddle pan. When hot, ladle 60 ml (21/4 fl oz) of the batter into the pan and cook until bubbles form around the edge and the underside is light golden brown (about 4–5 minutes). You might be able to cook 3 or 4 at a time, depending on the size of your pan. Turn the pancakes over and cook the other side until speckled brown (about another 2 minutes). Transfer to the warm plate in the oven and cover with a clean tea towel. Make the remaining pancakes in the same way.

Serve 3 pancakes per person, topping each serving with equal amounts of the melted coconut oil and fresh berries.

Nutritional analysis per serving:
calories 460, fat 39 g, saturated fat 19 g, cholesterol 225 mg,
fibre 10 g, protein 59 g, carbohydrate 20 g, sodium 580 mg

SALADS

Lemon-Dill Prawn and Avocado Salad

The classic flavour combination of bright lemon and refreshing dill make a creamy sauce for cooked prawns, served over an avocado half with crisp greens. With the items packed separately and kept cold, it transports easily for lunch away from home. Homemade mayonnaise makes this salad extra delicious.

Yield: 4 servings
Prep time: 20 minutes
Cook time: 0 minutes

- 550 g (1¼ lb) cooked prawns
- juice of 1 lemon
- 1 small shallot, finely chopped
- 2 celery sticks, finely chopped
- 3 tablespoons organic or homemade mayonnaise (page 332)
- 1 rounded tablespoon Dijon mustard
- 1 rounded tablespoon capers, rinsed and drained
- 2 tablespoons finely chopped fresh dill, plus a little extra for garnish (optional)
- 350 g (12 oz) salad greens, washed and dried
- 2 avocados, stoned and quartered
- 1 rounded tablespoon hemp seeds
- about 20 tiny tomatoes (e.g. tomberries), halved
- sea salt and ground black pepper, to taste
- 2 large spring onions, finely chopped

FOR THE VINAIGRETTE

- 3 tablespoons extra virgin olive oil
- 1½ tablespoons champagne or white wine vinegar
- 1 teaspoon Dijon mustard

Place the prawns in a bowl, toss with 1 tablespoon of the lemon juice, then set aside.

In another small bowl, combine the shallot, celery, mayonnaise, 4 teaspoons of the lemon juice, the mustard, capers and dill and mix well. Season to taste with a little salt and pepper.

Drain the prawns and add them to the bowl with the mayonnaise mixture. Toss gently to coat.

Make the vinaigrette by whisking together the olive oil, vinegar and mustard until smooth.

Divide the salad greens between 4 plates. Place 2 avocado quarters in the centre and top each serving with a quarter of the prawn mixture. Scatter 1 teaspoon of the hemps seeds over each salad and garnish with a little extra dill, if desired. Scatter the tomatoes around each plate. Drizzle the vinaigrette over the salad greens and serve.

Nutritional analysis per serving:
calories 520, fat 38 g, saturated fat 5 g, cholesterol 235 mg,
fibre 10 g, protein 34 g, carbohydrate 19 g, sodium 600 mg

ROAST CHICKEN, RASPBERRY AND WALNUT SALAD

Here's a fun and healthy twist on classic chicken salad. Roast the chicken a few days ahead to make assembly faster, or use leftover roast chicken, or a rotisserie chicken from the supermarket.

Yield: 4 servings
Prep time: 20 minutes

- 65 g (2½ oz) chopped walnuts
- 1 large celery stick, finely chopped
- 50 g (2 oz) organic or homemade mayonnaise (see page 332)
- 1 small shallot, finely chopped
- 2½ tablespoons chopped fresh herbs (dill, parsley, coriander, tarragon or thyme)
- 2 teaspoons fresh lemon juice
- 450 g (1 lb) roast chicken breast, chopped into bite-sized pieces
- sea salt and pepper
- 225 g (8 oz) salad greens (e.g. rocket, lamb's lettuce, romaine)
- 1 avocado, stoned and quartered
- 90 g (3½ oz) fresh raspberries

FOR THE VINAIGRETTE

- 2 tablespoons walnut oil
- 1 tablespoon vinegar (champagne, raspberry or red wine)
- sea salt and ground black pepper

Put the walnuts, celery, mayonnaise, shallot, herbs and lemon juice in a medium bowl and stir together until well combined. Add the chopped chicken breast and toss to coat evenly. Season with salt and pepper, as needed.

To assemble the dish, divide the salad greens between 4 plates. Whisk the oil and vinegar together, add a little seasoning, then drizzle the dressing over the greens. Top each plate with equal amounts of the chicken salad. Place an avocado quarter and some of the raspberries around the edge of each plate.

Nutritional analysis per serving:
calories 450, fat 34 g, saturated fat 4 g, cholesterol 55 mg, fibre 7 g, protein 26 g, carbohydrate 14 g, sodium 151 mg

CALIFORNIA KALE COBB SALAD

With artichoke hearts and avocado, this colourful and hearty kale salad will fill and fuel you with veggies, healthy fats and plenty of protein. To save prep time, wash and chop the kale and bake the bacon ahead of time.

Yield: 4 servings
Prep time: 20 minutes

- 4 slices turkey bacon
- 400 g (14 oz) kale
- 1 avocado, stoned and diced
- 100 g (4 oz) tomberries or cherry tomatoes, halved
- 1 x 400 g (14 oz) can water-packed artichoke heart quarters, drained
- 450 g (1 lb) cooked chicken, diced
- 4 spring onions, green parts thinly sliced for garnish

FOR THE DRESSING

- 100 g (4 oz) organic or homemade mayonnaise (see page 332)
- 2 tablespoons fresh lemon juice
- 2 tablespoons finely chopped flatleaf parsley
- 1 tablespoon Dijon mustard
- 1 garlic clove, finely chopped
- pinch of ground black or white pepper

Preheat the oven to 180°C/350°F/Gas mark 4. Line a rimmed baking sheet with foil, and place a wire rack on it if you wish; this will help the bacon you are going to cook to become crisp and brown.

When the oven is ready, place the bacon strips on the foil and bake for 9–10 minutes. Turn the strips and bake the other side for another 9–10 minutes, or until crisp and brown. Remove the bacon and chop into small pieces. Set aside.

While the bacon is baking, wash the kale leaves, cut out the central rib and chop leaves widthways into thin ribbons. Pile them onto 4 plates and top with equal amounts of the avocado, bacon, tomatoes, artichokes and chicken.

Put all the dressing ingredients into a small bowl and whisk until creamy and smooth.

Sprinkle each salad with the spring onions and serve with 2 tablespoons of creamy dressing on the side per serving.

Nutritional analysis per serving:
calories 540, fat 33 g, saturated fat 5 g, cholesterol 130 mg, fibre 9 g, protein 38 g, carbohydrate 28 g, sodium 490 mg

CURRIED EGG SALAD (AND HOW TO MAKE PERFECT HARD-BOILED EGGS)

Hard-boiled eggs keep for a week in the refrigerator, so you can have a supply of them ready to make this quick salad for lunch or a snack. This recipe, which includes the best technique for peeling eggs, gives a spicy Indian twist to standard egg salad.

A tip for finely zesting ginger: use a microplane grater.

Yield: 4 servings
Prep time: 25 minutes, including boiling time for the eggs
Cook time: 25 minutes, including boiling and cooling the eggs

- 8 large omega-3 eggs
- 3 tablespoons white vinegar
- 2 teaspoons sea salt
- 100 g (4 oz) organic or homemade mayonnaise (see page 332)
- 2 rounded tablespoons mild curry powder
- 2 tablespoons fresh lime juice
- 5-cm (2-in) piece of fresh ginger, peeled and finely grated
- ¼ teaspoon sea salt
- ¼ teaspoon ground black pepper
- ¼ teaspoon cayenne pepper, or to taste
- 2 large celery sticks, trimmed and finely chopped
- 1 small shallot, finely chopped
- 2 tablespoons finely chopped coriander leaves
- 250 g (9 oz) baby salad greens

Start by hard-boiling the eggs. Half-fill a medium saucepan with water (enough to cover the eggs once they are added). Place over a medium-high heat and bring almost to the boil. Add the vinegar and salt, then gently submerge the eggs in the water (to make it easy, use a slotted spoon or long-handled, flat mesh strainer). Turn the heat down to low and simmer the eggs for 15 minutes.

While the eggs are simmering, prepare an ice bath. Half-fill a medium bowl with ice, then fill three-quarters full of cold water. Set it by the stove to chill the eggs when they are done.

While the eggs are boiling and cooling, make the dressing. Put the mayonnaise in a medium bowl and stir in the curry powder, lime juice, ginger, salt and pepper and mix until smooth. Add the celery, shallots and coriander and stir again.

When the eggs have completely cooled in the ice bath, store in the refrigerator, or use straight away in the salad. To peel, crack them all over on the edge of the sink, then roll gently in your hands under running water. The shell should come off easily.

Cut the eggs into eighths, then chop. Add to the bowl with the dressing and mix gently. If the salad seems stiff (it will depend on the thickness of your mayonnaise), add a little water to make it softer and creamier. Start with 1–2 teaspoons, and continue adding until it is as creamy as you prefer.

Place a quarter of the salad greens on a plate, top with a quarter of the egg salad and serve. The leftovers can be stored in a covered container in the refrigerator for up to 3 days.

Nutritional analysis per serving:
calories 360, fat 33 g, saturated fat 6 g, cholesterol 495 mg,
fibre 2 g, protein 16 g, carbohydrate 8 g, sodium 350 mg

BISTRO FLANK STEAK SALAD WITH BABY GREEN BEANS

The classic French flavours of Dijon mustard and tarragon combine for a marinade and vinaigrette for this main course salad. Grill or griddle the steak in just minutes, and serve with oven-caramelized red onions (page 336) and tender baby beans, both of which can be prepared in advance if you wish.

Yield: 4 servings
Prep time: 10 minutes, plus 1 hour for marinating
Cook time: 20 minutes

- 4 tablespoons extra virgin olive oil
- 4 tablespoons red wine vinegar
- 4 tablespoons Dijon mustard
- 1 tablespoon chopped fresh tarragon or thyme leaves
- 550–750 g (1¼ –1½ lb) grass-fed flank steak
- ¼ teaspoon sea salt
- ¼ teaspoon ground black pepper
- ¼ teaspoon garlic granules
- 1 teaspoon avocado oil (for grill pan)
- 225 g (8 oz) fresh mixed baby greens or spinach
- 350 g (12 oz) cooked baby green beans (see page 251)

FOR THE VINAIGRETTE

- 2 tablespoons oil (extra virgin olive, walnut or avocado)
- 1 tablespoon vinegar (red wine or balsamic)
- 1 teaspoon Dijon mustard
- pinch of sea salt and ground black pepper

In a small bowl, whisk together the oil, vinegar, mustard and tarragon until smooth. Sprinkle the steak with the salt, pepper and garlic. Place the steak in a flat glass dish and cover with the marinade, coating both sides. Set aside to marinate at room temperature for 1 hour, or refrigerate overnight for more flavour. If marinating overnight, allow the steak to stand at room temperature for 1 hour before grilling.

Brush a griddle pan with the avocado oil and place over a medium-high heat. When hot, add the steak and griddle for 3–4 minutes per side. Flank steak is best cooked to medium-rare to maintain tenderness (the internal temperature should be about 50°C/125°F).

When the steak is done, transfer it to a cutting board and allow to stand for 10 minutes to redistribute the internal juices.

Meanwhile, put all the vinaigrette ingredients in a small bowl and whisk together.

To serve, pile the salad greens in the centre of 4 plates and scatter the green beans around the edges. (Note: green beans can be served warm, at room temperature or chilled.) Drizzle with the vinaigrette. Slice the steak thinly across the grain and arrange equal amounts on top of each salad. Serve straight away.

Nutritional analysis per serving:
calories 470, fat 32 g, saturated fat 7 g, cholesterol 105 mg,
fibre 3 g, protein 39 g, carbohydrate 8 g, sodium 500 mg

CHICKEN CHOPPED SALAD WITH PALM HEARTS AND CREAMY HERB DRESSING

Tender, ivory-coloured palm hearts are the edible part of buds from the cabbage palm. Their delicate flavour, a bit like that of mild artichokes, makes a nice addition to this salad. The chicken breasts can be poached

3–4 days ahead of time and refrigerated until needed, or cooked just before you tackle this recipe, as they take only 10 minutes. All the salad ingredients can be prepped ahead and assembled before serving, then dressed.

Yield: 4 servings
Prep time: 25 minutes

- 450–750 g (1–1½ lb) poached chicken breast (see page 298)
- 1 x 400-g (14-oz) can water-packed hearts of palm, drained
- 225 g (8 oz) leafy salad greens (e.g. lamb's lettuce, baby kale)
- 4 small plum tomatoes, quartered or sliced
- 1 avocado, stoned and diced or sliced
- 4 tablespoons raw sunflower seeds
- ¼ red onion, thinly sliced

FOR THE CREAMY DRESSING

- 100 g (4 oz) organic or homemade mayonnaise (see page 332)
- 3 tablespoons fresh lime juice
- 1 tablespoon chopped flat leaf parsley leaves
- 1 tablespoon chopped coriander leaves
- 3 large garlic cloves, finely chopped or grated
- pinch of sea salt
- pinch of ground black or white pepper

First make the dressing by putting all the ingredients for it in a small bowl and whisking together until smooth. If the mixture seems too thick, add another tablespoon of lime juice. Set aside.

Cut the poached chicken into 2.5-cm (1-in) chunks. Slice the artichoke hearts into 1-cm (1/2-in) pieces.

Divide the salad greens between 4 plates. Top with the chicken, palm hearts, tomatoes, avocado, seeds and onion. Serve with the dressing on the side – 2 tablespoons per person.

Nutritional analysis per serving:
calories 420, fat 34 g, saturated fat 6 g, cholesterol 60 mg,
fibre 9 g, protein 15 g, carbohydrate 17 g, sodium 625 mg

MEDITERRANEAN LAMB CHOP AND SPINACH SALAD WITH GREEK PESTO

This main-course salad, with its Greek-inspired flavours, gives you a taste of the Mediterranean. To save time, you can make the pesto in advance and keep it refrigerated. Once the remaining prep work is done, the lamb chops cook quickly, so this is a fast recipe to put together.

Yield: 4 servings
Prep time: 30 minutes
Cook time: 15 minutes

- 12 grass-fed double-rib lamb chops
- 1–2 teaspoons coconut oil (for greasing)

FOR THE PESTO

- 250 g (9 oz) fresh mint leaves
- 225 g (8 oz) fresh oregano leaves
- 6 garlic cloves, peeled
- 2 teaspoons lemon zest
- 120 ml (4 fl oz) fresh lemon juice
- 120 ml (4 fl oz) extra virgin olive oil
- 120 g (4½ oz) chopped walnuts
- optional: 2 tablespoons nutritional yeast
- ½ teaspoon sea salt
- ¼ teaspoon ground black pepper

FOR THE VINAIGRETTE

- 4 tablespoons extra virgin olive oil
- 2 tablespoons red wine vinegar
- sea salt and ground black pepper

FOR THE SALAD

- 350 g (12 oz) baby spinach leaves
- 100 g (4 oz) pitted Kalamata olives, rinsed and drained
- 100 g (4 oz) tiny tomatoes, halved
- 4 small cucumbers, preferably seedless type, chopped or sliced

First make the pesto. Place all the ingredients for it in a food processor and pulse until a smooth paste forms, scraping down the sides of the bowl as needed. Set aside.

Using about 120 g (4 1/2 oz) of the pesto, brush it thinly over each side of the lamb chops. Place the chops on a foil-lined baking sheet or large plate and leave to stand at room temperature for 30–40 minutes.

Meanwhile, make the vinaigrette by whisking the oil and vinegar together in a small bowl until combined. Season to taste with salt and pepper. Set aside.

Heat the grill or a large griddle pan until hot. Lower the heat to medium. Wipe the grill pan or griddle pan lightly with the coconut oil to prevent sticking. Place the chops on it and cook for 3–3 1/2 minutes per side. When done to your liking, allow to stand for 5–10 minutes to reabsorb the juices.

Divide the spinach leaves between 4 plates, add the olives, tomatoes and cucumbers, then drizzle with the vinaigrette. Add 3 lamb chops to each plate and serve with a tablespoon of pesto on top or on the side. Any leftover pesto can be refrigerated for future use, provided it has not touched the raw meat.

Nutritional analysis per serving:
calories 740, fat 56 g, saturated fat 10 g, cholesterol 130 mg,
fibre 5 g, protein 47 g, carbohydrate 16 g, sodium 710 mg

BASIC SALAD WITH VINAIGRETTE DRESSING

Adding a tossed green salad to any meal is a great way to increase your vegetable intake. Leafy salad greens, the darker the better, are packed with nutrition, so give the iceberg a miss and try some of the many other varieties now available. The amount of greens listed below is ideal for a main-course salad, so use a little less for a side salad. To increase the healthy fat content, add a wedge of avocado and a sprinkle of chopped nuts or seeds.

Yield: 4 servings
Prep time: 15 minutes

- 350 g (12 oz) dark leafy greens
- 1 avocado, stoned and sliced or diced
- 1 handful of chopped nuts or seeds

FOR THE VINAIGRETTE

- 3 tablespoons oil (e.g. extra virgin olive oil, or minimally refined flavoured oil, such as avocado, walnut, pumpkin seed or pistachio)
- 1 tablespoon vinegar (e.g. red or white wine, unseasoned rice, balsamic, apple cider or raspberry, or even lemon or lime juice)
- pinch of sea salt and ground black pepper
- optional: 1 garlic clove, finely chopped or grated
- optional: 1–2 teaspoons Dijon mustard

First make the vinaigrette. Whisk the oil and the vinegar together until combined, then season to taste with salt and pepper. For extra flavour, add the optional ingredients if you wish.

Divide the greens equally between 4 plates. Top with the avocado and nuts, and drizzle 1 tablespoon of the vinaigrette over each salad.

Nutritional analysis per serving:
calories 190, fat 18 g, saturated fat 3 g, cholesterol 0 mg,
fibre 5 g, protein 2 g, carbohydrate 7 g, sodium 150 mg

CHICKEN, TURKEY AND DUCK

SUN-DRIED TOMATO AND TURKEY BURGERS

You won't miss the bun with these moist and flavourful turkey burgers.

Yield: 4 servings
Prep time: 10 minutes
Cook time: 15 minutes

- 550 g (1¼ lb) minced dark turkey meat (ideally,15% fat, but if you can find only 7–10% fat content, add 2 teaspoons olive oil to the burger mix)
- 12 large oil-packed, sulphite-free sundried tomatoes, chopped
- 2 tablespoons finely chopped fresh basil or parsley leaves
- 1 rounded tablespoon, Dijon mustard
- ¼ teaspoon sea salt
- ¼ teaspoon ground black pepper
- optional: 2 pinches of dried red chilli flakes
- 1 teaspoon extra virgin olive oil
- 1 quantity Avocado Cream (see page 266)

Put the turkey meat in a medium bowl with the tomatoes, herbs, mustard, salt, pepper and chilli flakes (if using). Mix with wet hands (to prevent sticking) until well incorporated. Divide the mixture into 4 equal portions and shape into round burgers about 2 cm (3/4 in) thick. Using a 10-cm (4-in) ring mould makes light work of this.

Place the oil in a non-stick frying pan over a medium-low heat. When hot, add the burgers and cook until the underside forms a browned crust (3–4 minutes). Turn the burgers over, cover the pan with a lid and cook on a low heat for 7–8 minutes, or until a meat thermometer registers 75°C (165°F) when inserted in the centre.

Serve each burger with a quarter of the avocado cream on top. This goes nicely with a side salad and the Courgette Ribbon Salad (see page 339-40).

Nutritional analysis per serving:
calories 460, fat 38 g, saturated fat 8 g, cholesterol 135 mg,
fibre 4 g, protein 26 g, carbohydrate 26 g, sodium 470 mg

QUICK CHICKEN BREAST WITH SPANISH ROMESCO SAUCE

A classic sauce from the Catalonia region of Spain, romesco works beautifully over fish as well as this quick chicken. For an extra layer of flavour, use smoked paprika. Serve this with broccoli drizzled with 1 teaspoon of olive oil per person, and a tossed green side salad with a quarter of an avocado.

Yield: 4 servings
Prep time: 15 minutes
Cook time: 20 minutes

- 4 boneless, skinless chicken breasts (about 750 g/1½ lb in total)
- ¼ teaspoon sea salt
- ¼ teaspoon ground black pepper
- ¼ teaspoon garlic granules
- 1 tablespoon extra virgin olive oil
- 120 ml (4 fl oz) low-sodium chicken stock

FOR THE SAUCE

- 40 g (1½ oz) whole almonds
- 3 garlic cloves, peeled
- 225 g (8 oz) ready-made roasted red peppers, drained, seeded and roughly chopped
- 2 medium tomatoes, quartered and cored
- 40 g (1½ oz) finely chopped onion
- 3 tablespoons extra virgin olive oil
- 1½ teaspoons paprika, regular or smoked
- 1 teaspoon sherry vinegar or red wine vinegar
- ¼ teaspoon sea salt
- ¼ teaspoon ground black pepper

First make the sauce. Using a food processor, grind the almonds and garlic together for 20–30 seconds. Add all the remaining sauce ingredients and process until fairly smooth (1–2 minutes).

Sprinkle the chicken with the salt, pepper and garlic. Heat the oil in a large, heavy-based frying pan. When hot but not smoking, add the chicken breasts, smooth-side down, and cook over a medium heat until this side is golden (about 5 minutes).

Turn the chicken over, add the stock, then cover the pan with a tight-fitting lid. Cook over a low heat until a meat thermometer registers 75°C/165°F when inserted into the thickest part of the chicken (about 7–8 minutes).

Allow the chicken to rest for a few minutes, then slice across grain. Serve with 4 tablespoons of the romesco sauce per person. If refrigerated in separate airtight containers, any leftover chicken will keep for 3 days, and the sauce for 4–5 days.

Nutritional analysis per serving:
calories 460, fat 27 g, saturated fat 4 g, cholesterol 100 mg,
fibre 6 g, protein 43 g, carbohydrate 13 g, sodium 550 mg

POACHED CHICKEN BREAST

Poaching chicken breasts takes just minutes and the meat can be used for many different meals. For proper poaching, you'll need to use a large, heavy-based pan that will take all the breasts in a single layer without being squashed together. They can be prepared up to four days ahead, and refrigerated (well wrapped) for use during the busy week. The meat can be used chilled for salads, or warmed and enjoyed with one of the sauces. As a bonus, the poaching liquid can be saved and used for soups, so nothing goes to waste.

Yield: 4 servings
Prep time: 5 minutes
Cook time: 10 minutes

- 950 ml (32 fl oz) low- or no-sodium chicken stock
- 4 boneless, skinless chicken breasts (about 750 g/1½ lb in total)

Pour the stock into a large saucepan and bring to a simmer, with small bubbles breaking the surface. Turn the heat to low and test the temperature of the stock – it should be 70–80°C (160–180°F) for proper poaching.

Place the chicken breasts in the stock. If the liquid does not quite cover them, add a little more stock or water. Poach the chicken for 8–10 minutes, or until a meat thermometer registers 75°C/165°F when inserted into the thickest part of the chicken.

Using a slotted spoon, transfer the chicken to plates and serve while still hot or warm. Alternatively, allow to cool, then place in an airtight container and chill for use in a salad.

To save the poaching liquid for future use, bring it to the boil for 15 seconds, then set aside to cool in a metal or glass bowl, stirring occasionally. Do not leave it out for more than 1 hour. Set a timer to remind yourself, if needed.

When the stock is at 20°C (70°F) or cooler, place in an airtight container, adding a label with the amount and date. Refrigerate for a maximum of 3 days, or freeze for up to 3 months.

Nutritional analysis per serving (175 ml/6 fl oz): calories 170, fat 2 g, saturated fat 1 g, cholesterol 95 mg, fibre 0 g, protein 37 g, carbohydrate 2 g, sodium 590 mg

TURKEY LETTUCE WRAPS WITH CREAMY CASHEW LIME SAUCE

These wraps make a terrific, satisfying lunch, and are easily transportable for meals at the office or school. For a nut-free version, replace the chopped cashews with 6 tablespoons of hemp seeds and replace the cashew butter with tahini (sesame seed paste).

Tip: To grate ginger finely, use a microplane zester.

Yield: 4 servings
Prep time: 20 minutes
Cook time: 20 minutes

- 225 g (8 oz) sugarsnap peas
- 1 teaspoon sea salt
- 1 tablespoon coconut oil
- ½ medium onion, finely chopped
- 4 garlic cloves, finely chopped
- 5-cm (2-in) piece of fresh ginger, peeled and finely grated

- 450 g (1 lb) minced dark turkey meat
- 20 ml (1 tablespoon plus 1 teaspoon) low-sodium tamari
- 75 g (3 oz) cashew nuts, chopped, or 6 tablespoons hemp seeds
- 5 g (1 rounded teaspoon) chopped fresh coriander leaves
- 4 spring onions, finely chopped
- optional: 8–10 drops hot pepper sauce or dried red chilli flakes, to taste
- 16 soft lettuce leaves

FOR THE SAUCE

- 4 tablespoons raw creamy cashew butter, or tahini
- juice of 1 large lime
- 20 ml (1 tablespoon plus 1 teaspoon) low-sodium tamari
- 20 ml (1 tablespoon plus 1 teaspoon) unseasoned rice vinegar

Bring a large pan of water to the boil. Meanwhile, top the peas and pull off the side strings. When the water is boiling, add the salt and peas and boil for 2 minutes. Drain immediately. Chop the peas widthways into thin pieces and set aside.

Put the coconut oil in a large frying pan over a medium heat. When hot, add the onion and cook until soft but not brown, lowering the heat if necessary. Add the garlic and ginger and cook for 1 more minute. Add the turkey, breaking it up with a spatula or wooden spoon, and cook for 8–10 minutes, until no longer pink.

While the turkey is cooking, make the sauce. Put all the ingredients for it in a small bowl and stir until smooth. Set aside.

When the turkey is cooked, add the chopped peas and the tamari, then stir in the cashews, coriander, spring onions and pepper sauce (if using).

To serve, lay 4 lettuce leaves on each person's plate and top with a quarter of the turkey mixture. Add 1½ tablespoons of the sauce per plate.

Nutritional analysis per serving:
calories 470, fat 31 g, saturated fat 9 g, cholesterol 90 mg, fibre 5 g, protein 28 g, carbohydrate 20 g, sodium 540 mg

GREEK CHICKEN THIGHS WITH ARTICHOKES AND OLIVES

Mediterranean flavours of lemon, oregano, artichokes and olives make for a delicious dinner dish. You can buy pitted olives in jars or from deli counters. Serve them in shallow bowls with the vegetables and juices poured over the top. Accompany with a green salad plus a quarter of an avocado per person tossed with vinaigrette (see page 294).

Yield: 4 servings
Prep time: 15 minutes
Cook time: 25 minutes

- 8 bone-in, skin-on chicken thighs (about 1.25 kg/2½ lb in total)
- ¼ teaspoon sea salt
- ¼ teaspoon ground black pepper
- ¼ teaspoon garlic granules
- 1 medium onion
- 2½ tablespoons extra virgin olive oil
- 3 large garlic cloves, finely chopped
- 1 x 400-g (14-oz) can water-packed artichoke hearts, well drained
- 100 g (4 oz) mixed, pitted Greek olives
- 375 ml (13 fl oz) low-sodium chicken stock
- 2 tablespoons fresh chopped oregano leaves, or 2 teaspoons dried
- 1 large lemon (preferably Meyer), sliced into thin rounds
- optional: 1 tablespoon arrowroot mixed with 1 tablespoon filtered water

Trim any excess fat from the chicken thighs. Season the meat with the salt, pepper and garlic granules.

Place 11/2 tablespoons of the olive oil in a large, wide pan over a medium heat. When hot, add the chicken, skin-side down, and cook until crisp and golden brown (7–9 minutes). Transfer to a plate or rimmed baking sheet.

Put the onions into the empty pan and cook until softened (3–4 minutes). Add the chopped garlic and cook for 1 minute more. Add the artichoke hearts, olives, stock, remaining tablespoon of olive oil and the oregano and stir to combine.

Return the chicken thighs to the pan and top with the lemon slices. Bring to a strong simmer, cover with a lid, then simmer over a low heat for 12–13 minutes, or until a meat thermometer registers 75°C/165°F when inserted into the thickest part of the thighs without touching the bone.

To serve, divide the chicken thighs equally between 4 shallow bowls and pour the vegetables and juices over the top. If you prefer a thicker sauce, keep the juices in the pan and pour in the optional arrowroot paste. Stir and cook 1–2 minutes, until the liquid thickens to your liking. Pour it over the chicken and vegetables and serve straight away.

Nutritional analysis per serving:
calories 450, fat 25 g, saturated fat 4 g, cholesterol 160 mg,
fibre 4 g, protein 39 g, carbohydrate 24 g, sodium 690 mg

CRISPY SEARED DUCK BREAST WITH BLUEBERRY BALSAMIC SAUCE

If you have never cooked duck breasts, you will be amazed how easy and quick it is. The fruitiness of the blueberry sauce works well with the rich, crisp duck skin. Serve with asparagus, broccolini or green beans drizzled with olive oil, or spoon the rendered duck fat over the veggies.

Yield: 4 servings
Prep time: 15 minutes
Cook time: 20 minutes

- 4 boneless duck breasts (175 g/6 oz each)
- ¼ teaspoon sea salt
- ¼ teaspoon ground black pepper
- ¼ teaspoon garlic granules

FOR THE SAUCE

- 1 tablespoon extra virgin olive oil
- 1 small shallot, finely chopped (2 tablespoons)
- 1 garlic clove, finely chopped
- 200 g (7 oz) frozen blueberries, thawed
- 2 tablespoons balsamic vinegar
- 1 teaspoon chopped fresh thyme leaves

Preheat the oven to 220°C/425°F/Gas mark 7. Heat a large, ovenproof frying pan over a medium heat.

Meanwhile, place the duck breasts, skin-side up, on a chopping board and pat dry with kitchen paper. Turn them over and trim off any excess skin around the edges. Turn the breasts skin-side up again and use a sharp knife to score a diamond pattern over them, making the slashes 5 mm (1/4 in) apart without cutting into the flesh. Season with the salt, pepper and garlic.

Place the breasts, skin-side down, in the hot pan over a low heat. They should sizzle as they hit the surface. Sear the skin until crisp and golden brown (6–8 minutes), and the fat is rendered (released).

While the meat is searing, make the sauce (but keep your eye on the duck, peeking underneath occasionally to check the colour and crispness). Heat the olive oil in a small pan over medium-low heat. Add the shallot and cook until softened (about 2 minutes). Add the garlic and cook for another 30 seconds. Add the blueberries, vinegar and thyme, and turn the heat up to medium. Cook the blueberries, stirring, until a juicy sauce starts to form and the vinegar cooks down (about 3–4 minutes).

When the duck skin is golden brown, turn the breasts skin-side up and place the pan in the hot oven for 3–6 minutes, or until a meat thermometer registers 70°C/160°F when inserted into the thickest part of the meat. The timing depends on the thickness of the breasts. Remove the pan from the oven and set aside to rest for a few minutes.

Cut the duck breasts into thin, widthways slices. Properly cooked duck will still be pink in the middle. Take 1 tablespoon of the rendered duck fat from the pan and stir it into the blueberry sauce for added richness. Serve 1 sliced duck breast with 2 tablespoons of sauce per person.

Nutritional analysis per serving:
calories 370, fat 24 g, saturated fat 6 g, cholesterol 180 mg, fibre 2 g, protein 32 g, carbohydrate 8 g, sodium 260 mg

BRAISED CHICKEN WITH CREAMY CASHEW GRAVY

This crisp-skinned chicken with a creamy sauce will make you feel like you are eating at a French bistro. Cashew butter gives the sauce an amazingly smooth richness.

Yield: 4 servings
Prep time: 15 minutes
Cook time: 40 minutes

- 4 bone-in, skin-on chicken breasts (about 750 g/1½ lb in total)
- 1 tablespoon extra virgin olive oil
- ½ teaspoon sea salt
- ½ teaspoon garlic granules
- ¼ teaspoon ground black pepper
- 375 ml (13 fl oz) low- or no-sodium chicken stock
- 375 ml (13 fl oz) unsweetened almond milk
- 65 g (2½ oz) creamy raw cashew butter
- 2 tablespoons Dijon mustard
- 4 garlic cloves, finely chopped
- 1½ tablespoons chopped fresh thyme leaves
- 1 tablespoon arrowroot
- 2 tablespoons filtered water

Preheat the oven to 190°C/375°F/Gas mark 5.

Trim any excess fat from the top and sides of the chicken breasts. Using a heavy knife or poultry scissors, trim off the small side rib bones for a clean edge. Discard the ribs and excess fat.

Heat the olive oil in a flameproof casserole dish or frying pan large enough to hold all the chicken breasts in a single layer. Combine the salt, garlic and pepper in a small bowl and sprinkle this mixture over the chicken. Place the breasts, skin-side down, in the pan and cook until they have a golden brown crust (5–7 minutes). Turn the chicken over.

Pour the stock into a large bowl, add the almond milk, cashew butter, mustard and garlic and whisk until smooth. Pour this liquid around the chicken in the pan. Sprinkle with 1 tablespoon of the thyme, then cover and place in the oven. Cook for about 30 minutes, or until a meat thermometer registers 70–75°C (160–165°F) when inserted into the thickest part of the chicken without touching the bone. When ready, transfer the pieces to a plate, cover with foil and keep warm.

Combine the arrowroot and water in a small bowl and stir until smooth. Add this mixture to the pan juices and whisk until smooth. Simmer for 2–3 minutes to cook off the raw taste and allow the juices to thicken into a gravy.

Divide the chicken, vegetables and gravy equally between 4 plates and sprinkle with the remaining chopped thyme for added flavour and colour. This dish goes nicely with Braised Fennel (see page 334). Store any leftover sauce in an airtight container in the refrigerator for up to 5 days.

Nutritional analysis per serving:
calories 340, fat 23 g, saturated fat 6 g, cholesterol 65 mg,
fibre 1 g, protein 24 g, carbohydrate 10 g, sodium

BEEF AND LAMB

Beef and Veggie Stuffed Peppers

Sweet peppers make great containers for a spiced beef and vegetable filling. Prep them a day or two ahead, and refrigerate until you are ready to bake them. If you prefer, you can bake them up to 3 days ahead as they reheat well too. In this case, bring them to room temperature and bake as before.

Yield: 4 servings
Prep time: 20 minutes
Cook time: 55 minutes

- 2 tablespoons extra virgin olive oil
- 1 small onion, finely chopped
- 4 garlic cloves, finely chopped
- 1 rounded tablespoon ancho or other mild chilli powder
- 2 teaspoons ground cumin
- 2 teaspoons paprika
- 2 teaspoons dried oregano
- 1 small courgette, quartered lengthways and diced
- 450 g (1 lb) grass-fed minced beef (15% fat)
- 1 x 400-g (14-oz) can chopped tomatoes
- ½ teaspoon sea salt
- ¼ teaspoon ground black pepper
- 1 heaped tablespoon chopped coriander or flatleaf parsley leaves
- 4 large red, orange or yellow peppers, halved lengthways and seeded

Preheat the oven to 180°C/350°F/Gas mark 4.

Place the olive oil in a large frying pan over a medium heat. Add the onion and cook gently until it is soft and translucent (about 3 minutes), stirring occasionally. Add the garlic, chilli powder, cumin, paprika and oregano and cook for 1–2 minutes. Add the courgette and cook until it has softened (3–4 minutes).

Add the beef to the pan, breaking it up with a wooden spoon. Cook until it is no longer pink (8–10 minutes), stirring now and then to prevent burning. Add the tomatoes and simmer for another 8–10 minutes. Season with the salt and pepper, then fold in the fresh herbs.

Divide the filling equally between the 8 pepper halves. Place them in a large, heatproof baking dish, cover with foil and bake for about 30 minutes, or until a meat thermometer registers 75°C/165°F when inserted in the middle of the filling.

Serve 2 pepper halves per person, with a dollop of No-Cheese Sauce (see page 330), or add a green side salad with diced avocado and tomatoes.

If you want to make this dish in advance, place the peppers in a covered dish and refrigerate for up to 3 days. When ready to bake, bring them to room temperature and bake as above. Baked peppers or leftovers can be stored, cooled and covered, in a glass casserole dish or storage container with a lid for up to 3 days.

Nutritional analysis per serving (2 stuffed pepper halves):
calories 410, fat 25 g, saturated fat 8 g, cholesterol 75 mg,
fibre 6 g, protein 25 g, carbohydrate 21 g, sodium 390 mg

**Nutritional analysis per serving (2 stuffed pepper halves
with 1 tablespoon No-Cheese Sauce):**
calories 450, fat 28g, saturated fat 10g, cholesterol 75mg,
fibre 6g, protein 26g, carbohydrate 23g, sodium 425g

SPICED LAMB AND VEGETABLE SHEPHERD'S PIE

This easy casserole is made with minced lamb, but it also works with beef. Although the topping looks like traditional high-carb mashed potatoes, we used puréed cauliflower instead. You will love the switch! This dish can be made a day or two ahead and refrigerated until needed. Just remember to bring it back to room temperature before baking. Any leftovers will keep for up to three days if covered and refrigerated.

Yield: 4 servings
Prep time: 30 minutes
Cook time: 20 minutes

- 2 heads of cauliflower, or 900 g (2lb) frozen florets
- 60 ml (2 1/4 fl oz) extra virgin olive oil
- 1 medium onion, chopped
- 4 celery sticks, chopped
- 1 large red pepper, cored, seeded and chopped
- 3 garlic cloves, finely chopped
- 1/2 teaspoon sea salt
- 1/4 teaspoon ground black pepper
- pinch of garlic granules
- 450 g (1 lb) minced lamb (15% fat)
- 2 teaspoons paprika
- 1 teaspoon ground cumin
- 1 teaspoon ground coriander
- 1 teaspoon ground cinnamon
- dash of cayenne pepper
- optional: 1/4 teaspoon saffron strands
- 2 small courgettes (350g/12 oz in total), trimmed, quartered lengthways and diced
- 1 x 400-g (14-oz) can chopped tomatoes
- 3 tablespoons chopped fresh coriander leaves

Preheat the oven to 180°C/350°F/Gas mark 4.

Cut the core from the cauliflowers and break the heads into small florets. Pour a 5-cm (2-in) depth of water into a large saucepan and place a steamer basket inside. Cover and bring to the boil. When steam is coming out of the lid, add the cauliflower florets, replace the lid, and steam over a medium heat until very tender (12–14 minutes).

Meanwhile, put 2 tablespoons of the oil in another large pan over a medium heat. When hot, add the onion and celery and cook, stirring occasionally, until softened (about 4 minutes). Add the garlic and cook for another minute, stirring to ensure it does not brown. Add the lamb to the pan, breaking it up with a wooden spoon, and cook until it is no longer pink (about 4 minutes). Add the paprika and ground herbs, crushing the saffron strands between your fingers. Stir well and cook for 2–3 minutes so that the flavours develop.

When the cauliflower is tender, drain it and transfer to a food processor. Add the remaining 2 tablespoons oil, plus a pinch more salt, pepper and garlic granules. Purée until smooth.

Add the courgette to the lamb mixture, followed by the tomatoes. Stir in the fresh coriander and season again with salt and pepper. Cook for another 3–4 minutes.

Carefully tip the lamb and vegetable mixture into a large baking dish. Spoon the cauliflower purée evenly over the top and smooth with a spatula. Bake for 20 minutes, until the edges are lightly browned and a meat thermometer registers 75°C/165°F when inserted into the centre.

Nutritional analysis per serving:
calories 550, fat 39 g, saturated fat 14 g, cholesterol 85 mg, fibre 9 g, protein 26 g, carbohydrate 29 g, sodium 430 mg

SPICED BEEF TACO WRAPS WITH GUACAMOLE

For a great lunch that won't weigh you down, try these crisp lettuce leaves spread with creamy guacamole and topped with spicy beef, cool cabbage, tomato and coriander, and finished with squeezes of tart lime juice. If you use mini romaine leaves, you will need 6 leaves per person or about 3 mini heads.
Tip: The most nutrient-dense part of the avocado is just under the skin, so be sure to capture this slightly darker green flesh when peeling the fruit.

Yield: 4 servings
Prep time: 10 minutes
Cook time: 20 minutes

- 1 tablespoon extra virgin olive oil
- 1 small onion, chopped (225 g/8 oz)
- 4 garlic cloves, finely chopped
- 750 g (1½ lb) grass-fed minced beef (15% fat)
- 2½ teaspoons ancho or other mild chilli powder
- 1 tablespoon, plus 1 teaspoon, ground cumin
- 1½ teaspoons ground coriander
- optional: dash of fiery chipotle powder
- ¼ teaspoon sea salt
- ¼ teaspoon ground black pepper
- 1 large avocado, stoned and chopped
- 4 limes (2 juiced, 2 quartered), for garnish

- 12 soft or romaine lettuce leaves
- ¼ small head of green or red cabbage, grated or finely chopped
- 2 medium plum tomatoes, seeded and chopped
- 2 tablespoons chopped fresh coriander leaves

Place the olive oil in a large frying pan over a medium heat. When hot, add the chopped onion and cook until soft (1–2 minutes). Add the garlic and cook, stirring, for another 30 seconds. Add the beef, breaking it up with a wooden spatula or spoon, and cook until is it no longer pink (about 2 minutes). Add the ancho powder, 1 tablespoon of cumin, the coriander and chipotle powder. Cook for another 1–2 minutes, stirring, so that the flavours develop. Season with the salt and pepper, then transfer the meat to a bowl and set aside.

To make the guacamole, place the avocado in a small bowl. Add the lime juice and remaining teaspoon of cumin and mash with a fork until smooth. Add a pinch of sea salt and ground black pepper.

Divide the lettuce leaves equally between 4 plates. Spread the guacamole inside them. Top with the spicy beef, then with the chopped cabbage, tomatoes and fresh coriander. Serve with wedges of lime.

Nutritional analysis per serving:
calories 600, fat 43 g, saturated fat 15 g, cholesterol 110 mg,
fibre 9 g, protein 35 g, carbohydrate 25 g, sodium 290 mg

SEAFOOD

Coconut Curry Mussels with Courgette Noodles

This richly flavoured, Indian-inspired seafood dish, with flavours of curry, ginger, lime and coconut milk, comes together quickly. After eating the mussels, enjoy the flavourful broth like a soup. When buying fresh mussels, they should be closed or should close when you tap them, meaning they are alive. Avoid those with broken or cracked shells. Store the mussels in the refrigerator on ice covered with damp kitchen paper, and use within a day of purchase. Do not store them in a closed plastic bag or the mussels will suffocate. Wash the mussels just before cooking.

Yield: 4 servings
Prep time: 15 minutes
Cook time: 20 minutes

- 1.75 kg (4 lb) mussels
- 2 leeks
- 2 tablespoons coconut oil
- 4 garlic cloves, finely chopped
- 2 tablespoons curry powder
- 7.5-cm (3-in) piece of fresh ginger, peeled and finely grated
- 500 ml (17 fl oz) full-fat coconut milk
- 60 ml (21/4 fl oz) fresh lime juice
- 2 tablespoons chopped coriander or flatleaf parsley leaves
- sea salt and ground black pepper
- optional: pinch of dried red chilli flakes (for heat)

FOR THE COURGETTE NOODLES

- 4 large courgettes (about 900 g/2 lb)
- 1 teaspoon coconut oil

First make the noodles. Trim the courgettes and use a spiralizer to cut them into long thin strips. Place in a bowl and set aside.

Place the mussels in a colander in the sink and rinse well with cold water. Scrub to remove any exterior debris if they are not clean. Discard any with broken shells and allow the remaining mussels to drain. With your fingers, pull out and discard any stringy "beard" that appears between the shells.

Slice the leeks in half lengthways and hold under running cold water to dislodge any sand or dirt. Chop them widthways into thin pieces.

To cook the mussels all at once you will need a 9-litre (16-pint) pan with a tight-fitting lid, or two smaller ones of half that size. If cooking the mussels in two batches, be sure to divide all the other ingredients in half when adding them to the pans.

Place 4 teaspoons of the coconut oil in the pan over a medium-low heat. When hot, add the leeks and cook until they have softened (about 2 minutes). Add the garlic and cook for 1 more minute. Stir in the curry powder, ginger and chilli flakes (if using). Cook for 1–2 minutes, until the spices become fragrant. Add the coconut milk and lime juice. Cook for another 2 minutes to combine the flavours.

Add the mussels to the broth, cover the pan and increase the heat to medium-high. When steam starts escaping, turn the heat down to low and cook the mussels for about 5 minutes.

Meanwhile, preheat the oven to its lowest setting. Place 1 teaspoon of the coconut oil in a medium pan over a medium heat. When hot, add the courgette noodles and cook for about 3 minutes. Drain, cover and keep warm.

Check the mussel pan to see if the shellfish are open. If not, continue cooking for another minute or so. When the mussels have opened, sprinkle with the coriander and some seasoning. Using a slotted spoon, transfer the mussels to a large bowl, discarding any that have not opened. If cooking in batches, cover this first batch with foil and keep warm in the oven while you cook the remainder.

To serve, divide the courgette noodles equally between 4 wide, shallow bowls. Top with the mussels, then pour the cooking liquid over them. Be sure to provide a bowl for the discarded shells.

Nutritional analysis per serving:
calories 560, fat 38 g, saturated fat 29 g, cholesterol 65 mg,
fibre 4 g, protein 33 g, carbohydrate 30 g, sodium 690 mg

FIVE-SPICE SEARED SALMON WITH SAUTÉED SESAME CABBAGE

Here is an easy dinner with Asian flavours that come from Chinese five-spice powder, a blend that includes cinnamon, star anise, ginger, cloves and nutmeg. It works wonderfully against the richness of wild salmon. The sesame cabbage also makes a great accompaniment for basic poached chicken.

Yield: 4 servings
Prep time: 20 minutes
Cook time: 25 minutes

- 850 g (1¾ lb) wild salmon, skinned and cut into 4 fillets
- ½ teaspoon garlic granules
- ¼ teaspoon sea salt
- 1 rounded tablespoon Chinese five-spice powder
- 1 teaspoon coconut oil
- 1 tablespoon toasted sesame oil, for drizzling

FOR THE SESAME CABBAGE

- 2 tablespoons coconut oil
- 6 spring onions, finely chopped
- 4 garlic cloves, finely chopped
- 5-cm (2-in) piece of fresh ginger, peeled and finely grated
- 1 head of green cabbage (750 g/1½ lb), cut in half, cored and thinly sliced
- 1 tablespoon low-sodium tamari
- 2 tablespoons white or black sesame seeds
- 2 tablespoons chopped fresh coriander or parsley leaves

Preheat the oven to 220°C/425°F/Gas mark 7.

Lay the salmon fillets flesh-side up and use a sharp, thin knife to trim out any dark purple bloodline. (This will make the salmon taste milder.)

Sprinkle each fillet with equal amounts of the garlic granules, salt and five-spice powder. Set aside.

To cook the cabbage, put the coconut oil in a large frying pan over a medium heat. When hot, add the spring onions, garlic and ginger and cook, stirring, for about 1 minute. Lower the heat if necessary so that the garlic and ginger do not burn. Add the sliced cabbage to the pan;

it will seem like a huge amount, but will quickly reduce. Cook, stirring with a spatula, until it wilts and softens.

Stir in the tamari, sprinkle with the sesame seeds and fold in the coriander. Keep the cabbage warm while you cook the salmon.

Heat a large ovenproof frying pan over a medium heat until hot (4–5 minutes). Add the oil, then the salmon fillets, spice-side down. Cook until the underside is golden and crusted (4–5 minutes), being careful not to burn the spices. Turn the fillets spiced-side up and place the pan in the oven to finish cooking (2–3 minutes for fillets 2.5 cm/1 in thick).

Divide the cabbage equally between 4 plates, top each pile with a salmon fillet and drizzle with the sesame oil. Refrigerate any leftovers in airtight containers. Salmon is best finished the next day, but the cabbage will keep for up to 3 days.

Nutritional analysis per serving:
calories 440, fat 23 g, saturated fat 11 g, cholesterol 75 mg, fibre 5 g, protein 41 g, carbohydrate 15 g, sodium 440 mg

TERIYAKI BLACK COD WITH SESAME ASPARAGUS

Also called sablefish, black cod has rich, silky flesh and almost twice the healthy omega-3 fats of salmon. Ask for fillets cut from the thicker end of the piece, not the tail. Mirin is Japanese rice wine, available from most supermarkets. Choose a brand that is made with only water, rice, koji and sea salt, avoiding anything made with glucose syrup, corn syrup or other added sugar.

Yield: 4 servings
Prep time: 30 minutes, including marinating
Cook time: 10 minutes

- 4 black cod fillets (175 g/6 oz each)
- 3 tablespoons low-sodium tamari
- 3 tablespoons mirin
- 5-cm (2-in) piece of fresh ginger, peeled and finely grated
- 3 limes (2 juiced, 1 quartered)
- 2 garlic cloves, finely chopped or grated

- 450 g (1 lb) asparagus
- 1 tablespoon melted coconut oil
- pinch of sea salt and ground black pepper
- 20 ml (1 tablespoon plus 1 teaspoon) sesame oil
- 2 teaspoons white or black sesame seeds

Preheat the oven to 200°C/400°F/Gas mark 4.

Lay the fish fillets skin-side up in a glass or ceramic baking dish just large enough to hold them in a single layer. Combine the tamari, mirin, ginger, lime juice and garlic in a small bowl and whisk together. Pour this mixture over the fillets, lifting them so that it runs underneath too. Leave to marinate at room temperature for 30 minutes.

Meanwhile, snap the tough ends off the asparagus and place the spears in a foil-lined baking tin. Drizzle with 2 teaspoons of the coconut oil and sprinkle with the salt and pepper.

Drain the marinated fish, discarding the marinade. Place the remaining teaspoon coconut oil in a large, ovenproof pan over a medium heat. Spread it across the pan and, when hot, lay the fish in it skin-side down and sear for 2 minutes. Turn the fish and sear for another 2 minutes. Peel off and discard the skin. Return the fillets to the pan, top side up.

Add the asparagus to the fish, then place the pan in the oven for 3–5 minutes, or until a digital thermometer registers 65°C/145°F when inserted into the thickest part. (If you don't have a thermometer, fillets 4 cm/1½ in thick will take about 5 minutes.) The flesh will be just coming apart, almost flaking, and a pearly white colour inside. The asparagus is done if it is tender when pierced with the tip of a sharp knife.

To serve, place the fish and asparagus on plates and drizzle each fillet with 1 teaspoon of sesame oil. Sprinkle the sesame seeds equally over the asparagus. Serve with a lime wedge to squeeze over the fish.

Nutritional analysis per serving:
calories 480, fat 35 g, saturated fat 9 g, cholesterol 85 mg,
fibre 3 g, protein 27 g, carbohydrate 15 g, sodium 510 mg

ASIAN GINGER PRAWNS WITH CREAMY ALMOND DIPPING SAUCE

Fresh prawns make for a quick and easy dinner, and even indicate when they are cooked by turning pink. The creamy, lime-infused sauce makes a rich accompaniment for them. For an upgrade to your spice collection, try this with Szechuan pepper. Readers with nut allergies can replace the cashew butter with tahini.

Yield: 4 servings
Prep time: 20–30 minutes, including marinating
Cook time: 10 minutes

- 2 tablespoons freshly squeezed lime juice
- 2 tablespoons coconut oil, melted
- 5-cm (2-in) piece of fresh ginger, peeled and finely grated
- 3 garlic cloves, peeled and finely chopped
- ¼ teaspoon sea salt
- ¼ teaspoon ground black pepper
- 750 g (1½ lb) large fresh prawns, peeled and deveined

FOR THE SAUCE

- 75 ml (scant 3 fl oz), fresh lime juice
- 65 g (2½ oz) creamy raw almond butter
- 2 tablespoons full-fat coconut milk
- 20 ml (1 tablespoon plus 1 teaspoon) melted coconut oil
- 2 teaspoons unseasoned rice vinegar

In a bowl large enough to hold all the prawns, mix the lime juice, oil, ginger, garlic, salt and pepper until combined. (Note: in cool weather the coconut oil may solidify, making more of a paste than a liquid.) Add the prawns to the bowl and turn to coat in the marinade. Leave to stand at room temperature for 20–30 minutes.

Meanwhile, make the dipping sauce. Put the lime juice in a small bowl, add the almond butter, coconut milk, coconut oil and vinegar and mix until smooth.

Preheat the grill, placing the shelf about 13 cm (5 in) below the heat source. Place the prawns on a foil-lined baking tray in a single layer and grill on one side just until they turn pink (3–4 minutes). Turn them over and grill for about another minute, just until the second side turns pink. Prawns cook quickly, so do not leave them unattended. (Note: prawns can also be skewered for grilling, or griddling in a pan.)

Serve with the dipping sauce over Herbed Cauliflower "Rice" (see pages 335).

Nutritional analysis per serving (12 prawns, 2 tablespoons sauce):
calories 370, fat 23 g, saturated fat 13 g, cholesterol 275 mg,
fibre 2 g, protein 38 g, carbohydrate 7 g, sodium 390 mg

MACADAMIA-COCONUT CRUSTED FISH FILLETS

Buttery macadamia nuts and desiccated coconut make a delicious crunchy coating for baked fish fillets.

Yield: 4 servings
Prep time: 10 minutes
Cook time: 15 minutes

- 90 g (3½ oz) finely chopped raw macadamia nuts (use a food processor)
- 5 tablespoons, unsweetened shredded coconut
- 4 skinless halibut or cod fillets (175 g/6 oz each)
- 4 tablespoons organic or homemade mayonnaise (see page 332)
- ¼ teaspoon sea salt
- ¼ teaspoon ground black pepper
- ¼ teaspoon garlic granules
- 20 ml (1 tablespoon plus 1 teaspoon) melted coconut oil
- 1 lemon, quartered

Preheat the oven to 220°C/425°F/Gas mark 7.

Combine the macadamia nuts and coconut in a small bowl. Line a baking tray with foil, place a wire rack on top and brush with a little oil to prevent sticking. Place the fish on the rack. Spread each fillet with 1 tablespoon of the mayonnaise, then sprinkle equally with the salt, pepper and garlic. Pack the top of each fillet evenly with the macadamia-coconut mixture.

Bake the fish for about 12 minutes, or until a digital thermometer registers 65°C (145°F) when inserted into the thickest part. The top should be a light golden brown.

Serve the fish drizzled with 1 tablespoon of the melted coconut oil per serving, and a lemon wedge to squeeze over the top. Pair with sugarsnap peas or roast asparagus drizzled with melted coconut oil (see page 251).

Nutritional analysis per serving:
calories 500, fat 39 g, saturated fat 14 g, cholesterol 95 mg,
fibre 3 g, protein 33 g, carbohydrate 6 g, sodium 250 mg

GRILLED SCALLOPS WITH LEMON-CAPER VINAIGRETTE

Buy the largest scallops you can find for this easy, fast dinner. Look for "dry" scallops that are pearly white and uniform in size, with firm, slightly moist flesh. They should smell fresh, like the ocean, never fishy. If grilling them, you will need 4–8 bamboo or metal skewers. The vinaigrette also works well with chicken or fish as a sauce.

Yield: 4 servings
Prep time: 20 minutes (plus soaking time if using bamboo skewers)
Cook time: 15 minutes

- 750 g (1½ lb) large scallops
- 1 tablespoon extra virgin olive oil
- ¼ teaspoon sea salt
- ¼ teaspoon ground black pepper
- ¼ teaspoon garlic granules

FOR THE VINAIGRETTE

- 60 ml (2 1/4 fl oz) fresh lemon juice
- 60 ml (2 1/4 fl oz) extra virgin olive oil
- 1 tablespoon Dijon mustard
- 2 teaspoons finely chopped shallot
- 2 garlic cloves, finely chopped
- pinch of sea salt and ground black pepper
- 1 tablespoon finely chopped fresh parsley or coriander leaves

If using bamboo skewers, put them to soak in a shallow pan of warm water for about 20–30 minutes so that they don't burn.

Put all the vinaigrette ingredients into a small bowl and whisk together. Set aside.

Prepare the scallops by removing the small, tough muscle on the side that looks like a little tag (just tear it off with your fingers). Divide the scallops into 4 equal portions and thread them onto the skewers. If the scallops are large, using double skewers spaced a little apart will give them more stability when grilling. Brush the scallops lightly with olive oil, then sprinkle with the salt, pepper and garlic.

Heat the grill until very hot (about 5 minutes). Line a baking tray with foil, place a wire rack on top and brush with a little oil to prevent sticking. Place the skewered scallops on the rack, lower the heat to medium and grill for 2–3 minutes per side, depending on size.

If you prefer to cook the scallops on the hob, heat a non-stick pan over a high heat, then brush with 1–2 teaspoons olive oil. Place the scallops in the pan and cook until a good crust forms (3–4 minutes, depending on the size). Turn them over and cook for 1 minute longer.

Note: Scallops cook quickly, and are ready when they are barely opaque in the centre. Do not overcook or they will become rubbery.

Divide the hot scallops equally between 4 plates and drizzle 2 table-spoons of the vinaigrette over each serving. Pair with broccolini drizzled with 1 tablespoon extra vinaigrette or 2 teaspoons olive oil and a squeeze of lemon juice.

Nutritional analysis per serving:
calories 310, fat 19 g, saturated fat 3 g, cholesterol 55 mg,
fibre 0 g, protein 29 g, carbohydrate 6 g, sodium 40 mg

STEAMED SALMON FILLETS WITH LEMON AÏOLI

Steaming is a fast, easy and nutritious way to prepare salmon. It can be served warm or chilled, making it easily transportable to the office or other places away from home. You can steam and chill the salmon ahead of time.

Yield: 4 servings
Prep time: 20 minutes
Cook time: 10 minutes

- 4 skinless salmon fillets (175 g/6 oz each)
- ¼ teaspoon salt
- ¼ teaspoon ground black pepper

FOR THE STEAMING BROTH

- 1 litre (1¾ pints) filtered water
- 1 bay leaf
- 2 garlic cloves, crushed
- 3 sprigs of fresh thyme
- 1 carrot, roughly chopped
- 1 celery stick, roughly chopped
- ½ small onion, roughly chopped
- 1 large lemon, quartered

FOR THE LEMON AÏOLI

- 100 g (4 oz) organic or homemade mayonnaise (see page 332)
- juice and zest of 1 lemon
- 1 garlic clove, finely chopped or grated
- pinch of sea salt and white pepper

Put all the broth ingredients into a large wide pan, squeezing in the lemon quarters, then adding the rinds. Place a trivet or upturned saucer in the pan, ensuring the liquid is just below them. Bring to the boil, then cover and simmer for 15 minutes.

Meanwhile, combine all the aïoli ingredients in a small bowl and mix until smooth. Set aside.

Sprinkle the salmon fillets with the salt and pepper. Place them in a single layer on the steamer rack and replace the lid. Steam the salmon for 5–6 minutes, or until a digital thermometer registers 65°C (145°F) when inserted into the thickest part. The fillets should be a light pinky-orange colour.

Serve the salmon warm or cool with 2 tablespoons of the aïoli per person. Pair with Broccoli Slaw (see page 337). Any leftovers should be chilled and eaten within 2 days. If cooked in advance, it can be stored in the refrigerator for up to 2 days.

Nutritional analysis per serving:
calories 450, fat 31 g, saturated fat 5 g, cholesterol 125 mg,
fibre 0 g, protein 38 g, carbohydrate 2 g, sodium 310 mg

SOUPS AND STEWS

DR. HYMAN'S VEGGIE-BONE STOCK RECIPE

Yield: 1.75 litres (3 pints)
Prep time: 10 minutes
Cook time: 15 to 27 hours (depending on desired cooking time, including at least 3 hours cooling time)

- 1.75 kg (4 lb) soup bones from organic or grass-fed beef, lamb, venison, chicken, turkey or duck
- 2 tablespoons apple cider vinegar
- 2 carrots, roughly chopped
- 2 celery sticks, roughly chopped
- 1 medium onion, chopped
- 2 garlic cloves, crushed
- 2 bay leaves
- 75-g (3-oz) bunch of parsley
- 1 tablespoon sea salt
- 1 litre (1¾ pints) filtered water

Place the bones in a slow cooker and drizzle the vinegar all over them. Add the vegetables, herbs and salt. Pour in the water and stir to combine. Set the cooker on low and leave for 12–24 hours.

At the end of the cooking time, discard the bones, vegetables and herbs. Strain the liquid to remove and other solids, then refrigerate in a large airtight container overnight, or for at least 3 hours. It will become jelly-like and the fat will rise to the top and form an opaque white layer. At this point you can discard the fat, or leave it in if you like the stock "creamy".

To serve, heat the stock over a medium-low heat, stirring occasionally. Enjoy a mugful at a time as a savoury hot drink, or use it in recipes calling for chicken or beef stock.

Store any leftover stock in an airtight container in the refrigerator for up to 4 days, or in the freezer for 9–12 months.

Nutritional analysis per serving (250 ml/8 fl oz):
calories 72, fat 6 g, saturated fat 3 g, cholesterol 22 mg,
fibre 0 g, protein 6 g, carbohydrate 1 g, sodium 269 mg

SPICED CARIBBEAN TEMPEH STEW

Don't let the length of the ingredient list scare you away from making this recipe – many of the items are spices. Tempeh is a plant protein powerhouse made from fermented soya beans in cake form. It has a nutty flavour and texture that absorbs all the wonderful Caribbean flavours of this stew. Find it in the refrigerated dairy section of your supermarket, and be sure to buy only organic. To save time during the week, make a pot of this stew at the weekend, then cool and store it in portions for eating during the week. If you want to make them slightly juicier when reheating, add a little vegetable, chicken stock or water.

Yield: 4 servings
Prep time: 30 minutes
Cook time: 30 minutes

- 4 tablespoons coconut oil
- 250 g (8 oz) organic tempeh, cut into 2-cm (3/4-in) cubes
- 1 small onion
- 3 celery stick
- 1/2 small orange sweet potato, peeled (150 g/5 oz)
- 4 garlic cloves
- 2 red peppers
- optional: 1 jalapeño chilli pepper
- 1½ teaspoons ground cumin
- 1½ teaspoons ground coriander
- 1 teaspoon ground turmeric
- ¼ teaspoon ground allspice
- ¼ teaspoon ground nutmeg
- pinch of cayenne pepper
- 1 x 400-g (14-oz) can chopped tomatoes
- 3 limes (2 juiced, 1 quartered)
- 1 x 400-g (14-oz) can full-fat coconut milk
- 250 ml (8 fl oz) filtered water
- ¼ teaspoon sea salt
- ¼ teaspoon ground black pepper
- 50 g (2 oz) fresh coriander, chopped

Place 2 tablespoons of the coconut oil in a large pan over a medium heat. When hot, add the tempeh and cook until golden (7–10 minutes), stirring occasionally and lowering the heat if necessary. Transfer it to a bowl and set aside.

Meanwhile, chop the onion, celery and sweet potato into small pieces. Crush the garlic. Core, seed and chop the red peppers into small pieces. If using the jalapeño, remove the seeds and white membrane if you want less heat, then finely chop.

Add the remaining coconut oil to the pan in which you cooked the tempeh and place over a medium heat. When hot, add the onion, red peppers and celery and cook until softened (4–5 minutes). Stir in the jalapeño and garlic and cook for 1 minute longer. Add all the spices and cook for 1–2 minutes, stirring until fragrant.

Add the tomatoes, sweet potatoes and lime juice and stir well. Mix in the coconut milk and water, the reserved tempeh, salt and pepper, then cover and cook until bubbling. Lower the heat and cook gently for 15–20 minutes, or until the sweet potato is tender.

Serve the stew in shallow bowls with a wedge of lime, and garnish with the coriander.

Cool any leftovers and refrigerate in an airtight container for up to 5 days.

Nutritional analysis per serving:
calories 600, fat 37 g, saturated fat 25 g, cholesterol 0 mg,
fibre 7 g, protein 27 g, carbohydrate 34 g, sodium 250 mg

CLAM CHOWDER

Fresh steamed clams make this creamy chowder extra good, but canned clams work too. In the latter case, use 350 g (12 oz) raw canned clams (drained weight) and 475 ml (16 fl oz) low-sodium bottled clam juice. The clams can be steamed one day ahead and the meat removed and refrigerated to save time. For a dairy-free version, use olive oil or coconut oil instead of grass-fed butter. To increase the vegetable content, add 50–75 g (2–3 oz) cooked chopped baby green beans to the salad. This recipe yields 1.75 litres (3 pints), so you'll have a little left over for a treat.

Yield: 4 servings
Prep time: 25 minutes
Cook time: 20 minutes

- 750 ml (1¼ pints) filtered water
- juice of 2 lemons
- 2 bay leaves
- 4 large garlic cloves, lightly crushed
- 4 sprigs of fresh thyme
- ¼ teaspoons sea salt
- 1.75 kg (4 lb) fresh small clams

FOR THE CHOWDER

- 2 leeks
- 4 celery sticks
- 4 tablespoons unsalted grass-fed butter
- 4 large garlic cloves, finely chopped
- 4 tablespoons coconut flour
- ¼ teaspoon ground black pepper
- 2 teaspoons chopped fresh thyme leaves
- 2 x 400-g (14-oz) cans full-fat coconut milk
- 1 tablespoon freshly chopped tarragon or parsley leaves

Place the water, lemon juice, bay leaves, garlic, thyme and salt in a large saucepan with a tight-fitting lid. Bring to boil over high heat. When steam starts coming out, add all the clams and replace the lid. Leave to steam over a medium heat until all the shells have opened (about 5 minutes). Drain the clams through a colander, reserving the liquid in a large bowl. Discard any unopened clams, as well as the thyme, bay leaves and garlic. Remove the meat from the remaining clams, discarding the shells, and set aside.

To make the chowder, slice the leeks in half lengthways and hold under running cold water to dislodge any sand or dirt. Pat dry. Lay the leeks flat on a chopping board and cut widthways into thin pieces. You should have about 185 g (6½ oz).

Trim the celery and slice lengthwise into 4 or 6 thin strips. Chop widthways into small pieces. You should have about 200 g (7 oz).

Melt the butter in a large saucepan over a medium to medium-low heat. Add the leeks and celery and cook slowly, stirring occasionally, until soft (about 5 minutes). Add the garlic and cook for 1 more minute. Sprinkle in the coconut flour, then stir with the vegetables until the mixture has thickened (about 2 minutes). Stir in the pepper and thyme leaves. Add 500 ml (17 fl oz) of the reserved clam broth, stir well and heat until the soup is thick and saucy (3–4 minutes). Add the coconut milk and clams and heat the chowder through. Stir in the fresh herbs at the end.

Ladle into soup bowls and serve hot with a tossed green salad containing avocado, tomato and cucumber and your favourite healthy, full-fat, homemade dressing. Cool leftovers and refrigerate in an airtight container for up to 2 days. Reheat and enjoy!

Nutritional analysis per serving (about 375 g/13 oz):
calories 580, fat 42 g, saturated fat 35 g, cholesterol 75 mg, fibre 4 g, protein 25 g, carbohydrate 18 g, sodium 580 mg

BISTRO BEEF AND VEGETABLE STEW

This rich and hearty beef stew is full of flavour and vegetables. It includes Herbes de Provence, a classic mixture of dried thyme, savory, fennel, rosemary, marjoram, basil, lavender and tarragon. Ideally, use homemade stock. Failing that, buy good-quality organic stock that contains no sodium or additives.

Serves: 4
Prep time: 20 minutes
Cook time: 40 minutes

- 900 g (2 lb) top sirloin, trimmed of excess fat to 750 g (1½ lb)
- 2 tablespoons grass-fed butter or extra virgin olive oil
- 1 small onion, diced
- 3 celery sticks, chopped into small pieces
- 1 fennel bulb, chopped
- 1 leek, chopped into thick chunks
- 2½ teaspoons dried Herbes de Provence or dried thyme
- ¼ teaspoon sea salt

- ¼ teaspoon ground black pepper
- 2 medium carrots, cut into 2.5-cm (1-in) pieces
- 1 x 400-g (14-oz) can chopped tomatoes, drained
- 600 ml (1 pint) low- to no-sodium beef stock
- 2 tablespoons arrowroot
- 2 tablespoons cold filtered water
- 2 tablespoons finely chopped flatleaf parsley leaves, for garnish

Place the meat on a chopping board and use a sharp, heavy knife to trim off any excess fat. The trimmed piece should weigh about 750 g (1½ lb). Cut the meat into 2.5-cm (1-in) cubes.

Put 1 tablespoon of the butter into a large ovenproof casserole dish over a medium heat. When hot, add the meat and brown on all sides for 7–8 minutes. Transfer the meat and juices to a bowl and set aside.

Melt the remaining butter in the casserole dish. Add the onion, celery, fennel, leek and Herbes de Provence. Cook over medium-low heat, stirring occasionally, until the vegetables are soft but not brown (about 5 minutes). Add the salt and pepper, then return the meat to the pan, followed by the carrots, tomatoes and stock. Cover and simmer until the carrots are tender (20–25 minutes). The stew can be enjoyed as it is, or you can stir in a paste made from the arrowroot and water to thicken the stock into a gravy. Bring back almost to the boil and bubble for a minute to cook out the rawness.

To serve, ladle the stew into 4 serving bowls (about 2 ladlefuls per person) and garnish with the parsley. Pair with a tossed green salad with a full-fat dressing, olive oil vinaigrette and avocado. Cool any stew leftovers and refrigerate in an airtight container for up to 3 days. To reheat, place a portion in a small lidded pan and heat gently, stirring occasionally, until hot.

Nutritional analysis per serving (about 350 g/12 oz):
calories 410, fat 15 g, saturated fat 4 g, cholesterol 95 mg,
fibre 6 g, protein 40 g, carbohydrate 28 g, sodium 440 mg

CREAM OF MUSHROOM HERB SOUP

Rich and creamy, this mushroom soup gets a lift in flavour from herbs and brightness from lemon juice. Enjoy it chunky or smoothly puréed – it's up to you. A food processor and slicing disc make easy work of the prep. Serve this soup as an accompaniment to a salad with, say, chicken or beef, as a way of getting in your protein.

Yield: 4 servings
Prep time: 20 minutes
Cook time: 25 minutes

- 450 g (1 lb) firm white mushrooms
- 450 g (1 lb) firm chestnut mushrooms
- 3 large shallots, chopped
- 3 garlic cloves
- 2 tablespoons butter
- 1 tablespoon chopped fresh tarragon or 1 teaspoon dried
- 1 tablespoon fresh thyme leaves or 1 teaspoon dried
- 1 litre (1¾ pints) low- or no-sodium chicken stock
- ½ teaspoon sea salt
- ¼ teaspoon ground black pepper
- 250 ml (8 fl oz) full-fat coconut milk
- 2 lemons (1 juiced, 1 quartered)
- 1½ tablespoons chopped fresh parsley leaves

Clean the mushrooms by wiping them with damp kitchen paper. Using a knife or a food processor, cut them into slices about 5 mm (1/8-in) thick. Set aside.

Melt the butter in a large saucepan over a medium-low heat. Add the shallots and cook until softened (7–8 minutes). Stir in the garlic and cook for another minute. Add the sliced mushrooms and cook, stirring and turning them with a wooden spoon, until soft (7–8 minutes). Stir in the tarragon and thyme, then add the stock, salt and pepper. Bring almost to the boil, then turn off the heat and stir in the coconut milk and lemon juice.

This soup can be served as it is, or puréed to a smooth texture. If using a jug blender, purée it in small batches, filling the jug no more than half full as hot liquids expand when blended. Hold the lid on tight with a tea towel, and start blending on a slow speed, gradually increasing it.

Serve the soup immediately, garnished with a sprinkle of chopped parsley and a squeeze of fresh lemon juice to brighten the flavour.

Nutritional analysis per serving (425 ml/14 fl oz): calories 260, fat 15 g, saturated fat 11 g, cholesterol 20 mg, fibre 4 g, protein 9 g, carbohydrate 22 g, sodium 260 mg

SAUCES

No-Cheese Sauce

With its lovely yellow colour and creamy texture, you might think this sauce actually contains cheese, but there is no dairy involved. The savoury, cheesy flavour comes from nutritional yeast flakes, which might not sound appetizing but really do taste delicious. Dollop this sauce onto vegetables, chicken or fish, or use as a dip with raw veggies for a snack.

Yield: 300 ml (1/2 pint)
Prep time: 6–8 hours, including soaking time
Cook time: 5 minutes

- 65 g (2½ oz) raw cashew nuts
- 175 ml (6 fl oz) full-fat unsweetened coconut milk
- 3 tablespoons nutritional yeast flakes
- 2 teaspoons finely grated onion
- 1 teaspoon Dijon mustard
- ½ teaspoon garlic granules
- ½ teaspoon ground turmeric
- ¼ teaspoon sea salt
- ¼ teaspoon white pepper

Place the cashews in a medium bowl and cover them with at least twice their depth of water. Cover the bowl and set aside for 6–8 hours. Drain the softened nuts, discarding the water, then transfer to a blender. Add all the remaining ingredients and purée until smooth and creamy.

Refrigerate the sauce in a screwtop jar and consume within a week. If the sauce gets too thick, stir in a little water.

Nutritional analysis per serving (2 tablespoons):
calories 80, fat 6 g, saturated fat 4 g, cholesterol 0 mg,
fibre 1 g, protein 3 g, carbohydrate 4 g, sodium 70 mg

ALMOND SAUCE

This creamy sauce was created for the Ginger Prawn and the Raw Courgette Ribbon Salad recipes, but it's so versatile you will probably find more uses for it. Any leftovers have a way of disappearing quickly, but don't worry: this recipe is quick to make and the quantities can easily be doubled.

Yield: 100 g (4 oz)
Prep time: 10 minutes

- 75 ml (3 fl oz) fresh lime juice
- 120 g (4½ oz) creamy raw almond butter
- 2 tablespoons full-fat coconut milk
- 20 ml (1 tablespoon plus 1 teaspoon) melted coconut oil
- 2 teaspoons unseasoned rice vinegar

Combine all the ingredients in a small bowl and mix until smooth. Refrigerate the sauce in a screwtop jar and consume within a week.

Nutritional analysis per serving (1 tablespoon):
calories 80, fat 7 g, saturated fat 3 g, cholesterol 0 mg,
fibre 1 g, protein 2 g, carbohydrate 3 g, sodium 0 mg

EASY CREAMY BLENDER HOLLANDAISE

A classic French sauce, this creamy mixture is easy to make in a blender in just minutes. It can be made a day ahead or just before serving. Use it for topping eggs, vegetables, fish or just about anything. See notes for variations below.

Yield: 165 g (5½ oz)
Prep time: 5 minutes
Cook time: 10 minutes

- 12 tablespoons unsalted grass-fed butter
- 2 large omega-3 egg yolks
- 1 tablespoon fresh lemon juice

- ¼ teaspoon sea salt
- ¼ teaspoon white pepper
- pinch of cayenne pepper
- optional: few drops of hot pepper sauce, 1 tablespoon finely chopped tarragon leaves, 1 tablespoon finely chopped dill fronds, 2 teaspoons Dijon mustard

Melt the butter in a small pan and keep it at 80°C (175°F), using a digital thermometer.

Put the egg yolks in a blender, add the lemon juice, salt, pepper and cayenne pepper and pulse on low to combine. With the motor running slowly, drizzle in the melted butter very, very gradually so that an emulsion forms and the sauce becomes creamy. Taste and adjust the seasoning with more salt, pepper or lemon juice, as needed. Add any optional ingredients desired and stir to incorporate.

To keep sauce warm while you are making another dish, place it in a heatproof container in a small pan of warm water (a water bath) over a low heat. If it gets too thick, add a little more lemon juice or a few drops of warm water and whisk until smooth.

To store leftover sauce, refrigerate in an airtight container for up to a week. Rewarm the sauce using a warm water bath as instructed above.

Nutritional analysis per serving (3 tablespoons):
calories 340, fat 36 g, saturated fat 26 g, cholesterol 175 mg,
fibre 0 g, protein 1 g, carbohydrate 1 g, sodium 460 mg

RICH HOMEMADE MAYONNAISE

Once you make this creamy concoction, you will throw out any shop-bought mayo in your refrigerator! You will get a great arm workout making it by hand, but you can make it in a blender if you prefer. Use pasteurized eggs.

Yield: 165 g (5½ oz)
Prep time: 25 minutes

- 2 large omega-3 egg yolks
- 1 tablespoon fresh lemon juice

- 1 tablespoon white wine or champagne vinegar
- ¼ teaspoon Dijon mustard
- pinch of sea salt and white pepper
- 185 ml (6½ fl oz) avocado oil or extra virgin olive oil

To make the mayonnaise by hand, place the egg yolks, lemon juice, vinegar, mustard, salt and pepper in a medium bowl resting on a damp tea towel to prevent it sliding around. Using a balloon whisk, beat until everything is smoothly combined. Now whisk in the oil, a few drops at a time, until the mayonnaise starts to come together and thicken. As this happens, continue whisking vigorously while pouring the oil in a very thin stream. If you add it too quickly, the mayo will not thicken. You can stop for a moment to rest your arm or switch hands, if needed. Once all of the oil has been added and the mayonnaise is thick and creamy, taste and add salt, pepper or more lemon juice, as needed.

To make the mayonnaise in a blender, first whisk the yolks, lemon juice, vinegar, mustard, salt and pepper together in a small bowl until smooth. Transfer the mixture to a blender and blend on low for a few seconds. With the motor running, begin adding the oil very slowly, a few drops at a time. Once a smooth emulsion forms, add the remaining oil in a very slow, steady stream. Taste and add more salt, pepper or lemon juice, as needed.

(Tool Tip: a long, flexible silicone spatula makes it easier to get all the mayonnaise out of the blender.)

Refrigerate the mayonnaise in a screwtop jar and use within 4 days. If it gets too thick, whisk in 1–2 teaspoons warm water to thin.

Nutritional analysis per serving (1 tablespoon):
calories 100, fat 11 g, saturated fa: 2 g, cholesterol 25 mg,
fibre 0 g, protein 0 g, carbohydrate 0 g, sodium 10 mg

SIDE DISHES AND VEGETABLES

BRAISED SWEET FENNEL

Slow cooking brings out the natural sweetness of fennel. You can make this ahead of time and reheat it as a side dish for the Braised Chicken on page 304.

Yield: 4 servings
Prep time: 10 minutes
Cook time: 35 minutes

- 1 tablespoon extra virgin olive oil
- 3 large fennel bulbs, cut into wedges 1 cm (½ in) thick
- ¼ teaspoon sea salt
- ¼ teaspoon ground black pepper
- ¼ teaspoon garlic granules
- 185 ml (6½ fl oz) low- or no-sodium chicken stock
- 1 tablespoon chopped fresh thyme leaves

Put the olive oil into a wide frying pan over a medium heat. Place the fennel wedges flat in a single layer in the pan, sprinkle with the salt, pepper and garlic and cook until each side is golden brown (about 10 minutes). Lower the heat as necessary to avoid burning.

When the browning is done, add the chicken stock and stir in the thyme. Cover and simmer until the fennel is very tender when pierced with the tip of a knife (15–20 minutes).

Nutritional analysis per serving (about 75 g/3 oz):
calories 90, fat 4 g, saturated fat 1 g, cholesterol 0 mg,
fibre 5 g, protein 3 g, carbohydrate 13 g, sodium 250 mg

HERBED CAULIFLOWER "RICE"

You will never believe how much like rice this is! In fact, it's better than rice — and better for you, with no starchy carbs. It's a great way to get more veggies into your diet. This is a versatile dish that is easily changed using different herbs and spices, so experiment to find what you enjoy. You can grate the cauliflower ahead of time and keep it refrigerated until you are ready to cook it.

Yield: 4 servings
Prep time: 10 minutes
Cook time: 15 minutes

- 1 large head of cauliflower (900 g/2 lb)
- 20 ml (1 tablespoon plus 1 teaspoon) coconut oil
- 1 medium shallot, finely chopped
- 4 garlic cloves, finely chopped
- optional: 2 teaspoons finely grated ginger
- 35 g (1¼ oz) chopped fresh coriander, parsley, or a combination
- ¼ teaspoon sea salt
- ¼ teaspoon ground black pepper

Trim off and discard the cauliflower stalks and leaves. Cut the cauliflower into manageable pieces and grate over a plate or dish using the coarse side of a box grater.

Place the oil in a large non-stick frying pan over a medium-low heat. When hot, add the shallot and sauté until soft (1–2 minutes). Stir in the garlic and ginger (if using) and continue to cook for another minute. Add the cauliflower and cook, stirring, until hot (8–10 minute). Fold in the herbs, season with the salt and pepper and serve.

Nutritional analysis per serving (225 g/8 oz):
calories 110, fat 5 g, saturated fat 4 g, cholesterol 0 mg,
fibre 5 g, protein 5 g, carbohydrate 15 g, sodium: 220 mg

Oven Caramelized Red Onions

These onions are a sweet complement to many meals. Pile them on steak, chicken or salads, or add them to simple cooked green vegetables, such as asparagus or beans, to up your veggie consumption for the day.

Yield: 4 servings
Prep time: 10 minutes
Cook time: 40 minutes

- 2 tablespoons extra virgin olive oil
- 1 tablespoon Dijon mustard
- 2 teaspoons red wine vinegar
- 2 garlic cloves, finely chopped
- 1/4 teaspoon sea salt
- 1/4 teaspoon ground black pepper
- 2 large red onions (750–900 g/1½–1¾ lb in total)
- 1 tablespoon balsamic vinegar

Preheat the oven to 200°C/400°F/Gas mark 6.

Put the oil into a small bowl, add the mustard, red wine vinegar, garlic, salt and pepper and whisk together.

Cut the onions in half from top to bottom, then slice into half-moons 1 cm (1/2 in) wide. Place the onions in a large baking tray, add the vinaigrette and toss with your hands until all the pieces are well coated. The onions will come apart into slices. Spread them out into a single layer.

Roast for about 20 minutes, then stir and cook for another 15–20 minutes, or until they have shrivelled and the edges are starting to brown and crisp.

Serve the onions warm, at room temperature or cold, as a side dish or on top of a salad.

Nutritional analysis per serving (about 50 g/1 oz):
calories 90, fat 7 g, saturated fat 1 g, cholesterol 0 mg,
fibre 1 g, protein 1 g, carbohydrate 8 g, sodium 200 mg

Rosemary Garlic Sweet Potatoes

If you want a starchy vegetable to accompany dinner, look no further than this sweet and tasty side dish.

Yield: 4 servings
Prep time: 5 minutes
Cook time: 10 minutes

- 1 small sweet potato
- 3 tablespoons unsalted butter
- 1 tablespoon chopped fresh rosemary
- 1/4 teaspoon sea salt
- 1/4 teaspoon ground black or white pepper
- 1/4 teaspoon garlic granules

Peel the potato and chop into small cubes. Pour a 5-cm (2in) depth of water into a large pan, insert a steamer, then cover and bring to the boil over a medium-high heat. When steam starts escaping from the lid, add the potatoes and steam until completely tender when pierced with the tip of a sharp knife (4–5 minutes).

Drain the potatoes, then return them them to the hot pan. Add the butter, herbs and seasonings. Mash until as smooth or chunky as you like.

Nutritional analysis per serving (165 g (5½ oz):
calories 190, fat 10 g, saturated fat 8 g, cholesterol 25 mg,
fibre 4 g, protein 2 g, carbohydrate 25 g, sodium 300 mg

Lemony Broccoli Slaw

As cruciferous vegetables are amongst the healthiest things we can eat, this crunchy raw salad packs a nutritional punch. It's easy to make with a food processor and comes out light and fluffy. Top it with a small portion (100g/4 oz) of the chilled steamed salmon on page 320 for lunch, or add the optional cashews for extra crunch and healthy fat. For another lunch option, try it with a little chopped or shredded leftover chicken. Make the salad ahead and dress just before serving to keep it crunchy. Undressed salad will keep for a week in the refrigerator. For vegetarians and vegans, this dish works alone as a satisfying main course.

Yield: 4 servings
Prep time: 25 minutes

- 750 g (1½ lb) broccoli
- ½ small head of green cabbage (275 g/10 oz)
- 2 carrots
- optional: 100 g (4 oz) raw cashew nuts
- 4 tablespoons chopped Italian parsley
- 25 g (1 oz) chopped chives or spring onions
- 2 lemons, zested

FOR THE DRESSING

- 165 g (5½ oz) organic or homemade mayonnaise (see page 332)
- 2 tablespoons fresh lemon juice (use lemons from the salad)
- 2 tablespoons white wine vinegar
- ¼ teaspoon sea salt
- ¼ teaspoon ground black pepper

Cut off the broccoli stems, peel them with a vegetable peeler, then cut in half lengthways. Grate them in a food processor fitted with a coarse grating attachment.

Dump the grated stems onto double layers of kitchen paper and squeeze dry. It will probably take 3 lots of doubled paper as the stems are very wet. Place in a large wide bowl.

Repeat the grating and drying process with the broccoli florets. They are not as wet, so won't take as much paper to dry. Add them to the bowl with the stems.

Cut the cabbage into manageable chunks and grate in the food processor. Now grate the carrots. Combine all the vegetables in the bowl, and add the cashews (if using). Gently stir in the herbs and lemon zest.

Make the dressing by whisking all the ingredients for it in a small bowl.

Dress as much salad as you plan to use just before serving.

Nutritional analysis per serving (120 g/4½ oz, 2½ dressing): calories 380, fat 33 g, saturated fat 5 g, cholesterol 70 mg, fibre 8 g, protein 7 g, carbohydrate 19 g, sodium 270 mg

Nutritional analysis per serving (120 g/4½ oz, 1 tablespoon cashews, 2½ dressing):
calories 540, fat 45 g, saturated fat 7 g, cholesterol 70 mg, fibre 9g, protein 13 g, carbohydrate 27 g, sodium 135 mg

RAW COURGETTE RIBBON, TOMATO AND AVOCADO SALAD

Here is another recipe that uses a spiralizer, this time to make ribbons rather than noodles. Toss with creamy almond sauce, plus tomatoes, herbs and avocado and you have a fantastic vegetable salad, a nice alternative to ordinary greens. To save time, the ribbons can be made the night before use and refrigerated.

Yield: 4 servings
Prep time: 20 minutes

- 4 small courgettes, trimmed
- 60 ml (2 1/4 fl oz) Almond Sauce (see page 331)
- 20 ml (1 tablespoon plus 1 teaspoon) vinegar (white wine, champagne or unseasoned rice)
- 20 ml (1 tablespoon plus 1 teaspoon) extra virgin olive oil
- 3 tablespoons chopped parsley leaves
- 1 tablespoon finely chopped chives
- optional: 2–3 pinches of dried red chilli flakes
- 20 tomberries or cherry tomatoes, halved
- 1 avocado, stoned and quartered
- large pinch of sea salt and ground black pepper

Using a spiralizer fitted with a flat cutting blade, slice the courgettes into long ribbons. Set aside.

Place the almond sauce in a medium bowl, add the vinegar, oil, parsley, chives and red chilli flakes and whisk until combined. Add the courgette ribbons and toss until they are lightly coated with the dressing.

Divide the mixture between 4 plates, add equal amounts of the tomatoes and avocado to each serving, and lightly season with salt and pepper.

Nutritional analysis per serving (about 65 g/2½ oz):
calories 210, fat 17 g, saturated fat 4 g, cholesterol 90 mg,
fibre 7 g, protein 5 g, carbohydrate 15 g, sodium 95 mg

Acknowledgments

Anything I have done in life that truly mattered was done with the support and love of my community — of friends, family, mentors, teachers, collaborators, cocreators, supporters, work family, students, patients. In a thousand ways I am grateful for all those who have touched, inspired, helped, supported, and guided me. The list is almost too long to include everyone, and I fear I will leave many out. You know who you are. Thank you!

There are a few who have stood out in the creation of this book, which is among the hardest I have ever done because the subject of fat is slippery and the margin of error big.

I want to thank my publishing family: Richard Pine, my ever-encouraging cheerleader, agent, and guide. Tracy Behar, my editor from the start, who takes my words and makes them smarter, better, and thankfully fewer. Debra Goldstein, who helps me shape and massage the ideas into a clearer rendition of the truth. Sally Cameron, who created magically luscious recipes with joy. Sarah Jane Sandy, who helped me create a fat bible — a deep dive into the world of fat. Anahaḍ O'Connor, for our early conversations and for helping me dig up the hundreds of studies that uncovered the fat facts. Lauren Doscher, who helped me track down every reference.

And then to my home team, who allows me to be the doctor and teacher while they create magic, helping me share my work with millions online. Dhru Purohit, my partner, who sees the vision better than I do and rocks everything he touches. And my online team, who takes care of me and my community: Laurie Roman, Shibani Subramanya, Kaya Purohit, Farrell Feighan, Ben Tseitlin, John Baldwin, Amber

Cox, Holly Stillwell, and Susan Verity. And those who helped me greatly along the way: Lizzy Swick, Daffnee Cohen, and Tina Naser.

I would also like to thank a few very special people who reviewed the manuscript and provided invaluable and thoughtful feedback on how to get the science and the story right, including Jeffrey Bland, Pilar Gerasimo, Carrie Diulus, and Chris Kresser. My deepest gratitude goes out to David Ludwig for his guidance, wisdom, encouragement, and his introducing me to leading experts in the world of fat, but mostly for his friendship.

And, of course, Anne McLaughlin, the glue that holds my world together, and Dianna Galia, who fills in all the cracks and makes my world work better.

The deepest gratitude and love to my dearest friends and spiritual caretakers Alberto Villoldo and Marcella Lobos, at whose house in Chile I dove into the story of fat and wrote a big chunk of this book. And to Lauren Zander and the Handel community, who inspire, support, and love me, no matter what. There is often more "no matter what" than I would like!

To my team at The UltraWellness Center: Donna Doscher, Liz Boham, Todd Lepine, Maggie Ward, Denise Curtin, Jamie Delaney, Susan Wallingford, and everyone there who holds our world together while I am out spreading the wisdom of functional medicine.

There is no way I could have written this book without the tireless work of hundreds of researchers, scientists, doctors, thinkers, teachers, and experts, each of whom has inspired and instructed me, and helped with this book. To Walter Willett, Ronald Krauss, Barry Sears, Aseem Malholtra, Eric Ravussin, Kevin Hall, Joel Fuhrman, Neal Barnard, and Josh Axe. And especially to David Ludwig, an intellectual giant, who has helped me understand the biology of sugar, fat, and weight for decades and guided and protected me throughout all of it.

There is a long, long list of others who have helped me. David Perlmutter, Marc David, Jeffrey Bland, Nina Teicholz, Chris Kresser, Vani Hari, Nick Ortner, Kris Carr, Christiane Northrup, Dave Asprey, JJ Virgin, Tim Ryan, Deepak Chopra, Mike Roizen, Mehmet Oz, Daniel Amen, Rick Warren, Dee and Brett Eastman, Peter Attia, Gary

Taubes, Joseph Mercola, Pedram Shojai, Ken Cook, Heather White, Ann Louise Gittleman, John and Ocean Robbins, Alexandra Jamieson, Maria Shiver, Gunnar Lovelace and his team at Thrive Market, Joy Devins, and Ronald Gahler.

And now there is the whole community at Cleveland Clinic and the Institute of Functional Medicine that has allowed my dream to come true: to bring Functional Medicine to more people. Thank you for letting me do what I do! To Toby and Anita Cosgrove, who saw the future of health care and invited us into the center of the party. Thank you! And, of course, to Mary Curran, Linda McHugh, Tawny Jones, and the whole team at the Cleveland Clinic Center for Functional Medicine. We are building the future together! Without Laurie Hofmann and Patrick Hanaway and Christine Stead and Juliette Rogers, none of this would be possible.

I am very grateful for the love and support of my ever-growing community of family and friends, especially my children, Rachel and Misha, and my bonus children, Sarah and Ben.

And last but not least, this book would not have happened without the love and inspiration and endless conversations and delicious meals with the most magical, wise, and amazing human I know, Jody Levy. Thank you forever.

Resources

DR. MARK HYMAN AND FUNCTIONAL MEDICINE

Dr. Hyman on Social Media

www.drhyman.com
www.eatfatgetthin.com
Twitter: @markhymanmd
Instagram: @markhymanmd
Facebook: facebook.com/drmarkhyman

Books and Programs

The Blood Sugar Solution 10-Day Detox Diet (book and public television special)
The Blood Sugar Solution 10-Day Detox Diet Cookbook (book)
The Blood Sugar Solution (book and public television special)
The Blood Sugar Solution Cookbook (book)
The UltraMind Solution (book and public television special)
Six Weeks to an UltraMind (audio/DVD program)
The Daniel Plan (book)
The Daniel Plan Cookbook (book)
UltraCalm (audio program)
UltraMetabolism (book and public television special)
The UltraMetabolism Cookbook (book)
The UltraSimple Diet (book)
The UltraSimple Challenge (DVD coaching program)
The UltraThyroid Solution (e-book)
UltraPrevention (book)

The Five Forces of Wellness (audio program)
The Detox Box (audio/DVD program)

Finding a Functional Medicine Doctor

I am founder and director of two medical clinics where teams of experienced functional medicine physicians, nutritionists, nurses, and health coaches guide you through diet and lifestyle modifications, as well as provide specialized testing, nutritional supplementation, and medications.

The UltraWellness Center

55 Pittsfield Road, Suite 9
Lenox Commons
Lenox, MA 01240
(413) 637-9991
www.ultrawellnesscenter.com

Cleveland Clinic Center for Functional Medicine

9500 Euclid Avenue
Cleveland, OH 44195
(216) 445-6900 or toll-free at (844) 833-0126
http://my.clevelandclinic.org/services/center-for-functional-medicine

Institute for Functional Medicine

Additionally, I am the chairman of the board of the Institute for Functional Medicine, a 501(c)(3) nonprofit and the global leader in functional medicine education. Go to **www.functionalmedicine.org** to find a certified practitioner near you.

EAT FAT, GET THIN TOOLS AND RESOURCES

At www.eatfatgetthin.com, you will find all the resources listed below, and more, for support during and long after the twenty-one day *Eat Fat, Get Thin* Plan.

The Fat Summit: Separating Fat from Fiction

In my exclusive online conference, The Fat Summit: Separating Fat from Fiction, I interview more than thirty of the world's top experts on the topic of fat and what it really takes to lose weight, feel great, and reverse chronic disease naturally. Go to www.fatsummit.com to watch or listen to the conference.

The Eat Fat, Get Thin Supplements

When it comes to supplements, quality matters. In a sea of unregulated, poor-quality products that are not screened for potency or purity and that may not be bioavailable, we have screened and vetted a few ethical companies that focus on quality. We recommend that you choose the best supplements. After all, you have only one body.

Here are the daily recommendations for supplements and products that support the *Eat Fat, Get Thin 21-Day Plan*. For detailed descriptions of each item, see chapter 12, page 200.

- **Multivitamin and mineral supplement (high quality):** take as directed by manufacturer
- **Fish oil (purified):** 2 grams a day
- **Vitamin D$_3$:** 2,000 units a day
- **L-carnitine:** 300 to 400 milligrams twice a day
- **Coenzyme Q10:** 30 milligrams twice a day
- **Magnesium glycinate:** 100 to 150 milligrams a day (take 1 capsule twice a day)
- **PGX:** 2 to 5 grams a day (powder or capsule form), 3 times a day (take 15 minutes before each meal with a large glass of water)
- **Probiotics:** 10 to 20 billion CFUs a day
- **MCT (medium chain triglycerides) oil:** 1 to 2 tablespoons a day
- **Electrolytes:** 1 capful of E-lyte (a liquid electrolyte solution) in 8 ounces (200ml) of water, twice a day
- **Potato starch:** 1 to 2 tablespoons in 8 ounces (200ml) of water, twice a day

Please visit www.eatfatgetthin.com to find out where you can purchase these items.

Additional Supportive Supplements (depending on your needs)

- **Digestive enzymes:** 1 to 2 capsules with each meal to help with digestion
- **Magnesium citrate:** 150-milligram capsules or tablets, 2 to 3 capsules twice per day. Use this form of magnesium if you tend toward constipation.
- **Laxablend (an herbal laxative):** 2 to 3 capsules at night if you haven't had a bowel movement in a day or feel constipated.

- **Buffered ascorbic acid:** 500 mg capsules, 2 to 4 capsules twice a day to help with detoxification and constipation

Health and Testing Resources

- Basic lab testing guidelines
- Carbohydrate Intolerance Quiz and FLC (Feel Like Crap) Quiz
- *How to Work with Your Doctor to Get What You Need* downloadable e-book
- *Beyond Food: Other Causes of Obesity and Damaged Metabolism* downloadable e-book
- *The Fat Bible: Your Guide to Eating Fat* downloadable e-book
- Self-monitoring tools, including information on glucose monitors, Fitbit, Fitbit Wi-Fi Smart Scale and Withings scale, blood-pressure monitors, and personal movement and activity trackers
- Genetic testing, including information on at-home test kits for genomic testing
- Symptoms Tracking Chart (to test gluten and dairy)
- The *Eat Fat, Get Thin* Online Health Tracker

Eat Fat, Get Thin *Community Resources*

- The *Eat Fat, Get Thin* Online Course
- The *Eat Fat, Get Thin* Community pages
- Life coaching through the Handel Group (www.handelgroup.com)

Lifestyle Resources

- *Eat Fat, Get Thin* Online Journal
- *Eat Fat, Get Thin* Online Food Log
- Fitness resources
- *Restaurant Rescue Guide* downloadable e-book
- The *UltraCalm* guided audio-relaxation program
- Meditation resources
- Stress-busting tools

Sleep Resources

Blue Lights

www.lowbluelights.com
Products for naturally maximizing melatonin.

Spoonk Acupressure Mat

www.spoonkspace.com

Acupressure mats provide natural and powerful back-pain relief and body and mind relaxation, while improving blood circulation to every part of your body.

Earthing Sheet

www.earthing.com

Earthing sheets ground you to the earth and disconnect you from the electromagnetic frequencies (EMFs) that can affect your sleep.

GENERAL REFERENCES AND RESOURCES

Environmental Working Group

Environmental Working Group website, www.ewg.org

The Environmental Working Group empowers people to live healthier lives in a healthier environment, driving consumer choice, civic action, and an informed public with breakthrough research. Use this site to find: guides to making good food on a tight budget; the "Clean 15/Dirty Dozen" produce list; food scores to check your food for nutritional quality, ingredients, and level of processing; guides to healthy, sustainable low-mercury fish; a meat eater's guide to eating meat that is healthy for you and the planet; information on safe skin care and house-cleaning products; and more.

Food Essentials

Thrive Market

Online marketplace where you can shop for the best healthy, natural, non-GMO, organic, vegan, raw, Paleo, gluten-free, and non-toxic items from the top-selling brands at wholesale prices. This extraordinary company is changing the food landscape by providing access to real whole fresh foods at 25 to 50 percent off retail prices and shipping anywhere in the country, including food deserts. You can get a free three-month trial membership and 25 percent off your first order by going to www.thrivemarket.com/EFGT.

Grass-fed Meats

Mark's Daily Apple

    www.marksdailyapple.com/primal-resource-guide

    Online resources and blog

US Wellness Meats

    www.grasslandbeef.com

    A site offering 100 percent grass-fed beef treated humanely from birth to processing, using rotational grazing and never using herbicides, pesticides, or fertilizers

Seafood and Organic Frozen or Canned Fish

National Resources Defense Council

    http://www.nrdc.org/oceans/seafoodguide/

    Sustainably raised or harvested low-mercury fish sources

Vital Choice

    www.vitalchoice.com

    A selection of fresh, frozen, and canned wild salmon, sardines, black cod, and small halibut

Clean Fish

    www.cleanfish.com

    Sustainably-sourced (farmed or fished) seafood from artisan producers

Notes

Introduction

1. McCarthy M. US guideline may drop cholesterol limits but keep link between dietary saturated fats and trans fats and heart disease. *BMJ*. 2015 Feb 18;350:h835.

2. May AL, Kuklina EV, Yoon PW. Prevalence of cardiovascular disease risk factors among US adolescents, 1999–2008. *Pediatrics*. 2012 Jun;129(6):1035–41.

3. Mohindra D. Non-communicable diseases to cost $47 trillion by 2030, new study released today. World Economic Forum. http://www.weforum.org/news/non-communicable-diseases-cost-47-trillion-2030-new-study-released-today. Updated September 18, 2011.

Chapter 1

1. 2015 Dietary Guidelines Advisory Committee. Scientific report of the 2015 Dietary Guidelines Advisory Committee. Office of Disease Prevention and Health Promotion. http://www.health.gov/dietaryguidelines/2015-scientific-report/. February 2015.

2. Schulte EM, Avena NM, Gearhardt AN. Which foods may be addictive? The roles of processing, fat content, and glycemic load. *PLoS One*. 2015 Feb 18;10(2).

3. Allison DB. Liquid calories, energy compensation and weight: what we know and what we still need to learn. *Br J Nutr*. 2014 Feb;111(3):384–86.

4. Singh GM, Micha R, Khatibzadeh S, Lim S, Ezzati M, Mozaffarian D; Global Burden of Diseases Nutrition and Chronic Diseases Expert Group (NutriCoDE). Estimated global, regional, and national disease burdens related to sugar-sweetened beverage consumption in 2010. *Circulation*. 2015 Jun 29.

5. Iadecola C. Sugar and Alzheimer's disease: a bittersweet truth. *Nat Neurosci*. 2015 Apr;18(4):477–78.

6. Hession M, Rolland C, Kulkarni U, Wise A, Broom J. Systematic review of randomized controlled trials of low-carbohydrate vs. low-fat/low-calorie diets in the management of obesity and its comorbidities. *Obes Rev*. 2009 Jan;10(1):36–50.

7. Chowdhury R, Warnakula S, Kunutsor S, et al. Association of dietary, circulating, and supplement fatty acids with coronary risk: a systematic review and meta-analysis. *Ann Intern Med*. 2014 Mar 18;160(6):398–406.

8. Hamdy O. Nutrition revolution—the end of the high carbohydrates era for diabetes prevention and management. *US Endocrinol*. 2014;10(2)103–4.

9. Viguiliouk E, Kendall CW, Blanco Mejia S, et al. Effect of tree nuts on glycemic control in diabetes: a systematic review and meta-analysis of randomized controlled dietary trials. *PLoS One*. 2014 Jul 30;9(7):e103376.

10. Estruch R, Ros E, Salas-Salvadó J, et al; PREDIMED Study Investigators. Primary prevention of cardiovascular disease with a Mediterranean diet. *N Engl J Med*. 2013 Apr 4;368(14):1279–90.

11. Laing RD. *The Voice of Experience*. New York: Pantheon; 1982.

12. Ballard KD, Quann EE, Kupchak BR, et al. Dietary carbohydrate restriction improves insulin sensitivity, blood pressure, microvascular function, and cellular adhesion markers in individuals taking statins. *Nutr Res*. 2013 Nov;33(11):905–12.

13. Nickols-Richardson SM, Coleman MD, Volpe JJ, Hosig KW. Perceived hunger is lower and weight loss is greater in overweight premenopausal women consuming a low-carbohydrate/high-protein vs high-carbohydrate/low-fat diet. *J Am Diet Assoc*. 2005 Sep;105(9):1433–37.

14. Chowdhury R, Warnakula S, Kunutsor S, et al. Association of dietary, circulating, and supplement fatty acids with coronary risk: a systematic review and meta-analysis. *Ann Intern Med*. 2014 Mar 18;160(6):398–406.

15. Faghihnia N, Mangravite LM, Chiu S, Bergeron N, Krauss RM. Effects of dietary saturated fat on LDL subclasses and apolipoprotein CIII in men. *Eur J Clin Nutr*. 2012 Nov;66(11):1229–33.

16. Gardner CD, Kiazand A, Alhassan S, et al. Comparison of the Atkins, Zone, Ornish, and LEARN diets for change in weight and related risk factors among overweight premenopausal women: the A TO Z Weight Loss Study: a randomized trial. *JAMA*. 2007 Mar 7;297(9):969–77.

17. Margioris AN. Fatty acids and postprandial inflammation. *Curr Opin Clin Nutr Metab Care*. 2009 Mar;12(2):129–37. Review.

18. Wood RJ, Volek JS, Davis SR, Dell'Ova C, Fernandez ML. Effects of a carbohydrate-restricted diet on emerging plasma markers for cardiovascular disease. *Nutr Metab* (Lond). 2006 May 4;3:19.

19. Volek JS, Ballard KD, Silvestre R, et al. Effects of dietary carbohydrate restriction versus low-fat diet on flow-mediated dilation. *Metabolism*. 2009 Dec;58(12):1769–77.

20. Valls-Pedret C, Sala-Vila A, Serra-Mir M, et al. Mediterranean diet and age-related cognitive decline: a randomized clinical trial. *JAMA Intern Med*. 2015 May 11.

21. Accurso A, Bernstein RK, Dahlqvist A, et al. Dietary carbohydrate restriction in type 2 diabetes mellitus and metabolic syndrome: time for a critical appraisal. *Nutr Metab* (Lond). 2008 Apr 8;5:9.

22. Ramsden CE, Zamora D, Leelarthaepin B, et al. Use of dietary linoleic acid for secondary prevention of coronary heart disease and death: evaluation of recovered data from the Sydney Diet Heart Study and updated meta-analysis. *BMJ*. 2013 Feb 4;346:e8707. Patterson E, Wall R, Fitzgerald GF, Ross RP, Stanton C. Health implications of high dietary omega-6 polyunsaturated fatty acids. *J Nutr Metab*. 2012;2012:539426.

23. Volk BM, Kunces LJ, Freidenreich DJ, et al. Effects of step-wise increases in dietary carbohydrate on circulating saturated fatty acids and palmitoleic acid in adults with metabolic syndrome. *PLoS One*. 2014 Nov21;9(11):e113605. Forsythe CE, Phinney SD, Feinman RD, et al. Limited effect of dietary saturated fat on plasma saturated fat in the context of a low carbohydrate diet. *Lipids*. 2010 Oct;45(10):947–62.

24. Volk BM, Kunces LJ, Freidenreich DJ, et al. Effects of step-wise increases in dietary carbohydrate on circulating saturated fatty acids and palmitoleic acid in adults with metabolic syndrome. *PLoS One*. 2014 Nov21;9(11):e113605.

25. Richelsen B. Sugar-sweetened beverages and cardio-metabolic disease risks. *Curr Opin Clin Nutr Metab Care*. 2013 Jul;16(4):478–84.

26. Ameer F, Scandiuzzi L, Hasnain S, Kalbacher H, Zaidi N. De novo lipogenesis in health and disease. *Metabolism*. 2014 Jul;63(7):895–902.

27. Barclay AW, Petocz P, McMillan-Price J, et al. Glycemic index, glycemic load, and chronic disease risk—a meta-analysis of observational studies. *Am J Clin Nutr.* 2008 Mar;87(3):627–37. Review.
28. Castro-Quezada I, Sánchez-Villegas A, Estruch R, et al; PREDIMED Study Investigators. A high dietary glycemic index increases total mortality in a Mediterranean population at high cardiovascular risk. *PLoS One.* 2014 Sep 24;9(9):e107968.

Chapter 2

1. Ioannidis JPA. Implausible results in human nutrition research. *BMJ.* 2013;347:f6698.
2. Lesser LI, Ebbeling CB, Goozner M, Wypij D, Ludwig DS. Relationship between funding source and conclusion among nutrition-related scientific articles. *PLoS Med.* 2007 Jan;4(1):e5.
3. Schoeller DA. The energy balance equation: looking back and looking forward are two very different views. *Nutr Rev.* 2009 May;67(5):249–54.
4. Von Noorden C. Obesity. *Metabolism and practical medicine.* Vol 3: The pathology of metabolism. Von Noorden C, Hall I W, eds. Chicago: W T Keener, 1907: 693–715.
5. Pennington AW. A reorientation on obesity. *N Engl J Med.* 1953 Jun 4;248 (23):959–64.
6. Lewis SB, Wallin JD, Kane JP, Gerich JE. Effect of diet composition on metabolic adaptations to hypocaloric nutrition: comparison of high carbohydrate and high fat isocaloric diets. *Am J Clin Nutr.* 1977 Feb;30(2):160–70.
7. Willett WC. Dietary fat is not a major determinant of body fat. *Am J Med.* 2002;113(9B):47S–59S. Willett W. Dietary fat intake and the risk of coronary heart disease in women. *N Engl J Med.* 1997;337:1491–99.
8. DiNicolantonio JJ. The cardiometabolic consequences of replacing saturated fats with carbohydrates or Ω-6 polyunsaturated fats: do the dietary guidelines have it wrong? *Open Heart.* 2014 Feb 8;1(1):e000032.
9. Teicholz N. *The Big Fat Surprise.* New York: Scribner; 2014.
10. Food and Agriculture Organization of the United Nations. Fats and fatty acids in human nutrition: report of an expert consultation. 2010.
11. Yerushalmy J, Hilleboe HE. Fat in the diet and mortality from heart disease. *N Y State J Med.* 1957;57:2343–54.
12. Yudkin J. Dietary factors in arteriosclerosis: sucrose. *Lipids.* 1978 May;13(5):370–72.
13. Liu S, Willett WC, Stampfer MJ, et al. A prospective study of dietary glycemic load, carbohydrate intake, and risk of coronary heart disease in US women. *Am J Clin Nutr.* 2000;71:1455–61. Yang Q, Zhang Z, Gregg EW, Flanders WD, Merritt R, Hu FB. Added sugar intake and cardiovascular diseases mortality among US adults. *JAMA Intern Med.* 2014 Apr;174(4):516–24.
14. Malik VS, Schulze MB, Hu FB. Intake of sugar-sweetened beverages and weight gain: a systematic review. *Am J Clin Nutr.* 2006 Aug;84(2):274–88. Review.
15. Greenwood DC, Threapleton DE, Evans CE, et al. Association between sugar-sweetened and artificially sweetened soft drinks and type 2 diabetes: systematic review and dose-response meta-analysis of prospective studies. *Br J Nutr.* 2014 Sep 14;112(5):725–34.
16. Keys A, Menotti A, Aravanis C, et al. The Seven Countries Study: 2289 deaths in 15 years. *Prev Med.* 1984;13:141–54.
17. Menotti A, Kromhout D, Blackburn H, Fidanza F, Buzina R, Nissinen A. Food intake patterns and 25-year mortality from coronary heart disease: cross-cultural correlations in the Seven Countries Study. The Seven Countries Study Research Group. *Eur J Epidemiol.* 1999 Jul;15(6):507–15.

18. Gardner CD, Kiazand A, Alhassan S, et al. Comparison of the Atkins, Zone, Ornish, and LEARN diets for change in weight and related risk factors among overweight premenopausal women: the A TO Z Weight Loss Study: a randomized trial. *JAMA.* 2007 Mar 7;297(9):969–77.

19. Tobias, DK, et al., Effect of low-fat diet interventions versus other diet interventions on long-term weight change in adults: a systematic review and meta-analysis, *Lancet Diabetes Endocrinol.* 2015 Dec;3(12):968–79.

20. Create your plate. American Diabetes Association. http://www.diabetes.org/food-and-fitness/food/planning-meals/create-your-plate/?loc=ff-slabnav. Updated October 19, 2015.

21. Feinman RD, Pogozelski WK, Astrup A, et al. Dietary carbohydrate restriction as the first approach in diabetes management: critical review and evidence base. *Nutrition.* 2015 Jan;31(1):1–13.

22. Fagherazzi G, Vilier A, Saes Sartorelli D, Lajous M, Balkau B, Clavel-Chapelon F. Consumption of artificially and sugar-sweetened beverages and incident type 2 diabetes in the Etude Epidemiologique auprès des femmes de la Mutuelle Générale de l'Education Nationale—European Prospective Investigation into Cancer and Nutrition cohort. *Am J Clin Nutr.* 2013 Mar;97(3):517–23.

23. Swithers SE. Artificial sweeteners produce the counterintuitive effect of inducing metabolic derangements. *Trends Endocrinol Metab.* 2013 Sep;24(9):431–41.

24. Suez J, Korem T, Zeevi D, et al. Artificial sweeteners induce glucose intolerance by altering the gut microbiota. *Nature.* 2014 Oct 9;514(7521):181–86.

25. Nestle M. *Food Politics, How the Food Industry Influences Nutrition, and Health.* Oakland: University of California Press; 2007.

26. Astrup A, Dyerberg J, Elwood P, et al. The role of reducing intakes of saturated fat in the prevention of cardiovascular disease: where does the evidence stand in 2010? *Am J Clin Nutr.* 2011 Apr;93(4):684–88.

27. Chowdhury R, Warnakula S, Kunutsor S, et al. Association of dietary, circulating, and supplement fatty acids with coronary risk: a systematic review and meta-analysis. *Ann Intern Med.* 2014 Mar 18;160(6):398–406. Siri-Tarino PW, Sun Q, Hu FB, Krauss RM. Meta-analysis of prospective cohort studies evaluating the association of saturated fat with cardiovascular disease. *Am J Clin Nutr.* 2010 Mar;91(3):535–46.

28. Dreon DM, Fernstrom HA, Campos H, Blanche P, Williams PT, Krauss RM. Change in dietary saturated fat intake is correlated with change in mass of large low-density-lipoprotein particles in men. *Am J Clin Nutr.* 1998 May;67(5):828–36.

29. Krauss RM, Blanche PJ, Rawlings RS, Fernstrom HS, Williams PT. Separate effects of reduced carbohydrate intake and weight loss on atherogenic dyslipidemia. *Am J Clin Nutr.* 2006 May;83(5):1025–31.

30. Butler K. I went to the nutritionists' annual confab. It was catered by McDonald's. *MotherJones.*http://www.motherjones.com/environment/2014/05/my-trip-mcdonalds-sponsored-nutritionist-convention. Updated May 12, 2014.

31. Harper AE. Dietary goals—a skeptical view. *Am J Clin Nutr.* 1978 Feb;31(2):310–21. Review.

32. Harcombe Z, Baker JS, Cooper SM, Davies B, Sculthorpe N, DiNicolantonio JJ, Grace F. Evidence from randomised controlled trials did not support the introduction of dietary fat guidelines in 1977 and 1983: a systematic review and meta-analysis. *Open Heart.* 2015 Jan 29;2(1)

33. Ludwig DS, Willett WC. Three daily servings of reduced-fat milk: an evidence-based recommendation? *JAMA Pediatr.* 2013 Sep;167(9):788–89.

34. Datz T. Harvard serves up its own "plate." *Harvard Gazette.* http://news.harvard .edu/gazette/story/2011/09/harvard-serves-up-its-own-plate/?utm_content. Updated September 14, 2011.

35. Gornall J. Sugar's web of influence 2: biasing the science. *BMJ.* 2015 Feb 11;350:h215.

36. Schlanger Z. Report: the sugar lobby threatens organizations, buries science on health effects. *Newsweek.* http://www.newsweek.com/report-sugar-lobby-threatens-organizations-buries-science-health-effects-256529. Updated June 27, 2014.

37. WHO calls on countries to reduce sugars intake among adults and children. World Health Organization. http://www.who.int/mediacentre/news/releases/2015/sugar -guideline/en/. Updated March 4, 2015.

38. Office of Disease Prevention and Health Promotion. 2015 Dietary guidelines. http://health.gov/dietaryguidelines/2015/.

39. Mozaffarian D, Ludwig DS. The 2015 US Dietary Guidelines: lifting the ban on total dietary fat. *JAMA.* 2015;313(24):2421–2422.

40. Eckel RH, Jakicic JM, Ard JD, et al; American College of Cardiology/American Heart Association Task Force on Practice Guidelines. 2013 AHA/ACC guideline on lifestyle management to reduce cardiovascular risk: a report of the American College of Cardiology/American Heart Association Task Force on Practice Guidelines. *Circulation.* 2014;129:S76–S99.

41. Malhotra A. Saturated fat is not the major issue. *BMJ.* 2013;347:f6340.

42. Paoli A, Bianco A, Damiani E, Bosco G. Ketogenic diet in neuromuscular and neu-rodegenerative diseases. *Biomed Res Int.* 2014;2014:474296.

Chapter 3

1. Nutrition Science Initiative. www.nusi.org.

2. Hall KD, Hammond RA, Rahmandad H. Dynamic interplay among homeostatic, hedonic, and cognitive feedback circuits regulating body weight. *Am J Public Health.* 2014 Jul;104(7):1169–75.

3. Taubes G. The science of obesity: what do we really know about what makes us fat? An essay by Gary Taubes. *BMJ.* 2013 Apr 15;346:f1050.

4. Kraschnewski JL, Boan J, Esposito J, et al. Long-term weight loss maintenance in the United States. *Int J Obes* (Lond). 2010 Nov;34(11):1644–54.

5. Luo S, Romero A, Adam TC, Hu HH, Monterosso J, Page KA. Abdominal fat is associated with a greater brain reward response to high-calorie food cues in Hispanic women. *Obesity* (Silver Spring). 2013 Oct;21(10):2029–36.

6. Page KA, Seo D, Belfort-DeAguiar R, et al. Circulating glucose levels modulate neural control of desire for high calorie foods in humans. *J Clin Invest.* 2011 Oct;121(10):4161–69.

7. Gardner CD, Kiazand A, Alhassan S, et al. Comparison of the Atkins, Zone, Ornish, and LEARN diets for change in weight and related risk factors among overweight premenopausal women: the A TO Z Weight Loss Study: a randomized trial. *JAMA.* 2007 Mar 7;297(9):969–77.

8. Shai I, Schwarzfuchs D, Henkin Y, et al. Weight loss with a low-carbohydrate, Med-iterranean, or low-fat diet. *N Engl J Med.* 2008 Jul 17;359(3):229–41.

9. Larsen TM, Dalskov SM, van Baak M, et al; Diet, Obesity, and Genes (Diogenes) Project. Diets with high or low protein content and glycemic index for weight-loss maintenance. *N Engl J Med.* 2010 Nov 25;363(22):2102–13.

10. Yancy WS Jr, Olsen MK, Guyton JR, Bakst RP, Westman EC. A low-carbohydrate, ketogenic diet versus a low-fat diet to treat obesity and hyperlipidemia: a random-ized, controlled trial. *Ann Intern Med.* 2004 May 18;140(10):769–77.

11. Hession M, Rolland C, Kulkarni U, Wise A, Broom J. Systematic review of randomized controlled trials of low-carbohydrate vs. low-fat/low-calorie diets in the management of obesity and its comorbidities. *Obes Rev.* 2009 Jan;10(1):36–50.

12. Santos FL, Esteves SS, da Costa Pereira A, Yancy WS Jr, Nunes JP. Systematic review and meta-analysis of clinical trials of the effects of low carbohydrate diets on cardiovascular risk factors. *Obes Rev.* 2012 Nov;13(11):1048–66.

13. Pawlak DB, Kushner JA, Ludwig DS. Effects of dietary glycaemic index onadiposity, glucose homoeostasis, and plasma lipids in animals. *Lancet.* 2004 Aug 28–Sep 3;364(9436):778–85.

14. Kennedy AR, Pissios P, Otu H, et al. A high-fat, ketogenic diet induces a unique metabolic state in mice. *Am J Physiol Endocrinol Metab.* 2007 Jun;292(6):E1724–39.

15. Walsh CO, Ebbeling CB, Swain JF, Markowitz RL, Feldman HA, Ludwig DS. Effects of diet composition on postprandial energy availability during weight loss maintenance. *PLoS One.* 2013;8(3).

16. Ebbeling CB, Swain JF, Feldman HA, et al. Effects of dietary composition on energy expenditure during weight-loss maintenance. *JAMA.* 2012 Jun 27;307(24):2627–34.

17. Thomas DE, Elliott EJ, Baur L. Low glycaemic index or low glycaemic load diets for overweight and obesity. *Cochrane Database Syst Rev.* 2007 Jul 18;(3).

18. Tobias DK, Chen M, Manson JE, Ludwig DS, Willett W, Hu FB. Effect of low-fat diet interventions versus other diet interventions on long-term weight change in adults: a systematic review and meta-analysis. *Lancet Diabetes Endocrinol.* 2015 Dec;3(12):968–79.

19. Sumithran P, Proietto J. The defence of body weight: a physiological basis for weight regain after weight loss. *Clin Sci* (Lond). 2013 Feb;124(4):231–41.

20. Ochner CN, Barrios DM, Lee CD, Pi-Sunyer FX. Biological mechanisms that promote weight regain following weight loss in obese humans. *Physiol Behav.* 2013 Aug 15;120:106–13.

21. Wansink B, Shimizu M, Brumberg A. Association of nutrient-dense snack combinations with calories and vegetable intake. *Pediatrics.* 2013 Jan;131(1):22–29. doi: 10.1542/peds.2011–3895.

22. Rouhani MH, Kelishadi R, Hashemipour M, Esmaillzadeh A, Azadbakht L. Glycemic index, glycemic load and childhood obesity: a systematic review. *Adv Biomed Res.* 2014 Jan 24;3:47.

23. Ludwig DS. Dietary glycemic index and obesity. *J Nutr.* 2000 Feb;130(2S Suppl): 280S–283S. Review.

24. Ben-Gurion University of the Negev. Diet and Body Composition (CENTRAL). ClinicalTrials.gov. https://clinicaltrials.gov/ct2/show/NCT01530724. Updated September 29, 2015.

25. DeFronzo RA. The effect of insulin on renal sodium metabolism. A review with clinical implications. *Diabetologia.* 1981 Sep;21(3):165–71. Review.

Chapter 4

1. Fernando WM, Martins IJ, Goozee KG, Brennan CS, Jayasena V, Martins RN. The role of dietary coconut for the prevention and treatment of Alzheimer's disease: potential mechanisms of action. *Br J Nutr.* 2015 Jul 14;114(1):1–14.

2. Fallon S. Know your fats introduction. Weston A. Price Foundation. http://www.westonaprice.org/health-topics/know-your-fats-introduction/. February 24, 2009.

3. Wijga AH, Smit HA, Kerkhof M, et al; PIAMA. Association of consumption of products containing milk fat with reduced asthma risk in pre-school children: the PIAMA birth cohort study. *Thorax.* 2003 Jul;58(7):567–72.

4. Hämäläinen E, Adlercreutz H, Puska P, Pietinen P. Diet and serum sex hormones in healthy men. *J Steroid Biochem.* 1984 Jan;20(1):459–64.

5. Lawrence GD. Dietary fats and health: dietary recommendations in the context of scientific evidence. *Adv Nutr.* 2013 May 1;4(3):294–302.

6. Fallon S. Know your fats introduction. Weston A. Price Foundation. http://www.westonaprice.org/health-topics/know-your-fats-introduction/. February 24, 2009.

7. Fallon S. Know your fats introduction. Weston A. Price Foundation. http://www.westonaprice.org/health-topics/know-your-fats-introduction/. February 24, 2009.

8. European Food Information Council. Taking a closer look at saturated fat. http://www.eufic.org/article/en/diet-related-diseases/cardiovascular/artid/Saturated-fat-upclose/. March 2009.

9. Rioux V, Legrand P. Saturated fatty acids: simple molecular structures with complex cellular functions. *Curr Opin Clin Nutr Metab Care.* 2007;10:752–58.

10. Barnes DE, Yaffe K. The projected effect of risk factor reduction on Alzheimer's disease prevalence. *Lancet Neurol.* 2011 Sep;10(9):819–28.

11. Cordain L, Watkins BA, Florant GL, Kelher M, Rogers L, Li Y. Fatty acid analysis of wild ruminant tissues: evolutionary implications for reducing diet-related chronic disease. *Eur J Clin Nutr.* 2002 Mar;56(3):181–91. Review.

12. American Heart Association. Monounsaturated fats. http://www.heart.org/HEARTORG/GettingHealthy/NutritionCenter/HealthyEating/Monounsaturated-Fats_UCM_301460_Article.jsp. Updated August 5, 2014.

13. Body Ecology. The 6 benefits of monounsaturated fats (MUFAS). http://bodyecology.com/articles/6_benefits_monosaturated_fats.php#.VPdsfuGTvIU.

14. Fallon S, Enic MG. The great con-ola. Weston A. Price Foundation. http://www.westonaprice.org/health-topics/the-great-con-ola/. July 28, 2002.

15. Simopoulos AP. The importance of the ratio of omega-6/omega-3 essential fatty acids. *Biomed Pharmacother.* 2002;56(8):365–79.

16. Simopoulos AP. The importance of the ratio of omega-6/omega-3 essential fatty acids. *Biomed Pharmacother.* 2002;56(8):365–79.

17. Simopoulos AP. Evolutionary aspects of diet, the omega-6/omega-3 ratio and genetic variation: nutritional implications for chronic diseases. *Biomed Pharmacother.* 2006 Nov;60(9):502–7.

18. Good J. Smoke point of oils for healthy cooking. Baseline of Health Foundation. http://jonbarron.org/diet-and-nutrition/healthiest-cooking-oil-chart-smoke-points#.VPoxseGTvIU. April 17, 2012.

19. Ramsden CE, Ringel A, Feldstein AE, et al. Lowering dietary linoleic acid reduces bioactive oxidized linoleic acid metabolites in humans. *Prostaglandins Leukot Essent Fatty Acids.* 2012;87(4–5):135–41.

20. Ramsden CE, Hibbeln JR, Lands WE. Letter to the editor re: Linoleic acid and coronary heart disease, *Prostaglandins Leukot Essent Fatty Acids* (2008) by WS Harris. *Prostaglandins Leukot Essent Fatty Acids.* 2009 Jan;80(1):77; author reply, 77–78.

21. Leaf A. Dietary prevention of coronary heart disease: the Lyon Diet Heart Study. *Circulation.* 1999 Feb 16;99(6):733–35.

22. Stokel K. The beneficial omega-6 fatty acid. *Life Extension.* http://www.lef.org/magazine/2011/1/The-Beneficial-Omega-6-Fatty-Acid/Page-01. January 2011.

23. University of Maryland Medical System. Omega-3 fatty acids. http://umm.edu/health/medical/altmed/supplement/omega3-fatty-acids. Updated August 5, 2015.

24. Osher Y, Belmaker RH. Omega-3 fatty acids in depression: a review of three studies. *CNS Neurosci Ther.* 2009 Summer;15(2):128–33.

25. Jazayeri S, Tehrani-Doost M, Keshavarz SA, et al. Comparison of therapeutic effects of omega-3 fatty acid eicosapentaenoic acid and fluoxetine, separately and in combination, in major depressive disorder. *Aust N Z J Psychiatry.* 2008 Mar;42(3):192–98.

26. Kris-Etherton P, Eckel RH, Howard BV, St Jeor S, Bazzarre TL; Nutrition Committee Population Science Committee and Clinical Science Committee of the American Heart Association. AHA science advisory: Lyon Diet Heart Study. Benefits of a Mediterranean-style, National Cholesterol Education Program/American Heart Association Step I Dietary Pattern on Cardiovascular Disease. *Circulation.* 2001 Apr 3;103(13):1823–25.

27. Harvard School of Public Health. Shining the spotlight on trans fats. http://www.hsph.harvard.edu/nutritionsource/transfats/.

28. US Food and Drug Administration. Guidance for industry: trans fatty acids in nutritional labeling, nutrient content claims, health claims; small entity compliance guide. http://www.fda.gov/Food/GuidanceRegulation/GuidanceDocumentsRegulatoryInformation/LabelingNutrition/ucm053479.htm. August 2003. Updated May 29, 2015.

29. US Food and Drug Administration. FDA cuts trans fat in processed foods, http://www.fda.gov/ForConsumers/ConsumerUpdates/ucm372915.htm. Updated June 16, 2015.

30. US Food and Drug Administration. Trans fat at-a-glance. http://www.fda.gov/Food/IngredientsPackagingLabeling/LabelingNutrition/ucm079609.htm. Updated September 3, 2015.

31. US Food and Drug Administration. Trans fat at-a-glance. http://www.fda.gov/Food/IngredientsPackagingLabeling/LabelingNutrition/ucm079609.htm. Updated September 3, 2015.

32. Smith Y. Trans fat history. News Medical. http://www.news-medical.net/health/Trans-Fat-History.aspx. Updated June 14, 2015.

33. Harvard School of Public Health. Shining the spotlight on trans fats. http://www.hsph.harvard.edu/nutritionsource/transfats/.

34. Willett WC. Trans fatty acids and cardiovascular disease—epidemiological data. *Atheroscler Suppl.* 2006 May;7(2):5–8. Epub 2006 May 19. Review.

35. Wake Forest Baptist Medical Center. Trans fat leads to weight gain even on same total calories, animal study shows. http://www.wakehealth.edu/News-Releases/2006/Trans_Fat_Leads_To_Weight_Gain_Even_on_Same_Total_Calories,_Animal_Study_Shows.htm. 2006. Updated July 10, 2009.

36. Harvard School of Public Health. Shining the spotlight on trans fats. http://www.hsph.harvard.edu/nutritionsource/transfats/.

37. Slattery ML, Benson J, Ma KN, Schaffer D, Potter JD. Trans fatty acids and colon cancer. *Nutr Cancer.* 2001;39(2):170–75.

38. Walling E. A real killer: trans fat causes colon cancer. Natural News. http://www.naturalnews.com/025960_fat_trans_colon.html. March 30, 2009.

39. Chajes V, Thiébaut ACM, Rotival M, et al. Association between serum trans fatty acids and breast cancer. *Am J Epidemiol.* 2008;167(11):1312–20.

Chapter 5

1. Siri-Tarino PW, Chiu S, Bergeron N, Krauss RM. Saturated fats versus polyunsaturated fats versus carbohydrates for cardiovascular disease prevention and treatment. *Annu Rev Nutr.* 2015 Jul 17;35:517–43.

2. Estruch R, Ros E, Salas-Salvadó J, et al; PREDIMED Study Investigators. Primary prevention of cardiovascular disease with a Mediterranean diet. *N Engl J Med.* 2013 Apr 4;368(14):1279–90.

3. Ornish D. Does a Mediterranean diet really beat low-fat for heart health? Huffington Post. http://www.huffingtonpost.com/dr-dean-ornish/mediterraneandiet_b_2755940 .html. February 25, 2013. Updated April 27, 2013.

4. de Lorgeril M, Salen P, Martin JL, et al. Mediterranean diet, traditional risk factors, and the rate of cardiovascular complications after myocardial infarction: final report of the Lyon Diet Heart Study. *Circulation.* 1999;99:779–85.

5. Ball KP, Hanington E, McAllen PM, et al. Low-fat diet in myocardial infarction: a controlled trial. *Lancet.* 1965;2:501–4.

6. Howard BV, Van Horn L, Hsia J, et al. Low-fat dietary pattern and risk of cardiovascular disease: the Women's Health Initiative Randomized Controlled Dietary Modification Trial. *JAMA.* 2006;295:655–66.

7. Prentice RL, Caan B, Chlebowski RT, et al. Low-fat dietary pattern and risk of invasive breast cancer: the Women's Health Initiative Randomized Controlled Dietary Modification Trial. *JAMA.* 2006;295:629–42.

8. Beresford SA, Johnson KC, Ritenbaugh C, et al. Low-fat dietary pattern and risk of colorectal cancer: the Women's Health Initiative Randomized Controlled Dietary Modification Trial. *JAMA.* 2006;295:643–54.

9. Howard BV, Manson JE, Stefanick ML, et al. Low-fat dietary pattern and weight change over 7 years: the Women's Health Initiative Dietary Modification Trial. *JAMA.* 2006;295:39–49.

10. Multiple risk factor intervention trial. Risk factor changes and mortality results. Multiple Risk Factor Intervention Trial Research Group. *JAMA.* 1982;248: 1465–77.

11. Oh K, Hu FB, Manson JE, Stampfer MJ, Willett WC. Dietary fat intake and risk of coronary heart disease in women: 20 years of follow-up of the nurses' health study. *Am J Epidemiol.* 2005 Apr 1;161(7):672–79.

12. Hooper L, Summerbell CD, Thompson R, et al. Reduced or modified dietary fat for preventing cardiovascular disease. *Cochrane Database Syst Rev.* 2011 Jul 6;(7).

13. Ascherio A, Rimm EB, Giovannucci EL, Spiegelman D, Stampfer M, Willett WC. Dietary fat and risk of coronary heart disease in men: cohort follow up study in the United States. *BMJ.* 1996 Jul 13;313(7049):84–90.

14. Chowdhury R, Warnakula S, Kunutsor S, et al. Association of dietary, circulating, and supplement fatty acids with coronary risk: a systematic review and meta-analysis. *Ann Intern Med.* 2014 Mar 18;160(6):398–406.

15. Mozaffarian D, Micha R, Wallace S. Effects on coronary heart disease of increasing polyunsaturated fat in place of saturated fat: a systematic review and meta-analysis of randomized controlled trials. *PLoS Med.* 2010 Mar 23;7(3).

16. Siri-Tarino PW, Sun Q, Hu FB, Krauss RM. Meta-analysis of prospective cohort studies evaluating the association of saturated fat with cardiovascular disease. *Am J Clin Nutr.* 2010 Mar;91(3):535–46.

17. Hoenselaar R. Saturated fat and cardiovascular disease: the discrepancy between the scientific literature and dietary advice. *Nutrition.* 2012 Feb;28(2):118–23.

18. Harcombe Z, Baker JS, Cooper SM, et al. Evidence from randomised controlled trials did not support the introduction of dietary fat guidelines in 1977 and 1983: a systematic review and meta-analysis. *Open Heart.* 2015 Jan 29;2(1).

19. Dias CB, Garg R, Wood LG, Garg ML. Saturated fat consumption may not be the main cause of increased blood lipid levels. *Med Hypotheses.* 2014 Feb;82(2):187–95.

20. Dias CB, Phang M, Wood LG, Garg ML. Postprandial lipid responses do not differ following consumption of butter or vegetable oil when consumed with omega-3 polyunsaturated fatty acids. *Lipids.* 2015 Apr;50(4):339–47.

21. Forsythe CE, Phinney SD, Feinman RD, et al. Limited effect of dietary saturated fat on plasma saturated fat in the context of a low carbohydrate diet. *Lipids*. 2010 Oct;45(10):947–62.

22. Surette ME, Whelan J, Broughton KS, Kinsella JE. Evidence for mechanisms of the hypotriglyceridemic effect of n-3 polyunsaturated fatty acids. *Biochim Biophys Acta*. 1992 Jun 22;1126(2):199–205.

23. Fernandez ML, West KL. Mechanisms by which dietary fatty acids modulate plasma lipids. *J Nutr*. 2005 Sep;135(9):2075–78. Review.

24. Marina A, von Frankenberg AD, Suvag S, et al. Effects of dietary fat and saturated fat content on liver fat and markers of oxidative stress in overweight/obese men and women under weight-stable conditions. *Nutrients*. 2014 Oct 28;6(11):4678–90.

25. Koren MS, Purnell JQ, Breen PA, Matthys CC, Callahan HS, Weigle DS. Plasma C-reactive protein concentration is not affected by isocaloric dietary fat reduction. *Nutrition*. 2006 Apr;22(4):444–48.

26. Nanji AA, Jokelainen K, Tipoe GL, Rahemtulla A, Dannenberg AJ. Dietary saturated fatty acids reverse inflammatory and fibrotic changes in rat liver despite continued ethanol administration. *J Pharmacol Exp Ther*. 2001 Nov;299(2):638–44.

27. Yamagishi K, Iso H, Tsugane S. Saturated fat intake and cardiovascular disease in Japanese population. *J Atheroscler Thromb*. 2015 May 20;22(5):435–39.

28. Wang L, Folsom AR, Zheng ZJ, Pankow JS, Eckfeldt JH; ARIC Study Investigators. Plasma fatty acid composition and incidence of diabetes in middle-aged adults: the Atherosclerosis Risk in Communities (ARIC) Study. *Am J Clin Nutr*. 2003 Jul;78(1):91–98.

29. Wang L, Folsom AR, Eckfeldt JH. Plasma fatty acid composition and incidence of coronary heart disease in middle aged adults: the Atherosclerosis Risk in Communities (ARIC) Study. *Nutr Metab Cardiovasc Dis*. 2003 Oct;13(5):256–66.

30. Volk BM, Kunces LJ, Freidenreich DJ, et al. Effects of step-wise increases in dietary carbohydrate on circulating saturated fatty acids and palmitoleic acid in adults with metabolic syndrome. *PLoS One*. 2014;9(11).

31. Wood AC, Kabagambe EK, Borecki IB, Tiwari HK, Ordovas JM, Arnett DK. Dietary carbohydrate modifies the inverse association between saturated fat intake and cholesterol on very low-density lipoproteins. *Lipid Insights*. 2011;2011(4):7–15.

32. Siri-Tarino PW, Sun Q, Hu FB, Krauss RM. Saturated fat, carbohydrate, and cardiovascular disease. *Am J Clin Nutr*. 2010 Mar;91(3):502–9. doi: 10.3945/ajcn.2008.26285. Epub 2010 Jan 20. Review.

33. Parks EJ, Parks EJ. Changes in fat synthesis influenced by dietary macronutrient content. *Proc Nutr Soc*. 2002 May;61(2):281–86. Review.

34. Krauss RM. Atherogenic lipoprotein phenotype and diet-gene interactions. *J Nutr*. 2001 Feb;131(2):340S–43S. Review.

35. Hudgins LC, Hellerstein MK, Seidman CE, Neese RA, Tremaroli JD, Hirsch J. Relationship between carbohydrate-induced hypertriglyceridemia and fatty acid synthesis in lean and obese subjects. *J Lipid Res*. 2000 Apr;41(4):595–604.

36. Mensink RP, Zock PL, Kester AD, Katan MB. Effects of dietary fatty acids and carbohydrates on the ratio of serum total to HDL cholesterol and on serum lipids and apolipoproteins: a meta-analysis of 60 controlled trials. *Am J Clin Nutr*. 2003;77:1146–55.

37. Prado KB, Shugg S, Backstrand JR. Low-density lipoprotein particle number predicts coronary artery calcification in asymptomatic adults at intermediate risk of cardiovascular disease. *J Clin Lipidol*. 2011;5:408–13.

Notes **361**

38. Image adapted from Attia, P. The straight dope on cholesterol—part V. The Eating Academy blog. http://eatingacademy.com/nutrition/the-straight-dope-on-cholesterol-part-v. May 23, 2012.

39. Schwarz JM, Noworolski SM, Wen MJ, et al. Effect of a high-fructose weight-maintaining diet on lipogenesis and liver fat. *J Clin Endocrinol Metab.* 2015 Jun;100(6):2434–42.

40. Eckel RH, Jakicic JM, Ard JD, et al; American College of Cardiology/American Heart Association Task Force on Practice Guidelines. 2013 AHA/ACC guideline on lifestyle management to reduce cardiovascular risk: a report of the American College of Cardiology/American Heart Association Task Force on Practice Guidelines. *J Am Coll Cardiol.* 2014 Jul 1;63(25 Pt B):2960–84.

41. Fernandez ML. Rethinking dietary cholesterol. *Curr Opin Clin Nutr Metab Care.* 2012 Mar;15(2):117–21.

42. 2015 Dietary Guidelines Advisory Committee. Scientific report of the 2015 Dietary Guidelines Advisory Committee. Office of Disease Prevention and Health Promotion. http://www.health.gov/dietaryguidelines/2015-scientific-report/06-chapter-1/d1-2.asp#endnote-ref-35. February 2015.

43. Hansson GK. Inflammation, atherosclerosis, and coronary artery disease. *N Engl J Med.* 2005 Apr 21;352(16):1685–95. Review.

44. Barter P, Gotto AM, LaRosa JC, et al; Treating to New Targets Investigators. HDL cholesterol, very low levels of LDL cholesterol, and cardiovascular events. *N Engl J Med.* 2007 Sep 27;357(13):1301–10.

45. Ridker PM, Danielson E, Fonseca FA, et al; JUPITER Study Group. Rosuvastatin to prevent vascular events in men and women with elevated C-reactive protein. *N Engl J Med.* 2008 Nov 20;359(21):2195–207.

46. Abramson J, Wright JM. Are lipid-lowering guidelines evidence-based? *Lancet.* 2007 Jan 20;369(9557):168–69.

47. Abramson J, Wright JM. Are lipid-lowering guidelines evidence-based? *Lancet.* 2007 Jan 20;369(9557):168–69.

48. Brown BG, Taylor AJ. Does ENHANCE diminish confidence in lowering LDL or in ezetimibe? *N Engl J Med* 358:1504, April 3, 2008. Editorial.

49. Schatz IJ, Masaki K, Yano K, Chen R, Rodriguez BL, Curb JD. Cholesterol and all-cause mortality in elderly people from the Honolulu Heart Program: a cohort study. *Lancet.* 2001 Aug 4;358(9279):351–55.

50. Hansson GK. Inflammation, atherosclerosis, and coronary artery disease. *N Engl J Med.* 2005 Apr 21;352(16):1685–95. Review.

51. Ganga HV, Slim HB, Thompson PD. A systematic review of statin-induced muscle problems in clinical trials. *Am Heart J.* 2014 Jul;168(1):6–15.

52. Kelley BJ, Glasser S. Cognitive effects of statin medications. *CNS Drugs.* 2014 May;28(5):411–19. Review.

53. Davis R, Reveles KR, Ali SK, Mortensen EM, Frei CR, Mansi I. Statins and male sexual health: a retrospective cohort analysis. *J Sex Med.* 2015 Jan;12(1):158–67.

54. Ahmad Z. Statin intolerance. *Am J Cardiol.* 2014 May 15;113(10):1765–71.

55. Mansi I, Frei CR, Wang CP, Mortensen EM. Statins and new-onset diabetes mellitus and diabetic complications: a retrospective cohort study of US healthy adults. *J Gen Intern Med.* 2015 Apr 28.

56. Culver AL, Ockene IS, Balasubramanian R, et al. Statin use and risk of diabetes mellitus in postmenopausal women in the Women's Health Initiative. *Arch Intern Med.* 2012 Jan 23;172(2):144–52.

57. Sachdeva A, Cannon CP, Deedwania PC, et al. Lipid levels in patients hospitalized with coronary artery disease: an analysis of 136,905 hospitalizations in Get with the Guidelines. *Am Heart J.* 2009 Jan;157(1):111–17.

58. Jansen H, Samani NJ, Schunkert H. Mendelian randomization studies in coronary artery disease. *Eur Heart J.* 2014 Aug 1;35(29):1917–24.

59. Abramson JD, Rosenberg HG, Jewell N, Wright JM. Should people at low risk of cardiovascular disease take a statin? *BMJ.* 2013 Oct 22;347:f6123.

60. Pencina MJ, Navar-Boggan AM, D'Agostino RB Sr, et al. Application of new cholesterol guidelines to a population-based sample. *N Engl J Med.* 2014 Apr 10;370(15):1422–31.

61. D'Agostino RB Sr, Ansell BJ, Mora S, Krumholz HM. Clinical decisions. The guidelines battle on starting statins. *N Engl J Med.* 2014 Apr 24;370(17):1652–58.

62. Taylor F, Ward K, Moore TH, et al. Statins for the primary prevention of cardiovascular disease. *Cochrane Database Syst Rev.* 2011 Jan 19;(1).

63. Newman D. Statin drugs given for 5 years for heart disease prevention (without known heart disease). NNT. http://www.thennt.com/nnt/statins-for-heart-disease-prevention-without-prior-heart-disease/. Updated July 17, 2015.

64. Newman D. Statin drugs given for 5 years for heart disease prevention (without known heart disease). NNT. http://www.thennt.com/nnt/statins-for-heart-disease-prevention-with-known-heart-disease/. Updated July 17, 2015.

65. Mozaffarian D, Wilson PW, Kannel WB. Beyond established and novel risk factors: lifestyle risk factors for cardiovascular disease. *Circulation.* 2008;117(23):3031–38.

66. Menke A, Muntner P, Batuman V, Silbergeld EK, Guallar E. Blood lead below 0.48 micromol/L (10 microg/dL) and mortality among US adults. *Circulation.* 2006 Sep 26;114(13):1388–94.

67. Ford ES, Bergmann MM, Kröger J, Schienkiewitz A, Weikert C, Boeing H. Healthy living is the best revenge: findings from the European Prospective Investigation into Cancer and Nutrition-Potsdam study. *Arch Intern Med.* 2009 Aug 10;169(15):1355–62.

68. Yusuf S, Hawken S, Ounpuu S, et al; INTERHEART Study Investigators. Effect of potentially modifiable risk factors associated with myocardial infarction in 52 countries (the INTERHEART study): case-control study. *Lancet.* 2004;364 (9438):937–52.

69. American College of Preventive Medicine. *Lifestyle Medicine—Evidence Review.* http://www.acpm.org/?page=LifestyleMedicine. June 30, 2009. Accessed September 18, 2009.

70. Ludvigsson JF, Montgomery SM, Ekbom A, Brandt L, Granath F. Small-intestinal histopathology and mortality risk in celiac disease. *JAMA.* 2009 Sep 16;302(11): 1171–8. Ganguly P, Alam SF. Role of homocysteine in the development of cardiovascular disease. *Nutr J.* 2015 Jan 10;14:6.

Chapter 6

1. 2015 Dietary Guidelines Advisory Committee. Scientific report of the 2015 Dietary Guidelines Advisory Committee. Office of Disease Prevention and Health Promotion. http://www.health.gov/dietaryguidelines/2015-scientific-report/. February 2015.

2. Gerrior S, Bente L. *Nutrient Content of the U.S. Food Supply, 1909–1999: A Summary Report.* Washington, DC: US Department of Agriculture, Center for Nutrition Policy and Promotion, 2002.

3. Ramsden CE, Hibbeln JR, Majchrzak-Hong SF. All PUFAs are not created equal: absence of CHD benefit specific to linoleic acid in randomized controlled trials and prospective observational cohorts. *World Rev Nutr Diet.* 2011;102:30–43.

4. Ramsden CE, Hibbeln JR, Majchrzak SF, Davis JM. N-6 fatty acid-specific and mixed polyunsaturated dietary interventions have different effects on CHD risk: a meta-analysis of randomized controlled trials. *Br J Nutr.* 2010 Dec;104(11):1586–1600.

5. Dietary supplementation with n-3 polyunsaturated fatty acids and vitamin E after myocardial infarction: results of the GISSI-Prevenzione trial. Gruppo Italiano per lo Studio della Sopravvivenza nell'Infarto miocardico. *Lancet.* 1999 Aug 7;354 (9177):447–55.

6. Ramsden CE, Zamora D, Leelarthaepin B, et al. Use of dietary linoleic acid for secondary prevention of coronary heart disease and death: evaluation of recovered data from the Sydney Diet Heart Study and updated meta-analysis. *BMJ.* 2013 Feb 4;346.

7. Ravnskov U, DiNicolantonio JJ, Harcombe Z, Kummerow FA, Okuyama H, Worm N. The questionable benefits of exchanging saturated fat with polyunsaturated fat. *Mayo Clin Proc.* 2014 Apr;89(4):451–53.

8. Calder PC. The American Heart Association advisory on n-6 fatty acids: evidence based or biased evidence? *Br J Nutr.* 2010 Dec;104(11):1575–76.

9. Hibbeln JR, Nieminen LR, Blasbalg TL, Riggs JA, Lands WE. Healthy intakes of n-3 and n-6 fatty acids: estimations considering worldwide diversity. *Am J Clin Nutr.* 2006 Jun;83(6 Suppl):1483S–93S.

10. Patterson E, Wall R, Fitzgerald GF, Ross RP, Stanton C. Health implications of high dietary omega-6 polyunsaturated fatty acids. *J Nutr Metab.* 2012;2012:539426.

11. Maingrette F, Renier G. Linoleic acid increases lectin-like oxidized LDL receptor-1 (LOX-1) expression in human aortic endothelial cells. *Diabetes.* 2005 May;54(5): 1506–13.

12. Hibbeln JR, Nieminen LR, Lands WE. Increasing homicide rates and linoleic acid consumption among five Western countries, 1961–2000. *Lipids.* 2004;39:1207–13.

13. IBD in EPIC Study Investigators, Tjonneland A, Overvad K, et al. Linoleic acid, a dietary n-6 polyunsaturated fatty acid, and the aetiology of ulcerative colitis: a nested case-control study within a European prospective cohort study. *Gut.* 2009 Dec;58(12):1606–11.

14. Adoption of genetically engineered crops in the U.S. USDA Economic Research Service. http://www.ers.usda.gov/data-products/adoption-of-genetically-engineered-crops-in-the-us/recent-trends-in-ge-adoption.aspx. July 14, 2014. Updated July 9, 2015.

15. GMO Health Risks. Institute for Responsible Technology. http://responsibletech nology.org/gmo-education/health-risks/. December 20, 2013.

16. GMO Health Risks. Institute for Responsible Technology. http://responsibletech nology.org/gmo-education/health-risks/. December 20, 2013.

17. Ayyadurai VAS, Deonikar P. Do GMOs accumulate formaldehyde and disrupt molecular systems equilibria? Systems biology may provide answers. *Agricultural Sciences.* 2015;6:630–62.

18. Velimirov A, Binter C, Zentek J. Biological effects of transgenic maize fed in long term reproduction studies in mice. *Biosicherheit.de.* http://www.biosicherheit.de/ pdf/aktuell/zentek_studie_2008.pdf. November 11, 2008.

19. Markaverich B, Mani S, Alejandro MA, et al. A novel endocrine-disrupting agent in corn with mitogenic activity in human breast and prostatic cancer cells. *Environ Health Perspect.* 2002;110(2):169–77.

20. Guyton KZ, Loomis D, Grosse Y, et al; International Agency for Research on Cancer Monograph Working Group, IARC, Lyon, France. Carcinogenicity of tetrachlorvinphos, parathion, malathion, diazinon, and glyphosate. *Lancet Oncol.* 2015 May;16(5):490–91.

21. Pollack A. Weed killer, long cleared, is doubted. *New York Times.* http://www.nytimes.com/2015/03/28/business/energy-environment/decades-after-monsantos-roundup-gets-an-all-clear-a-cancer-agency-raises-concerns.html?_r=1. March 27, 2015.

22. Labeling around the world. Just Label It. http://www.justlabelit.org/right-to-know-center/labeling-around-the-world/.

23. Argentina: 30,000 doctors and health professionals demand ban on glyphosate. Sustainable Pulse. http://sustainablepulse.com/2015/04/19/argentina-30000-doctors-and-health-professionals-demand-ban-on-glyphosate/#.VTQd263BzGd. April 19, 2015.

24. Broze D. World Health Organization won't back down from study linking Monsanto to cancer. Global Research. http://www.globalresearch.ca/world-health-organization-wont-back-down-from-study-linking-monsanto-to-cancer/5439840. March 31, 2015.

Chapter 7

1. Shrank WH, Patrick AR, Brookhart MA. Healthy user and related biases in observational studies of preventive interventions: a primer for physicians. *J Gen Intern Med.* 2011 May;26(5):546–50.

2. Key TJ, Thorogood M, Appleby PN, Burr ML. Dietary habits and mortality in 11,000 vegetarians and health conscious people: results of a 17 year follow up. *BMJ.* 1996 Sep 28;313(7060):775–79.

3. Rohrmann S, et al. Meat consumption and mortality—results from the European Prospective Investigation into Cancer and Nutrition. *BMC Med.* 2013 Mar 7; 11:63.

4. Guyenet S. Does dietary saturated fat increase blood cholesterol? An informal review of observational studies. Whole Health Source. http://wholehealthsource.blogspot.com/2011/01/does-dietary-saturated-fat-increase.html. January 13, 2011.

5. Cordain L, Eaton SB, Sebastian A, et al. Origins and evolution of the Western diet: health implications for the 21st century. *Am J Clin Nutr.* 2005 Feb;81(2):341–54. Review.

6. O'Dea K. Marked improvement in carbohydrate and lipid metabolism in diabetic Australian aborigines after temporary reversion to traditional lifestyle. *Diabetes.* 1984 Jun;33(6):596–603.

7. Binnie MA, Barlow K, Johnson V, Harrison C. Red meats: time for a paradigm shift in dietary advice. *Meat Sci.* 2014 Nov;98(3):445–51.

8. Jönsson T, Granfeldt Y, Erlanson-Albertsson C, Ahrén B, Lindeberg S. A paleolithic diet is more satiating per calorie than a Mediterranean-like diet in individuals with ischemic heart disease. *Nutr Metab* (Lond). 2010 Nov 30;7:85.

9. Koeth RA, Wang Z, Levison BS, et al. Intestinal microbiota metabolism of L-carnitine, a nutrient in red meat, promotes atherosclerosis. *Nat Med.* 2013 May;19(5): 576–85.

10. Gregory JC, Buffa JA, Org E, et al. Transmission of atherosclerosis susceptibility with gut microbial transplant. *J Biol Chem.* 2015 Feb 27;290(9):5647–60.

11. Siri-Tarino PW, Sun Q, Hu FB, Krauss RM. Saturated fat, carbohydrate, and cardiovascular disease. *Am J Clin Nutr.* 2010;91(3):502–509.

12. Micha R, Wallace SK, Mozaffarian D. Red and processed meat consumption and risk of incident coronary heart disease, stroke, and diabetes: A systematic review and meta-analysis. *Circulation.* 2010;121(21):2271–2283.

13. Pan A, Sun Q, Bernstein AM, et al. Red meat consumption and mortality: results from two prospective cohort studies. *Arch Intern Med.* 2012;172(7):555–563.

14. Key TJ, Appleby PN, Davey GK, Allen NE, Spencer EA, Travis RC. Mortality in British vegetarians: review and preliminary results from EPIC-Oxford. *Am J Clin Nutr.* 2003 Sep;78(3 Suppl):533S–538S. Review.

15. Lee JE, McLerran DF, Rolland B, et al. Meat intake and cause-specific mortality: a pooled analysis of Asian prospective cohort studies. *Am J Clin Nutr.* 2013 Oct;98(4):1032–41.

16. Turnbaugh PJ, Ridaura VK, Faith JJ, Rey FE, Knight R, Gordon JI. The effect of diet on the human gut microbiome: A metagenomic analysis in humanized gnotobiotic mice. *Sci Trans Med.* 2009;1(6):6ra14.

17. Zhang AQ, Mitchell SC, Smith RL. Dietary precursors of trimethylamine in man: a pilot study. *Food Chem Toxicol.* 1999 May;37(5):515–20.

18. He K, Song Y, Daviglus ML, et al. Accumulated evidence on fish consumption and coronary heart disease mortality: a meta-analysis of cohort studies. *Circulation.* 2004 Jun 8;109(22):2705–11.

19. Pan A, Sun Q, Bernstein AM, et al. Red meat consumption and risk of type 2 diabetes: 3 cohorts of US adults and an updated meta-analysis. *Am J Clin Nutr.* 2011 Oct;94(4):1088–96.

20. Lindeberg S, Jonsson T, Granfeldt Y, et al. A Paleolithic diet improves glucose tolerance more than a Mediterranean-like diet in individuals with ischaemic heart disease. *Diabetologia.* 2007 Sep;50(9):1795–807.

21. Jonsson T, Granfeldt Y, Ahren B, et al. Beneficial effects of a Paleolithic diet on cardiovascular risk factors in type 2 diabetes: a randomized cross-over pilot study. *Cardiovasc Diabetol.* 2009 Jul 16;8:35.

22. Mellbergy C, Sandberg S, Ryberg M, et al. Long-term effects of a Paleolithic-type diet in obese postmenopausal women: a 2-year randomized trial. *Eur J Clin Nutr.* 2014 Mar;68(3):350–57.

23. Alexander DD, Cushing CA. Red meat and colorectal cancer: a critical summary of prospective epidemiologic studies. *Obes Rev.* 2011 May;12(5):e472–93.

24. Bellavia A, Larsson SC, Bottai M, Wolk A, Orsini N. Differences in survival associated with processed and with nonprocessed red meat consumption. *Am J Clin Nutr.* 2014 Sep;100(3):924–29.

25. Kim E, Coelho D, Blachier F. Review of the association between meat consumption and risk of colorectal cancer. *Nutr Res.* 2013 Dec;33(12):983–94.

26. Skog KI, Johansson MA, Jägerstad MI. Carcinogenic heterocyclic amines in model systems and cooked foods: a review on formation, occurrence and intake. *Food Chem Toxicol.* 1998 Sep–Oct;36(9–10):879–96. Review.

27. Sugimura T, Wakabayashi K, Nakagama H, Nagao M. Heterocyclic amines: mutagens/carcinogens produced during cooking of meat and fish. *Cancer Sci.* 2004;95:290–99.

28. Phillips DH. Polycyclic aromatic hydrocarbons in the diet. *Mutat Res.* 1999 Jul 15;443(1–2).

29. Uribarri J, Woodruff S, Goodman S, et al. Advanced glycation end products in foods and a practical guide to their reduction in the diet. *J Am Diet Assoc.* 2010 Jun;110(6):911–16.

30. Hodgson JM, Ward NC, Burke V, Beilin LJ, Puddey IB. Increased lean red meat intake does not elevate markers of oxidative stress and inflammation in humans. *J Nutr.* 2007 Feb;137(2):363–67.

31. Pischon T, Hankinson SE, Hotamisligil GS, Rifai N, Willett WC, Rimm EB. Habitual dietary intake of n-3 and n-6 fatty acids in relation to inflammatory markers among US men and women. *Circulation.* 2003 Jul 15;108(2):155–60.

32. Baines S, Powers J, Brown WJ. How does the health and well-being of young Australian vegetarian and semi-vegetarian women compare with non-vegetarians? *Public Health Nutr.* 2007 May;10(5):436–42.
33. Craig WJ. Nutrition concerns and health effects of vegetarian diets. *Nutr Clin Pract.* 2010 Dec;25(6):613–20.
34. Daley CA, Abbott A, Doyle PS, Nader GA, Larson S. A review of fatty acid profiles and antioxidant content in grass-fed and grain-fed beef. *Nutr J.* 2010 Mar 10;9:10.
35. Nakamura YK, Flintoff-Dye N, Omaye ST. Conjugated linoleic acid modulation of risk factors associated with atherosclerosis. *Nutr Metab.* 2008;5:22.
36. Castro-Webb N, Ruiz-Narváez EA, Campos H. Cross-sectional study of conjugated linoleic acid in adipose tissue and risk of diabetes. *Am J Clin Nutr.* 2012 Jul;96(1):175–81.
37. Ochoa JJ, Farquharson AJ, Grant I, Moffat LE, Heys SD, Wahle KW. Conjugated linoleic acids (CLAs) decrease prostate cancer cell proliferation: different molecular mechanisms for cis-9, trans-11 and trans-10, cis-12 isomers. *Carcinogenesis.* 2004 Jul;25(7):1185–91.
38. Leheska JM, Thompson LD, Howe JC, et al. Effects of conventional and grass-feeding systems on the nutrient composition of beef. *J Anim Sci.* 2008 Dec; 86(12):3575–85.
39. Daley CA, Abbott A, Doyle PS, Nader GA, Larson S. A review of fatty acid profiles and antioxidant content in grass-fed and grain-fed beef. *Nutr J.* 2010 Mar 10;9:10.

Chapter 8

1. Shin JY, Xun P, Nakamura Y, He K. Egg consumption in relation to risk of cardiovascular disease and diabetes: a systematic review and meta-analysis. *Am J Clin Nutr.* 2013;98(1):146–59.
2. Kern F Jr. Normal plasma cholesterol in an 88-year-old man who eats 25 eggs a day. Mechanisms of adaptation. *N Engl J Med.* 1991 Mar 28;324(13):896–99.
3. Djoussé L, Gaziano JM. Egg consumption in relation to cardiovascular disease and mortality: the Physicians' Health Study. *Am J Clin Nutr.* 2008 Apr;87(4):964–69.
4. Ratliff J, Leite JO, de Ogburn R, Puglisi MJ, VanHeest J, Fernandez ML. Consuming eggs for breakfast influences plasma glucose and ghrelin, while reducing energy intake during the next 24 hours in adult men. *Nutr Res.* 2010 Feb;30(2):96–103.
5. Mutungi G, Waters D, Ratliff J, et al. Eggs distinctly modulate plasma carotenoid and lipoprotein subclasses in adult men following a carbohydrate-restricted diet. *J Nutr Biochem.* 2010 Apr;21(4):261–67.
6. Bier DM. Saturated fats and cardiovascular disease: interpretations not as simple as they once were. *Crit Rev Food Sci Nutr.* 2015 Mar 16:0. Lawrence GD. Dietary fats and health: dietary recommendations in the context of scientific evidence. *Adv Nutr.* 2013 May 1;4(3):294–302.
7. Givens DI. Milk in the diet: good or bad for vascular disease? *Proc Nutr Soc.* 2012 Feb;71(1):98–104.
8. Wennberg M, Vessby B, Johansson I. Evaluation of relative intake of fatty acids according to the Northern Sweden FFQ with fatty acid levels in erythrocyte membranes as biomarkers. *Public Health Nutr.* 2009 Sep;12(9):1477–84. Wolk A, Vessby B, Ljung H, Barrefors P. Evaluation of a biological marker of dairy fat intake. *Am J Clin Nutr.* 1998;68:291–95. Khaw KT, Friesen MD, Riboli E, Luben R, Wareham N. Plasma phospholipid fatty acid concentration and incident coronary heart disease in men and women: the EPIC-Norfolk prospective study. *PLoS Med.* 2012;9:e1001255.

9. German JB, Dillard CJ. Saturated fats: a perspective from lactation and milk composition. *Lipids.* 2010 Oct;45(10):915–23.

10. Gertosio C, Meazza C, Pagani S, Bozzola M. Breast feeding: gamut of benefits. *Minerva Pediatr.* 2015 May 29.

11. Owen CG, Whincup PH, Cook DG. Breast-feeding and cardiovascular risk factors and outcomes in later life: evidence from epidemiological studies. *Proc Nutr Soc.* 2011 Nov;70(4):478–84.

12. Robinson J. Super natural milk. EatWild.com. http://www.eatwild.com/articles/superhealthy.html.

13. Pasture butter. OrganicValley.com. http://www.organicvalley.coop/products/butter/pasture/.

14. Watson SJ, Bishop G, Drummond JC, Gillam AE, Heilbron IM. The relation of the colour and vitamin A content of butter to the nature of the ration fed: the influence of the ration on the yellow colour of the butter. II. The carotenoid and vitamin A contents of the butter. *Biochem J.* 1934;28(3):1076–85.

15. Sisson M. Is all butter created equal? MarksDailyApple.com. http://www.marksdailyapple.com/grass-fed-butter/#axzz3WCaqOwnK. August 3, 2010.

16. Gunnars K. Why grass-fed butter is good for you. AuthorityNutrition.com. http://authoritynutrition.com/grass-fed-butter-superfood-for-the-heart/. November 2013.

17. Kaunitz H, Dayrit CS. Coconut oil consumption and coronary heart disease. *Philippine J Coconut Studies.* 1992;17:18–20. Prior IA, Stanhope JM, Evans JG, Salmond CE. The Tokelau Island migrant study. *Int J Epidemiol.* 1974 Sep;3(3):225–32.

18. Lipoeto NI, Agus Z, Oenzil F, Wahlqvist M, Wattanapenpaiboon N. Dietary intake and the risk of coronary heart disease among the coconut-consuming Minangkabau in West Sumatra, Indonesia. *Asia Pac J Clin Nutr.* 2004;13(4):377–84.

19. Lindeberg S, Nilsson-Ehle P, Terént A, Vessby B, Scherstén B. Cardiovascular risk factors in a Melanesian population apparently free from stroke and ischaemic heart disease: the Kitava study. *J Intern Med.* 1994 Sep;236(3):331–40.

20. Prior IA, Davidson F, Salmond CE, Czochanska Z. Cholesterol, coconuts, and diet on Polynesian atolls: a natural experiment: the Pukapuka and Tokelau island studies. *Am J Clin Nutr.* 1981 Aug;34(8):1552–61.

21. Müller H, Lindman AS, Brantsaeter AL, Pedersen JI. The serum LDL/HDL cholesterol ratio is influenced more favorably by exchanging saturated with unsaturated fat than by reducing saturated fat in the diet of women. *J Nutr.* 2003 Jan;133(1):78–83. Feranil AB, Duazo PL, Kuzawa CW, Adair LS. Coconut oil is associated with a beneficial lipid profile in pre-menopausal women in the Philippines. *Asia Pac J Clin Nutr.* 2011;20(2):190–95.

22. Lindeberg S, Eliasson M, Lindahl B, Ahrén B. Low serum insulin in traditional Pacific Islanders—the Kitava Study. *Metabolism.* 1999 Oct;48(10):1216–19.

23. St-Onge MP, Ross R, Parson WD, Jones PJ. Medium-chain triglycerides increase energy expenditure and decrease adiposity in overweight men. *Obes Res.* 2003 Mar;11(3):395–402.

24. Seaton TB, Welle SL, Warenko MK, Campbell RG. Thermic effect of medium-chain and long-chain triglycerides in man. *Am J Clin Nutr.* 1986 Nov;44(5):630–34.

25. Assunção ML, Ferreira HS, dos Santos AF, Cabral CR Jr, Florêncio TM. Effects of dietary coconut oil on the biochemical and anthropometric profiles of women presenting abdominal obesity. *Lipids.* 2009 Jul 44(7):593–601.

26. Ogbolu DO, Oni AA, Daini OA, Oloko AP. In vitro antimicrobial properties of coconut oil on Candida species in Ibadan, Nigeria. *J Med Food.* 2007 Jun 10(2):384–87.

27. Verall-Rowell VM, Dillague KM, Syah-Tjundawan BS. Novel antibacterial and emollient effects of coconut and virgin olive oils in adult atopic dermatitis. *Dermatitis.* 2008 Nov–Dec 19(6):308–15.

28. Prior IA, Davidson F, Salmond CE, Czochanska Z. Cholesterol, coconuts and diet in Polynesian atolls—a natural experiment; the Pukapuka and Toklau island studies. *Am J Clin Nutr.* 1981;34:1552–61.

29. Boon CM, Ng MH, Choo YM, Mok SL. Super, red palm and palm oleins improve the blood pressure, heart size, aortic media thickness and lipid profile in spontaneously hypertensive rats. *PLoS One.* 2013;8(2):e55908.

30. Odia OJ, Ofori S, Maduka O. Palm oil and the heart: a review. *World J Cardiol.* 2015 Mar 26;7(3):144–49.

31. Fattore E, Bosetti C, Brighenti F, Agostoni C, Fattore G. Palm oil and blood lipid-related markers of cardiovascular disease: a systematic review and meta-analysis of dietary intervention trials. *Am J Clin Nutr.* 2014 Jun;99(6):1331–50.

32. Covas MI, Nyyssonen K, Poulsen HE, et al. EUROLIVE Study Group. The effect of polyphenols in olive oil on heart disease risk factors: a randomized trial. *Ann Intern Med.* 2006 Sep 5;145(5):333–41.

33. Castaner O, Fito M, Lopez-Sabater MC, et al. The effect of olive oil polyphenols on antibodies against oxidized LDL. A randomized clinical trial. *Clin Nutr.* 2011 Mar 2.

34. de Roos B, Zhang X, Rodriguez Gutierrez G, et al. Anti-platelet effects of olive oil extract: in vitro functional and proteomic studies. *Eur J Nutr.* 2011 Jan 1.

35. Torres N, Guevara-Cruz M, Velázquez-Villegas LA, Tovar AR. Nutrition and atherosclerosis. *Arch Med Res.* 2015 Jul;46(5):408–26.

36. Terés S, Barcelo-Coblijn G, Benet M, et al. Oleic acid content is responsible for the reduction in blood pressure induced by olive oil. *Proc Natl Acad Sci USA.* 2008 Sep 16;105(37):13811–16.

37. Moreno-Luna R, Muñoz-Hernandez R, Miranda ML, et al. Olive oil polyphenols decrease blood pressure and improve endothelial function in young women with mild hypertension. *Am J Hypertens.* 2012 Dec;25(12):1299–304.

38. Hashim YZ, Eng M, Gill C, et al. Components of olive oil and chemoprevention of colorectal cancer. *Nutr Rev.* 2005 Nov;63(11):374–86.

39. Romero C, Medina E, Vargas J, Brenes M, Castro AD. In vitro activity of olive oil polyphenols against Helicobacter pylori. *J Agr Food Chem.* 2007 Feb 7;55(3):680–86.

40. Berr C, Portet F, Carriere I, et al. Olive oil and cognition: results from the three-city study. *Dement Geriatr Cogn.* 2009 Oct;28(4):357–64. Published online 2009 October 30. doi: 10.1159/000253483.

41. Elnagar AY, Sylvester PW, El Sayed KA. (-)-Oleocanthal as a c-Met inhibitor for the control of metastatic breast and prostate cancers. *Planta Med.* 2011 Feb 15. [Epub ahead of print]. Escrich E, Solanas M, Moral R, et al. Modulatory effects and molecular mechanisms of olive oil and other dietary lipids in breast cancer. *Curr Pharm Design.* 2011;17(8):813–30.

42. Machowetz A, Poulsen HE, Gruendel S, et al. Effect of olive oils on biomarkers of oxidative DNA stress in Northern and Southern Europeans. *FASEB J.* 2007 Jan;21(1):45–52. Epub 2006 Nov 16. PMID:17110467.

43. D'Imperio M, Gobbino M, Picanza A, et al. Influence of harvest method and period on olive oil composition: an NMR and statistical study. *J Agr Food Chem.* 2010 Oct 5. [Epub ahead of print].

44. Blechman N. Extra virgin suicide: the adulteration of Italian olive oil. *New York Times*, Opinion, Food Chains. January 24, 2014. http://www.nytimes.com/interactive/2014/01/24/opinion/food-chains-extra virgin-suicide.html.

45. Grosso G, Yang J, Marventano S, Micek A, Galvano F, Kales SN. Nut consumption on all-cause, cardiovascular, and cancer mortality risk: a systematic review and meta-analysis of epidemiologic studies. *Am J Clin Nutr.* 2015 Apr;101(4):783–93.

46. Hshieh TT, Petrone AB, Gaziano JM, Djoussé L. Nut consumption and risk of mortality in the Physicians' Health Study. *Am J Clin Nutr.* 2015 Feb;101(2):407–12.

47. Jiang R, Manson JE, Stampfer MJ, Liu S, Willett WC, Hu FB. Nut and peanut butter consumption and risk of type 2 diabetes in women. *JAMA.* 2002 Nov 27;288(20):2554–60.

48. Guasch-Ferré M et al; PREDIMED study group. Frequency of nut consumption and mortality risk in the PREDIMED nutrition intervention trial. *BMC Med.* 2013 Jul 16;11:164.

49. Jenkins DJ, Wong JM, Kendall CW, et al. Effect of a 6-month vegan low-carbohydrate ("Eco-Atkins") diet on cardiovascular risk factors and body weight in hyperlipidaemic adults: a randomised controlled trial. *BMJ Open.* 2014 Feb 5;4(2):e003505.

50. Kelly JH Jr, Sabaté J. Nuts and coronary heart disease: an epidemiological perspective. *Br J Nutr.* 2006 Nov;96 Suppl 2:S61–67. Review.

51. Kelly JH Jr, Sabate J. Nuts and coronary heart disease: an epidemiological perspective. *Br J Nutr.* 2006 Nov;96 Suppl 2:S61–67.

52. Bes-Rastrollo M, Sabate J, Gomez-Gracia E, Alonso A, Martinez JA, Martinez Gonzalez MA. Nut consumption and weight gain in a Mediterranean cohort: the SUN study. *Obesity.* 2007 Jan;15(1):107–16. PMID:17228038.

53. Howell E MD. *Food Enzymes for Health & Longevity.* Twin Lakes, WI: Lotus Press; 1994.

Chapter 9

1. Accurso A, Bernstein RK, Dahlqvist A, et al. Dietary carbohydrate restriction in type 2 diabetes mellitus and metabolic syndrome: time for a critical appraisal. *Nutr Metab* (Lond). 2008 Apr 8;5;9.

2. Feinman RD, Pogozelski WK, Astrup A, et al. Dietary carbohydrate restriction as the first approach in diabetes management: critical review and evidence base. *Nutrition.* 2015 Jan;31(1):1–13.

3. Action to Control Cardiovascular Risk in Diabetes Study Group, Gerstein HC, Miller ME, Byington RP, et al. Effects of intensive glucose lowering in type 2 diabetes. *N Engl J Med.* 2008 Jun 12;358(24):2545–59.

4. Bredesen DE. Reversal of cognitive decline: a novel therapeutic program. *Aging* (Albany NY). 2014 Sep;6(9):707–17.

5. Roberts RO, Roberts LA, Geda YE, et al. Relative intake of macronutrients impacts risk of mild cognitive impairment or dementia. *J Alzheimers Dis.* 2012;32(2):329–39.

6. Barberger-Gateau P, Raffaitin C, Letenneur L, et al. Dietary patterns and risk of dementia: the three-city cohort study. *Neurology.* 2007 Nov 13;69(20):1921–30.

7. Su KP, Wang SM, Pae CU. Omega-3 polyunsaturated fatty acids for major depressive disorder. *Expert Opin Investig Drugs.* 2013 Dec;22(12):1519–34.

8. Hibbeln JR, Gow RV. The potential for military diets to reduce depression, suicide, and impulsive aggression: a review of current evidence for omega-3 and omega-6 fatty acids. *Mil Med.* 2014 Nov;179(11 Suppl):117–28.

9. Bos DJ, Oranje B, Veerhoek ES, et al. Reduced symptoms of inattention after dietary omega-3 fatty acid supplementation in boys with and without attention deficit/hyperactivity disorder. *Neuropsychopharmacology.* 2015 Mar 19.

10. van Elst K, Bruining H, Birtoli B, Terreaux C, Buitelaar JK, Kas MJ. Food for thought: dietary changes in essential fatty acid ratios and the increase in autism spectrum disorders. *Neurosci Biobehav Rev.* 2014 Sep;45:369–78.

11. Michael-Titus AT, Priestley JV. Omega-3 fatty acids and traumatic neurological injury: from neuroprotection to neuroplasticity? *Trends Neurosci.* 2014 Jan;37(1):30–38.

12. Hussain G, Schmitt F, Loeffler JP, Gonzalez de Aguilar JL. Fatting the brain: a brief of recent research. *Front Cell Neurosci.* 2013 Sep 9;7:144.

13. Lima PA, Sampaio LP, Damasceno NR. Neurobiochemical mechanisms of a ketogenic diet in refractory epilepsy. *Clinics* (Sao Paulo). 2014 Dec;69(10):699–705.

14. Paganoni S, Wills AM. High-fat and ketogenic diets in amyotrophic lateral sclerosis. *J Child Neurol.* 2013 Aug;28(8):989–92.

15. Schwartz K, Chang HT, Nikolai M, et al. Treatment of glioma patients with ketogenic diets: report of two cases treated with an IRB-approved energy-restricted ketogenic diet protocol and review of the literature. *Cancer Metab.* 2015 Mar 25;3:3.

16. Simopoulos AP. Omega-3 fatty acids in inflammation and autoimmune diseases. *J Am Coll Nutr.* 2002 Dec;21(6):495–505. Review.

17. Belch JJ, Hill A. Evening primrose oil and borage oil in rheumatologic conditions. *Am J Clin Nutr.* 2000 Jan;71(1 Suppl):352S–356S. Review.

18. Nosaka N, Suzuki Y, Nagatoishi A, Kasai M, Wu J, Taguchi M. Effect of ingestion of medium-chain triacylglycerols on moderate- and high-intensity exercise in recreational athletes. *J Nutr Sci Vitaminol* (Tokyo). 2009 Apr;55(2):120–25.

19. Brennan SF, Woodside JV, Lunny PM, Cardwell CR, Cantwell MM. Dietary fat and breast cancer mortality: a systematic review and meta-analysis. *Crit Rev Food Sci Nutr.* 2015 Feb 18.

20. Schwab U, Lauritzen L, Tholstrup T, et al. Effect of the amount and type of dietary fat on cardiometabolic risk factors and risk of developing type 2 diabetes, cardiovascular diseases, and cancer: a systematic review. *Food Nutr Res.* 2014 Jul 10;58.

21. Moyad MA. Dietary fat reduction to reduce prostate cancer risk: controlled enthusiasm, learning a lesson from breast or other cancers, and the big picture. *Urology.* 2002 Apr;59(4 Suppl 1):51–62. Review.

22. Moy KA, Yuan JM, Chung FL, et al. Urinary total isothiocyanates and colorectal cancer: a prospective study of men in Shanghai, China. *Cancer Epidemiol Biomarkers Prev.* 2008 Jun;17(6):1354–59.

23. Yang M, Kenfield SA, Van Blarigan EL, et al. Dairy intake after prostate cancer diagnosis in relation to disease-specific and total mortality. *Int J Cancer.* 2015 May 20.

24. Triff K, Kim E, Chapkin RS. Chemoprotective epigenetic mechanisms in a colorectal cancer model: modulation by n-3 PUFA in combination with fermentable fiber. *Curr Pharmacol Rep.* 2015 Feb;1(1):11–20.

25. Devi KP, Rajavel T, Russo GL, Daglia M, Nabavi SF, Nabavi SM. Molecular targets of omega-3 fatty acids for cancer therapy. *Anticancer Agents Med Chem.* 2015 Apr 24.

26. Witte TR, Hardman WE. The effects of omega-3 polyunsaturated fatty acid consumption on mammary carcinogenesis. *Lipids.* 2015 May;50(5):437–46.

27. Lin PH, Aronson W, Freedland SJ. Nutrition, dietary interventions and prostate cancer: the latest evidence. *BMC Med.* 2015 Jan 8;13:3.

28. Bozzetti F, Zupec-Kania B. Toward a cancer-specific diet. *Clin Nutr.* 2015 Jan 23. pii: S0261-5614(15)00035-7.

29. Allen BG, Bhatia SK, Anderson CM, et al. Ketogenic diets as an adjuvant cancer therapy: history and potential mechanism. *Redox Biol.* 2014 Aug 7;2C:963–70.

Chapter 10

1. Jenkins DJ, Wong JM, Kendall CW, et al. Effect of a 6-month vegan low-carbohydrate ("Eco-Atkins") diet on cardiovascular risk factors and body weight in

hyperlipidaemic adults: a randomised controlled trial. *BMJ Open*. 2014 Feb 5;4(2):e003505.

2. Ludwig DS, Willett WC. Three daily servings of reduced-fat milk: an evidence-based recommendation? *JAMA Pediatr*. 2013 Sep;167(9):788–89.

3. Ludvigsson JF, Reutfors J, Osby U, Ekbom A, Montgomery SM. Coeliac disease and risk of mood disorders—a general population-based cohort study. *J Affect Disord*. 2007 Apr;99(1–3):117–26.

4. Millward C, Ferriter M, Calver S, Connell-Jones G. Gluten- and casein-free diets for autistic spectrum disorder. *Cochrane Database Syst Rev*. 2004;(2):CD003498. Review.

5. Ludvigsson JF, Osby U, Ekbom A, Montgomery SM. Coeliac disease and risk of schizophrenia and other psychosis: a general population cohort study. *Scand J Gastroenterol*. 2007 Feb;42(2):179–85.

6. Hu WT, Murray JA, Greenaway MC, Parisi JE, Josephs KA. Cognitive impairment and celiac disease. *Arch Neurol*. 2006 Oct;63(10):1440–46.

7. Ludvigsson JF, Montgomery SM, Ekbom A, Brandt L, Granath F. Small-intestinal histopathology and mortality risk in celiac disease. *JAMA*. 2009 Sep 16;302(11): 1171–78.

8. Green PH, Neugut AI, Naiyer AJ, Edwards ZC, Gabinelle S, Chinburapa V. Economic benefits of increased diagnosis of celiac disease in a national managed care population in the United States. *J Insur Med*. 2008;40(3–4):218–28.

9. Cortés-Giraldo I, Girón-Calle J, Alaiz M, Vioque J, Megías C. Hemagglutinating activity of polyphenols extracts from six grain legumes. *Food Chem Toxicol*. 2012 Jun;50(6):1951–54.

10. Sandberg AS. Bioavailability of minerals in legumes. *Br J Nutr*. 2002 Dec;88 Suppl 3:S281–85. Review.

11. Sinha R, Cross AJ, Graubard BI, Leitzmann MF, Schatzkin A. Meat intake and mortality: a prospective study of over half a million people. *Arch Intern Med*. 2009 Mar 23;169(6):562–71.

12. Hasselbalch AL. Genetics of dietary habits and obesity—a twin study. *Dan Med Bull*. 2010 Sep;57(9):B4182.

13. Bossé Y, Pérusse L, Vohl MC. Genetics of LDL particle heterogeneity: from genetic epidemiology to DNA-based variations. *J Lipid Res*. 2004 Jun;45(6):1008–26.

Chapter 12

1. Basch CE. Executive summary: healthier students are better learners. *J School Health* 2011;81(10):591–92.

2. Basch CE. Healthier students are better learners: a missing link in school reforms to close the achievement gap. *J School Health* 2011;81(10):593–98.

3. Ley RE. Obesity and the human microbiome. *Curr Opin Gastroenterol*. 2010 Jan;26(1):5–11.

4. Birt DF, Boylston T, Hendrich S, et al. Resistant starch: promise for improving human health. *Adv Nutr*. 2013 Nov 6;4(6):587–601.

5. Tarantino G. Gut microbiome, obesity-related comorbidities, and low-grade chronic inflammation. *J Clin Endocrinol Metab*. 2014 Jul;99(7):2343–46.

6. Foster JA, McVey Neufeld KA. Gut-brain axis: how the microbiome influences anxiety and depression. *Trends Neurosci*. 2013 May;36(5):305–12.

7. Roberfroid M, Gibson GR, Hoyles L, et al. Prebiotic effects: metabolic and health benefits. *Br J Nutr*. 2010 Aug;104 Suppl 2:S1–63.

8. Cummings JH, Macfarlane GT, Englyst HN. Prebiotic digestion and fermentation. *Am J Clin Nutr.* 2001 Feb;73(2 Suppl):415S–420S. Review.

9. Johnston KL, Thomas EL, Bell JD, Frost GS, Robertson MD. Resistant starch improves insulin sensitivity in metabolic syndrome. *Diabet Med.* 2010 Apr;27(4): 391–97.

10. Behall KM, Scholfield DJ, Hallfrisch JG, Liljeberg-Elmståhl HG. Consumption of both resistant starch and beta-glucan improves postprandial plasma glucose and insulin in women. *Diabetes Care.* 2006 May;29(5):976–81.

11. Raben A, Tagliabue A, Christensen NJ, Madsen J, Holst JJ, Astrup A. Resistant starch: the effect on postprandial glycemia, hormonal response, and satiety. *Am J Clin Nutr.* 1994 Oct;60(4):544–51. Robertson MD, Bickerton AS, Dennis AL, Vidal H, Frayn KN. Insulin-sensitizing effects of dietary resistant starch and effects on skeletal muscle and adipose tissue metabolism. *Am J Clin Nutr.* 2005 Sep;82(3):559–67.

12. Maki KC, Pelkman CL, Finocchiaro ET, et al. Resistant starch from high-amylose maize increases insulin sensitivity in overweight and obese men. *J Nutr.* 2012 Apr;142(4):717–23.

13. Higgins JA. Resistant starch and energy balance: impact on weight loss and maintenance. *Crit Rev Food Sci Nutr.* 2014;54(9):1158–66.

14. Udayappan SD, Hartstra AV, Dallinga-Thie GM, Nieuwdorp M. Intestinal microbiota and faecal transplantation as treatment modality for insulin resistance and type 2 diabetes mellitus. *Clin Exp Immunol.* 2014 Jul;177(1):24–29.

15. Brand-Miller JC, Atkinson FS, Gahler RJ. Kacinik V, Lyon MR, Wood S. Effects of added PGX®, a novel functional fibre, on the glycaemic index of starchy foods. *Br J Nutr.* 2012 Jul;108(2)245–48.

16. Solah VA, Brand-Miller JC, Atkinson FS, Gahler RJ, Kacinik V, Lyon MR, Wood S. Dose response effect of a novel functional fibre, PolyGlycopleX(®), PGX(®), on satiety. *Appetite.* 2014 Jun;77:72–76.

17. Reimer RA, Yamaguchi H, Eller LK, Lyon MR, Gahler RJ, Kacinik V, Juneja P, Wood S. Changes in visceral adiposity and serum cholesterol with a novel viscous polysaccharide in Japanese adults with abdominal obesity. *Obesity* (Silver Spring). 2013 Sep;21(9):E379–87.

Chapter 13

1. Rosenfeld CS. Microbiome disturbances and autism spectrum disorders. *Drug Metab Dispos.* 2015 Apr 7.

2. Lecomte V, Kaakoush NO, Maloney CA, et al. Changes in gut microbiota in rats fed a high fat diet correlate with obesity-associated metabolic parameters. *PLoS One.* 2015 May 18;10(5).

3. Goedert JJ, Hua X, Yu G, Shi J. Diversity and composition of the adult fecal microbiome associated with history of cesarean birth or appendectomy: analysis of the American Gut Project. *EBioMedicine.* 2014 Dec 1;1(2–3):167–72.

4. Bäckhed F, Roswall J, Peng Y, et al. Dynamics and stabilization of the human gut microbiome during the first year of life. *Cell Host Microbe.* 2015 May 13;17(5):690–703.

5. Versini M, Jeandel PY, Bashi T, Bizzaro G, Blank M, Shoenfeld Y. Unraveling the hygiene hypothesis of helminthes and autoimmunity: origins, pathophysiology, and clinical applications. *BMC Med.* 2015 Apr 13;13:81.

6. Halton TL, Hu FB. The effects of high protein diets on thermogenesis, satiety and weight loss: a critical review. *J Am Coll Nutr.* 2004 Oct;23(5):373–85. Review.

Index

About the Author

Mark Hyman, MD, believes that we all deserve a life of vitality—and that we have the potential to create it for ourselves. That's why he is dedicated to tackling the root causes of chronic disease by harnessing the power of functional medicine to transform health care. Dr. Hyman and his team work every day to empower people, organizations, and communities to heal their bodies and minds, and improve our social and economic resilience.

Dr. Hyman is a practicing family physician, a nine-time #1 *New York Times* bestselling author, and an internationally recognized leader, speaker, educator, and advocate in his field. He is the Pritzker Foundation Chair in Functional Medicine at Cleveland Clinic and the director of the Cleveland Clinic Center for Functional Medicine. He is also the founder and director of The UltraWellness Center, chairman of the board of the Institute for Functional Medicine, and a medical editor of *The Huffington Post*, and he has been a regular medical contributor on many television shows and networks, including *CBS This Morning, Today, Good Morning America,* CNN, *The View, Katie,* and *The Dr. Oz Show.*

Dr. Hyman works with individuals and organizations, as well as policy makers and influencers. He has testified before both the White House Commission on Complementary and Alternative Medicine and the Senate Working Group on Health Care Reform on Functional Medicine. He has consulted with the surgeon general on diabetes prevention, and participated in the 2009 White House Forum on Prevention and Wellness. Senator Tom Harkin of Iowa nominated Dr. Hyman for the President's Advisory Group on Prevention, Health Promotion, and Integrative and Public Health. In addition, Dr. Hyman has worked with President Clinton, presenting at the Clinton Foundation's Health Matters, Achieving Wellness in Every Generation conference, and the Clinton Global Initiative, as well as with the World Economic Forum on global health issues. He is the winner of the Linus Pauling Award and the Nantucket Project Award, was inducted into the Books for a Better Life Hall of Fame, and received the Christian Book of the Year Award for *The Daniel Plan*.

Dr. Hyman also works with fellow leaders in his field to help people and communities thrive—with Rick Warren, Dr. Mehmet Oz, and Dr. Daniel Amen, he created the Daniel Plan, a faith-based initiative that helped the Saddleback Church collectively lose 250,000 pounds. He is as an advisor and guest cohost on *The Dr. Oz Show* and is on the board of Dr. Oz's HealthCorps, which tackles the obesity epidemic by educating American students about nutrition. With Dr. Dean Ornish and Dr. Michael Roizen, Dr. Hyman crafted and helped introduce the Take Back Your Health Act of 2009 to the United States Senate to provide for reimbursement of lifestyle treatment of chronic disease. And with Tim Ryan in 2015, he helped introduce the ENRICH Act into Congress to fund nutrition in medical education. Dr. Hyman plays a substantial role in a major film produced by Laurie David and Katie Couric, released in 2014, called *Fed Up*, which addresses childhood obesity. Please join him in helping us all take back our health at www.drhyman.com, and follow him on Twitter, Facebook, and Instagram.